MANAGING YOUR OWN HEALTH CRISIS

MANAGING YOUR OWN HEALTH CRISIS

A Holistic Guide to Energised Living and Longevity

DR JOHN RYAN AND JEANIE RYAN

Contents

ABOUT THE AUTHORS

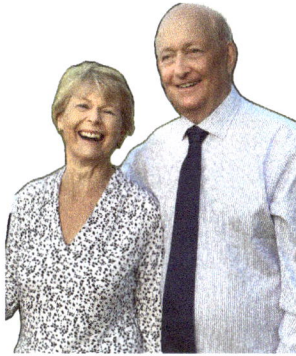

John and Jeanie

John Ryan

John gained qualifications in General Practice (Australia and UK), Paediatrics (Ireland), Acupuncture (Australia and USA) and Nutrition (Master's UK). He served on the National Examination Board of the Australian College of General Practitioners, and for three terms on the national Therapeutic Goods Administration (TGA) Committee formed to advise Government on the safety of products in natural medicine. He served also on Brisbane's Canossa Hospital Board and then on the Brisbane Mater Hospital Health Committee reviewing medical research.

John was a Government appointed Council Member of the Endeavour College of Natural Health (ECNH), the largest Australasian College of Natural Medicine. For 30 years he helped supervise the quality of teaching and was its Inaugural Ethics Chair.

In this book, John shares his experience helping patients including those in the "too hard basket' of general medicine. Examples include those who are exhausted or the women who don't get much of a hearing when their hormones go awry. The same applies to many others, including the elderly and those brave enough to seek a second opinion.

Jeanie Ryan

Hlth. Sc. Nutrition and Dietetics (QUT), RN (QLD), Cert Integrative Med., UQ.

Jeanie completedd her Nursing Degree in Ireland and receiving the gold medal as Dux of her course. Jeanie headed to Australia, where she met John while completing a Midwifery Course at the Mater Hospital in Brisbane. Managing the roles of wife, mother and medical practice manager, Jeanie then completed studies for a Bachelor of Nutrition and Dietetics at Queensland University of Technology (QUT). She concurrently studied Natural Medicine at the Australian College of Natural Medicine.

She became very well-known for her expertise in allergies and sensitivities. High on Jeanie's list of patients were those with Autism and ADHD. She was invited to present lectures at home and abroad.

ACKNOWLEDGEMENTS

The stimulus for this book was Dr James Joseph Ryan (1910–1974), without his inspiration, this book would certainly never have been born. We also acknowledge the guidance of Dr John's eldest brother Dr Barry Ryan, a medical doctor and clinical ecologist, who helped bring the management of food and chemical allergies and sensitivities to a new level in Australia.

We reflect and give thanks to our daughter Juliette and the many family members, colleagues and patients who encouraged us to lay down in a practical way the wisdom that have come our way in the years of involvement in traditional, nutritional and environmental medicine. We thank our niece and gifted journalist, Siobhain Ryan, who freely gave many months while hibernating in Salt Lake City until mid-2019.

We acknowledge also a great family friend and corporate educator, Angela Gifford of On Purpose Partners who assisted editing original manuscript.
Much of the book was written in Ireland where guidance and professional input was afforded by our family friend and professional colleague Denise Deighan.

You can see we have been blessed abundantly along the way.

John and Jeanie Ryan

Chapter 1

INFLAMMATION

"All things are a poison, and nothing is without poison, the dosage alone makes it so the thing is a poison."

THEOPHRASFUS VON HOHENHEIM (PARACELSUS)

Inflammation marks the starting point; it's where many health issues originate. Often, it creeps in gradually, unnoticed and painless.

For centuries, we've recognised inflammation's role in various diseases. But only recently have we grasped its damaging impact when left uncontrolled. Amidst staying home, Zooming with loved ones, and practising social distancing to avoid potential contagion, we've witnessed the toll that long-term inflammatory conditions and weakened immunity can take as we age.

The harsh truth is that the state of your immune system reflects your body's defences against potential threats. Everyday choices regarding diet and lifestyle can either bolster these defences or weaken them. You have the power to halt inflammation before it becomes chronic, or you can continue down the same path and witness its unchecked spread.

HOW INFLAMMATION SPREADS

In the delicate dance of health and disease, it's important to recognise inflammation's dual nature—its protective role and its potential for harm—which can guide us through its complexities. We're all bound to encounter the 'itis' club at some point, with conditions like sinusitis, dermatitis, bronchitis, periodontitis, and conjunctivitis being quite common. Yet, inflammation's influence reaches far beyond these familiar names. It plays a role in major diseases like asthma, heart disease, dementia, depression and cancer, sometimes subtly affecting us without our knowing. In fact, inflammation has evolved into a chronic state for many, playing a pivotal role in over ninety auto-immune diseases.

The COVID-19 pandemic has thrust the role of inflammation in disease into the spotlight. Those most severely affected by the virus often had preexisting medical conditions, compromised immunity or inflammatory disorders. Obesity emerges as a significant driver of inflammation, as fat cells not only store fat but also release inflammatory chemicals, signalling distress as they expand. Chronic stress also fans the flames of inflammation, paving the way for metabolic diseases like diabetes, heart disease, and hypertension.

Features of Inflammation

Redness (*rubor*)
Swelling *(tumour)*
Heat (*calor*)
Pain (*dolor*)
Loss of function *(functio laesa).*

The essence of inflammation was eloquently captured by Roman nobleman Cornelius Celsus over two millennia ago, identifying redness, swelling, heat, pain, and loss of function as its hallmark features. While 'functio laesa' didn't fit the Latin summary, we medical students aptly dubbed it 'kaput' in German. Across languages and centuries, these five features endure. Tissues flush red as blood cells mobilise to combat injury or infection, swelling ensues as fluid accumulates, heat rises with increased blood flow, and pain and loss of function follow suit. Normally, inflammation marks the initial step in the healing journey, but when derailed, it sets the stage for disease progression.

Inflammation: Acute vs. Chronic

Your immune system, a network of cells and tissues, stands as the body's defences against invaders from infections to allergens. From embryonic development onward, it learns to discern and neutralise threats, with gut microbes shaping its responses. In a well-functioning immune system, inflammation is a brief and beneficial response to assaults on the body.

In acute inflammation, the immune system springs into action, triggering symptoms like phlegm production to expel viruses or painful swelling to heal injuries. Ideally, once the threat is vanquished, immune cells deactivate, restoring equilibrium.

In chronic inflammation, immune cells may persistently target healthy tissues or fail to deactivate after eliminating the initial threat. Symptoms get worse over time and fatigue, muscle aches, and joint pains are the result. When inflammation becomes chronic, it transcends its role in the immune system's repertoire, becoming the lynch pin of diseases like cancer, arthritis, multiple sclerosis, and Parkinson's disease.

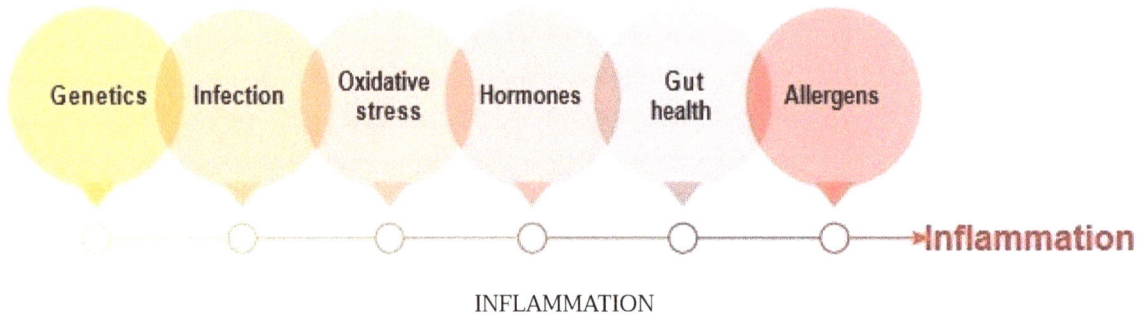

INFLAMMATION

In our quest to understand inflammation, we must broaden our perspective to encompass its genetic and environmental influences. Only by understanding the cause can we hope to mitigate or halt the progression of inflammatory diseases.

Many diseases and afflictions find their roots in genetics. Consider Crohn's disease, Type 1 diabetes mellitus, systemic lupus erythematosus (SLE), and autoimmune thyroiditis (Hashimoto's disease), among others. Families bearing histories of rheumatoid arthritis or multiple sclerosis often carry a genetic predisposition, rendering them more susceptible to autoimmune disorders.

Yet, beyond genetics lie the common triggers of autoimmunity. Your capacity to evade or confront these triggers, coupled with your overall health, dictate whether genetic destiny reigns supreme. Autoimmune culprits range from infections and oxidative stress to hormonal imbalances, unhealthy gut conditions, toxins, and lifestyle factors such as stress, sedentary habits, and poor dietary choices.

Common Inflammatory Triggers

- **Infection:** Is it viral, bacterial, fungal, or parasitic?
- **Allergies or intolerance:** Could food sensitivities or environmental irritants be at play?
- **Toxins:** Have you encountered substances like lead, mercury, aluminum, fluoride, or pesticides?
- **Radiation exposure:** From UV rays or medical procedures like CT scans or anti-cancer radiotherapy?
- **Medication reactions:** Could certain drugs be exacerbating inflammation?
- **Hormonal factors:** Are imbalances in adrenal and thyroid function contributing?
- **Diet and weight management:** Is your nutritional intake or blood sugar regulation problematic?
- **Past trauma:** Could spinal issues or nerve compression be triggering inflammation?

Infection, Oxidative Stress and Tissue Damage: Infection, pollution and psychological stress may result in oxidative stress, leading to cellular and tissue damage from free radicals. If left unchecked, these culminate in hyperinflammation or the dreaded 'cytokine storm' as witnesses in severe cases of COVID-19 or influenza.

The Role of Hormonal Imbalances: Hormones wield significant influence over inflammation, with oestrogen typically enhancing immune response. However, imbalances, whether from fluctuating levels or exposure to environmental oestrogenic compounds can tip the scales toward inflammation, particularly in those predisposed to auto-immune ailments.

Gut Health and Immunity: Gut health, a linchpin of natural immunity, hinges on adequate stomach acid to break down dietary proteins. Failure in this process can lead to incomplete digestion of proteins which become the catalyst for an inflammatory response.

Navigating Allergens and Medications: Allergens, both environmental and dietary, not only provoke immediate reactions but can also incite chronic inflammatory conditions. Meanwhile, medications and toxic substances in our environment further enhance the burden of autoimmune disease, with examples ranging from asbestos to smoking-related risks.

SIMPLE TESTS

On physical examination, an inflammatory disease may have all the usual features: redness, heat, swelling, pain and impaired function. But this is not always the case.

Blood tests are essential: You can check levels of inflammation and markers for cancer and autoimmune disease, viruses and allergy. Your levels of antibodies can be too low or high. If they're too low, they leave you more open to infection. If they're too high, they may point to an overactive immune response.

One major test for inflammation and toxicity is CRP (C-reactive protein), another is ESR (erythrocyte sedimentation rate). A test for viruses will reveal whether they are current or of past origin. The results should help with diagnosis, isolate some of the triggers and lead to lifestyle advice. In the meantime, ask your family members if they have allergies, sensitivities or autoimmune disorders. Genetics can play a big role.

INFLAMMATION

ACTION PLAN – CHECKLIST

- Measure inflammation markers.
- Support immunity with vitamins A, C, D, and minerals zinc and selenium.
- Use the Mediterranean diet. (More on this in Chapter 30.)
- Exercise and get fit.
- Get adequate sleep.
- Reduce stress; seek counselling if necessary.
- Reduce alcohol, caffeine, sugar and other environmental toxins.
- Aim for ideal waist and weight measurements.

References:

Rosenblum, M. D., Remedios, K. A., & Abbas, A. K. (2015). Mechanisms of human auto-immunity. *The Journal of clinical investigation*, *125*(6), 2228–2233. https://doi.org/10.1172/JCI78088

Zenewicz, L. A., Abraham, C., Flavell, R. A., & Cho, J. H. (2010). Unraveling the genetics of autoimmunity. *Cell*, *140*(6), 791–797. https://doi.org/10.1016/j.cell.2010.03.003

Chapter 2

ALLERGIES

"Let food be thy medicine and medicine be thy food."

AUTHOR UNKNOWN

Australia has some of the highest allergy rates in the world. Gradual exposure to our furry friends from an early age can help build tolerance against pet dander and other pet allergens as a person ages. Adequate Vitamin D and a diverse gut microbiome also contribute to long-term protection.

In the upcoming chapters, we'll delve into addressing the root causes rather than just the symptoms of common conditions like asthma, eczema, and migraines, often triggered by allergies and sensitivities.

MECHANICS OF AN ALLERGY REACTION

Allergies occur when our immune system produces antibodies, perceiving a threat. Mast cells, found in various body parts like the skin, mouth, nose, lungs, and digestive tract, defend against these perceived threats.

In an overactive immune system, allergens such as grass or certain foods interact with antibodies on mast cells, triggering the release of chemicals like histamine. This leads to allergic reactions such as runny nose, itchy throat, wheezing, skin flushing, hives, headache, abdominal discomfort, vomiting, and/or diarrhea. In very severe cases, life-threatening anaphylaxis can occur, necessitating immediate medical intervention.

Allergic predisposition may be inherited or develop later in life, influenced by genetic factors and environmental triggers. Young children, with less mature gut microbe populations, are more susceptible to allergies, although sensitivity often diminishes by adolescence. However, allergies can resurface or emerge in adulthood, often associated with stress, infections, and poor gut health.

Environmental Allergies are Common: Environmental allergens such as dust mites, pollens, moulds, insect stings, animal hair and skin and saliva, cockroaches, smoke, exhaust fumes and other chemicals can cause a sensitive immune system to overreact. You can desensitise your immune system to the irritant but it can take 3-5 years. About 60% of those desensitised have permanent benefits, but avoidance it if possible.

Mould allergies may cause an extensive range of symptoms apart from the usual cough, runny nose or itchy eyes or skin. Mould toxins may also cause fatigue, cognitive problems, muscle pains or headaches and may require more definitive supporting tests. Damp spaces need to be treated aggressively both inside and outside the home. It's an issue to consider when nothing else seems to be working. In Chapter 27 (When All Else

Fails) we go into much more detail on the treatment and eradication of mould should it cause health issues.

Dust Mites thrive in warm, humid climates which cause wheezing, asthma, sinus problems, and itchy eyes and skin. You can limit dust mites in the home by avoiding the use of carpets, cleaning your bedding often, and using tea tree or eucalyptus oil when washing bed linen. Soak bedding in a mix of four parts eucalyptus oil to one-part concentrated dishwashing detergent for 30 minutes before washing in hot water to reduce the number of live dust mites up to 97%.

Cat Saliva and dander are difficult to eradicate. Particles can remain in a room several weeks after a cat has left, so furniture really needs to be cleaned thoroughly.

Pollen allergies manifest seasonally, causing symptoms like itchy eyes and respiratory discomfort. Identifying specific pollen triggers can aid in managing symptoms effectively. Itchy eyes, skin rashes and a tight chest can appear on windy days. This can commonly occur at the end of summer or winter when pollen is released by grasses, shrubs and trees. Getting itchy while sitting on grass, having a rash or wheeze can develop when you are in a particular area and might help you pinpoint the cause. The following is a list of some of common pollens which can cause allergic reactions.

Chronic allergic sinus infections are common for those with a history of environmental allergies. Sinus infections can be the forerunner to asthma, respiratory infections, the common cold and immune problems.

Common Pollen Polluters

Flowering Plants: Chrysanthemums, sunflowers, dahlias, marigolds, daisies.

Trees & Shrubs: Wattle, pine /Cyprus, elm, oak, beach, willow, birch, privet, olive, maple, brunfelsia.

Herbs: Chamomile, wormwood, feverfew, echinacea, dandelion, Milk thistle.

Weeds: Paterson's curse, Plantago (asthma weed), ragweed, nettle, dock.

Grass: Rye, Bahia grass, Bermuda (couch) grass, canary grass, Johnson grass, Kentucky blue, Timothy grass.

Chronic allergic sinus infections are common for those with a history of environmental allergies. Sinus infections can be the forerunner to asthma, respiratory infections, the common cold and immune problems.

- **Strengthen your guard** against sinus infections with quercetin, which stabilise mast cells that release histamine to give you a runny nose. While the best source of natural quercetin is onion; you might want to use a quercetin supplement (400 mg) three times per day during the allergy season. If you find quercetin in a liquid form, you can reduce the dose to 250 mg three times per day.
- **Use a nasal irrigation solution** if you have missed the boat and your sinuses are in free flow. To make the solution, dilute 3 teaspoons of salt (iodine free) plus 1 teaspoon of baking soda in a cup (300ml) of warm water which has been previously boiled. The easiest way to use the solution is to tip the head back when having a shower.
- **Desensitisation Methods:** Desensitisation approaches involve sublingual drops, tablets, or immunotherapy injections, gradually increasing tolerance to specific

allergens over time. It takes time to change the immune system, so expect to be on the medications for years rather than months.

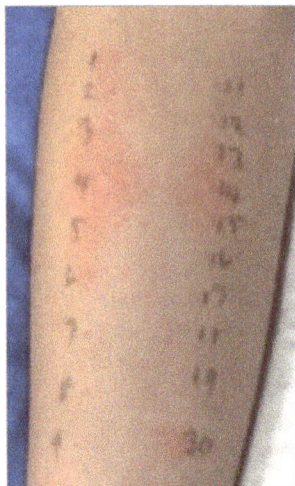

Skin Prick Tests

Testing for Food and Environmental Allergies: In a **skin prick test,** a drop of each suspected allergen is placed on the skin (usually the forearm or back). A special lancet pricks the skin so the solution can get under its surface. If positive to the allergen an itchy red weal develops at the site within twenty minutes. The size of the weal reflects the intensity of the reaction.

If those tests are inconclusive, you may still have a sensitivity (an intolerance), rather than an allergy. The photo here was taken in our office showing red weals from a positive skin prick test.

For the RAST blood test, a sample of blood is taken to check if it contains the antibody specific to an allergen such as milk, egg and peanuts, etc. (dust mites, mould, pollens can also be tested this way).

Sensitivities generally produce less immediate and less alarming symptoms, making them much more difficult to diagnose. It's hard to isolate specific intolerances in infants because of their immature digestive systems. Unaided, some people spend years trying to work out what's causing their symptoms, especially if multiple foods and/or food additives are involved.

It's rare for a small taste of a food to cause sensitivities, but true food allergies only require minute particles to cause problems. In cases of suspected severe reactions, the food challenges are undertaken with the immunologist or within a hospital setting. That said, it is much easier to diagnose a food allergy than a food intolerance.

FOOD ALLERGY VS FOOD INTOLERANCE

Food Allergy	Food Intolerance
Age of onset: Infants mostly sensitised by milk, soy or eggs.	**Onset:** Any age.
Symptoms: May present as infantile eczema, particularly on the face.	**Symptoms:** Often presents as:
Recurs with contact causing:	· irritable behaviour/sleep disturbance · (colic and screaming in babies) · irritable bowel (loose stools), reflux · recurrent mouth ulcers · eczema and/or non-specific rashes · nappy rash · recurrent hives and swelling · congested upper airways, · headaches · leg aches and pains
· rash about mouth · facial swelling · generalised hives · vomiting · respiratory distress · anaphylactic reactions.	
Timing of Reaction: Immediate, seconds or minutes after every contact.	**Timing of Reaction:** Delayed (in minutes or up to two days later). Not at every contact because the reaction depends on how much is consumed over time.
Mechanism: Immune system response (IgE). Infants are sensitised by prior exposure.	**Mechanism:** Non-immune response. Symptoms depend on the dose, rather than prior exposure.

Food Triggers: Peanut, egg, milk, nuts, soy, fish, shellfish.	**Food Triggers:** Milk, wheat, foods high in salicylates, amines, glutamates, preservatives and colours.
Amount for Trigger: A few grams, milligrams or even less.	**Amount for Trigger:** Depends on the person. Symptoms can be triggered by a mouthful, a full meal or several days' consumption.
Diagnosis: Skin prick tests and blood tests.	**Diagnosis:** No blood or skin tests. Trigger food must be eliminated from the diet, then reintroduced to check for symptoms.
Change Required: Need to completely avoid trigger food.	**Change required:** Need to limit the intake of the trigger food.
Prognosis: May resolve over time. But some allergies (nuts and fish) can be lifelong	**Prognosis:** Variable. Symptoms can flare up and then settle down over a lifetime. As children mature, they tend to react less to food triggers.
Associated Problems: People with food allergies also tend to suffer asthma or hay fever when exposed to environmental triggers.	**Associated Problems:** People with food sensitivities are also prone to attention deficit hyperactivity disorder (ADHD), irritable bowel, glue ears and blocked nose, headaches.
Genetics: People with food allergies tend to come from families with histories of reactions.	**Genetics:** People with food sensitivities tend to come from families with histories of irritable bowel, ADHD, sinusitis, mood changes, congestion, headaches and reactivity to food.

LET'S TALK ABOUT MILK

Milk boasts a rich composition of enzymes, vitamins and minerals, including vital fat-soluble vitamins such as A, D, E, and K essential for various bodily functions like bone health, vision, and immunity. However, it also contains proteins like casein and carbohydrates like lactose, which can provoke adverse reactions in certain individuals.

Infant Reactions to Milk: Babies in particular may exhibit adverse reactions to milk. Approximately 2% of infants develop dairy allergies. Presenting symptoms being facial swelling, abdominal discomfort, diarrhea, wheezing, or other inflammatory responses following milk consumption. Casein, a milk protein, can coagulate in the acidic stomach environment, slowing digestion and potentially causing constipation. Upon breakdown, it releases beta-casomorphine 7 (BCM7), a peptide that may trigger histamine release, impacting the skin, gastrointestinal tract, or respiratory system.

Testing for Milk Allergies: If you suspect milk as the culprit behind your child's reactions, it's advisable to explore allergy testing. A dietitian may recommend switching to a non-dairy formula for a brief period to assess any improvements. Rice or coconut milk are not recommended substitutes over a lengthy period due to their inferior nutritional profiles. Encouragingly, only a small percentage of children with positive milk allergy tests retain sensitivities into their teenage years.

Adult Intolerance to Lactose: Conversely, adults are more prone to lactose intolerance, an inability to digest the milk sugar lactose, unrelated to allergy. This intolerance stems from insufficient lactase enzyme levels required for lactose digestion, leading to symptoms like bloating and diarrhea after milk consumption. Certain populations, such as East Asians or Native Americans, exhibit higher lactose intolerance rates due to reduced lactase enzyme production. Lactase levels may also decline with age or following infections. You might replace milk with kale, since one cup of kale has about the same amount of calcium as dairy and is well absorbed when cooked.

Lactose Content of Milk

Source: Dairy Australia: https://www.dairy.com.au/dairy-matters/you-ask-we-answer/what-is-the-lactose-content-of-different-dairy-products.

Milk (regular) 250 ml (1 cup)	15.75 g
Yoghurt 200 g	10.0 g
Ice cream 50 g	1.65 g
Cream 20 ml	0.6 g
Cheddar cheese 2 tablespoons	0.04 g
Soy milk/beverage 250 ml	0 g

ALL YOU CAN'T EAT

Unlocking Food Sensitivities: Delving into the world of food sensitivities unveils the complexity of naturally occurring and added chemicals in our diet. Among these, amines and salicylates stand out as common triggers, abundantly present in fruits, vegetables, and aged or fermented foods.

Exploring Amines and Their Effects: Amines are the byproducts of amino acid which breakdown during digestion, they accumulate as food ages or when foods ferment. The rule of thumb holds true: the older and more pungent the food, the higher its amine content. Headaches, fatigue, mood swings, and even behavioural issues in children may signal amine sensitivity. For a peaceful night's rest, consider steering clear of high-amine foods after 4 PM.

Foods High in Amines

Chocolate	All forms
Cheese	Aged, strong cheeses such as Gouda, cheddar, Stilton, blue cheese, parmesan, Brie, Camembert and Roquefort.
Fruit	Citrus fruit, olives, overripe banana and avocado, dates and pineapple.
Fish	Dried, cured or smoked oysters, anchovies, smoked or pickled fish (e.g. herring), fish roe (including caviar), tuna, flake, smoked or canned salmon, shrimp paste (Terasi), fish sauce and leftover fish.
Meat	Pork, dried and cured meats (e.g. salami), chicken liver pâté and vacuum-packed meats.
Vegetables	Tomato sauce and paste, pickled cabbage and sauerkraut, aubergine (eggplant), spinach, all legumes, miso, tempeh and soy sauce.
Alcohol	Red wine, beer and champagne.
Other	Marmite, Vegemite, soup mixes, stock cubes and sauces.

Navigating Histamine Sensitivity: For some, histamine sensitivity adds another layer of complexity. This chemical is present in various foods and can unleash a cascade of symptoms affecting the skin, gut, brain, and cardiovascular system. We explore mast cells and address these challenges in Chapter 27 (When All Else Fails).

Understanding Salicylates and Their Effects: Salicylates, plant-based compounds abundant in fruits, vegetables, and herbs, offer a unique insight into dietary sensitivities. These chemicals thrive in plant sources, particularly in younger fruits, albeit diminishing slightly as they ripen. The repercussions of salicylate sensitivity manifest in various forms, from skin rashes to respiratory distress and occasional gastric disturbances. Cooking does little to diminish the salicylate content. Headaches, fatigue and central nervous system issues, notably hyperactivity, can arise from salicylate exposure echoing the challenges posed by amines.

Connecting the Dots: Aspirin Sensitivity: For some individuals, a reaction to aspirin serves as the initial clue to salicylate sensitivity. Moreover, adverse responses to non-steroidal anti-inflammatory drugs (NSAIDs) are commonplace. Medications like Nurofen, Celebrex, Voltaren, and Naprosyn fall under this category, warranting caution.

Salicylate Content of Foods; Source: Swain, et al (1985).

Food	Salicylate Content	Food	Salicylate Content
Apricots	2.58 mg	Curry powder	218 mg.
Fresh dates	3.73 mg	Pepper (dry)	6.2 mg
Dried dates	4.50 mg	Oregano	66 mg
Oranges	2.39 mg	Green olives	1.29 mg
Pineapples (fresh)	2.10 mg	Tomatoes	0.13 mg
Strawberries	1.36 mg	Worcestershire sauce	64.3 mg
Apples (Granny Smith)	5.9 mg	Mustard	26 mg
Apples (Golden Delicious)	0.8 mg	Peppermint	9.4 mg
Pears	0.27 mg	Cayenne	17.6 mg
Gherkins (canned)	6.1 mg	Almonds	3.0 mg

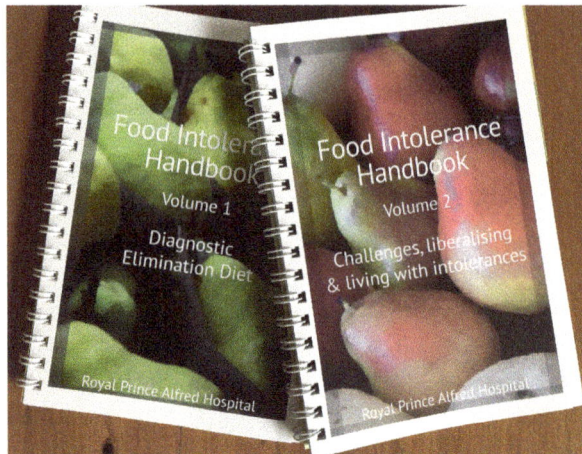

RPAH Food Intolerance Handbooks
https://www.slhd.nsw.gov.au/rpa/allergy/resources/foodintol/ff-handbooks.html

Unveiling the Impact of Additives: While amines and salicylates naturally find their way into our diets, processed foods often harbor an array of additives —colors, preservatives, flavor enhancers, and antioxidants. These synthetic compounds, meant to enhance taste, appearance, and shelf life, can wreak havoc on sensitive systems. For some individuals, additives spell trouble, triggering a range of symptoms from headaches and gastrointestinal distress to skin issues, fatigue, and even exacerbating behavioral problems, particularly in children.

Much of our understanding of additive sensitivities stems from the pioneering work of the allergy unit at Sydney's Royal Prince Alfred Hospital. Their research has shed light on the intricate relationship between additives and adverse reactions, guiding treatment strategies for chemical sensitivities. For comprehensive information on allergens beyond additives, including tree nuts and insect stings. The Australian Society of Clinical Immunology and Allergy's website serves as an invaluable resource.

Additives Most Likely to be a Problem

Food additive	Number	Foods
Yellows	102, 107, 110	Added to sweets, cakes, buns and biscuits, custard mixes, sauces, commercial jellies, savoury snacks, cordials and ice cream.
Reds	122-129	
Blues	131, 132	
Green	142	
Black	151	
Browns	154, 155	
Cochineal	120	Sourced from Mexican scale insects. Added to drinks, bakery products, some cheeses, sauces and sweets.
Annatto	160B	From seeds of the Central American plant. Added to cereals, snack foods and dairy products.
Food preservatives	Number	Foods
Sorbates	200-203	Added to cheese products, dried fruits, fruit juices, yoghurts with fruit or nuts, licorice, low-sugar jams, soft drinks.

Sulphites	220-228	Naturally fermented in many wines and vinegar. Added to dried fruits, potato products, prawns and meats to keep their colour.
Benzoates	210-228	Naturally found in berries and other fruit. Added to cordials, fruit drinks, soft drinks and marinades.
Nitrates and nitrites	249-252	Added to cured meats and cheeses.
Propionates	280-283	Naturally produced when bacteria ferments fibre in the large intestine. Added to bread crumbs, dressings, and fruit and vegetable juices to stop fungal growth.
Flavour enhancers	Number	Foods
Glutamates	N/A	Occur naturally in strong cheeses (parmesan, camembert, brie and gruyere), soy sauce, oyster sauce, black bean sauce, tomato sauce, miso, TVP, HVP, yeast extracts, mushrooms, plums and spinach.

Monosodium glutamate (MSG) and similar flavour compounds	621, 620, 622, 623	Used in fast foods, instant noodles, potato crisps, sauces.
Ribonucleotides	627, 631, 635	Used in instant noodles, snack foods, crackers, chips and sauces.
Antioxidants	**Number**	**Foods**
Vitamin C (ascorbic acid)	300-304	Added to flours and juice to stop discolouring.
Gallates	310-312	Used to prevent fats and oils from rancidity. Added to chewing gum, butter blends, peanut paste, desserts, peanut paste, snack foods, chips, battered fish and doughnuts.
Tertiary butylhydroquinone (TBHQ)	319	TBHQ is used to extend shelf life and prevent rancidity. TBHQ protects foods with iron from discoloration and is used in vegetable and animal fats. Its use is controversial. It is often used together with two other antioxidants, BHA and BHT.
BHA	320	

PROTOCOLS FOR ELIMINATION DIETS

When guiding individuals through elimination diets to address food sensitivities, our approach typically involves removing suspect foods or additives from the diet for a duration of three to four weeks, or until they've been symptom-free for approximately five consecutive days. Subsequently, we employ a systematic 'challenge' process, re-introducing one food or chemical at a time into their diet for a period of three to five days. Chemicals have a cumulative effect, so even if there is no reaction, the food/chemical is withdrawn form the diet until the end of the challenges.

Interpreting Reactions: The timing and nature of any reactions during the challenge phase provide crucial insights. If a reaction occurs on day one or two, it suggests a low tolerance to the food or additive. Conversely, if no noticeable reaction emerges until days three or four, it indicates a higher tolerance, prompting consideration for reducing intake rather than complete elimination.

Tailored Management: Identifying trigger foods is just the beginning; personalised strategies for managing sensitivities are essential. Recognising that each individual's response varies, there's no universal solution. Adhering to personal tolerance thresholds plays a pivotal role in symptom management.

Considering Gut Health and Immunity: The health of your gut microbiome significantly influences immune responses. Promoting a diverse array of "friendly" microbes through dietary measures, including prebiotics and probiotics, fosters the production of antimicrobial and anti-inflammatory molecules crucial for combating disease. Chapter 20 offers detailed guidance on optimising gut health, emphasising the importance of nutrient-rich diets and identifying potential deficiencies, such as zinc, that may hinder progress.

Exploring Conventional Treatments: While conventional treatments like antihistamines, corticosteroids, and decongestants effectively alleviate allergic reactions, understanding their appropriate use is paramount. Nasal saline rinses provide relief from naso-respiratory related symptoms, while corticosteroid creams address skin rashes.

Various antihistamines cater to different needs, with sedating options offering night-time relief and non-sedating alternatives suitable for daytime use, many of which are available without a prescription. In severe cases, oral or injectable steroids may be necessary, and individuals at risk of life-threatening reactions such as anaphylaxis require access to EpiPens for immediate intervention.

Implementing Action Plans: For comprehensive allergy management, resources from organisations like the Australasian Society for Clinical Immunology and Allergy (ASCIA) and booklets from the Royal Prince Alfred Allergy Unit in Sydney offer invaluable guidance. These sources provide detailed action plans for managing allergies and anaphylaxis, readily accessible for printing and reference.

ALLERGY

ACTION PLAN – CHECKLIST

- Check the allergy load with blood tests and skin prick or patch tests.
- Identify the allergen trigger – be it food, chemical or environmental.
- Determine the severity.
- Remove the triggers.
- Desensitise where possible.
- Manage the symptoms.
- Improve the gut microbiome.
- Support the immune system with vitamins A, C and E.
- Add zinc and quercetin for added protection.

References:

Australian Society of Clinical Immunology and Allergy. (2019). *Food Allergy.* ASCIA. https://www.allergy. org.au/patients/food-allergy/food-allergy

Swain, A. R., Dutton, S. P., & Truswell, A. S. (1985). Salicylates in foods. *Journal of the American Dietetic Association, 85*(8), 950–960.

Tovey, E. R.,& McDonald, L.G. (1997). A simple washing procedure with eucalyptus oil for controlling house dust mites and their allergens in clothing and bedding. *Journal of Allergy and Clinical Immunology, 100*, 464–466.

Chapter 3

AUTOIMMUNE DISEASES

"The natural healing force within each of us is the greatest force in getting well."

HIPPOCRATES

Autoimmune diseases are identified via their symptoms, signalling the body's misdirected immune response. Understanding these signals is essential for early detection and targeted intervention. Getting what these signals mean early on is key for getting the right help. And it's not just about our white cells, skin, airways, and tummy doing their thing – our genes, surroundings, and all those little critters living in our gut are part of the conversation too. They can either lend a hand to our immune system or make the pathway to wellness quite demanding.

Common Symptoms of Autoimmune Disease

· Muscle aches and pains
· Abdominal pain, bloating and other digestive issues
· Fatigue
· Poor concentration
· Fever
· Swollen glands
· Hair loss
· Rashes

Lots of factors, such as genetics and environment can contribute to health issues. Sensitivities to foods, stress, or having had infections needing antibiotics can interfere with the immune system. When this happens, it can lead to autoimmune diseases. Common diseases include rheumatoid arthritis, thyroid issues like Hashimoto's disease, multiple sclerosis, type 1 diabetes, lupus, and psoriasis. There are over ninety autoimmune diseases, and diagnosing them can be tricky because we often can't find specific antibodies in the blood for many of them.

PROTOCOLS FOR MANAGEMENT: A COMPREHENSIVE APPROACH

Treating autoimmune conditions involves a mix of approaches to tackle both causes and symptoms. There are common triggers that can initiate autoimmunity and there are genetic markers that predispose people to certain conditions. But having the gene doesn't always mean you'll get the condition. Targeting the root cause, measuring and reducing the antibody load is the cornerstone of autoimmune management.

Find the Cause and Trigger of Autoimmunity

Genetic links: Many diseases come through inheritance. Coeliac disease is well known. Inflammatory bowel disease (IBD) - Crohn's disease and ulcerative colitis are both associated with the IL-23 genes. Rheumatoid arthritis (RA) and multiple sclerosis (MS) also have a genetic link.

Environmental factors: Infections such as the Epstein Barr virus (EBV) causes infectious mononucleosis (glandular fever). EBV often persists and can be associated with lupus, Crohn's disease, eczema, Graves' disease may be linked to rheumatoid arthritis. Chlamydial infections have been linked to Multiple Sclerosis, Alzheimer's and Parkinson's disease. Periodontal infections and smoking have also been linked to rheumatoid arthritis. Between 40% and 70% of those with hepatitis C may develop at least one inflammatory disorder. So there are not many viruses or infections that don't have consequences.

Chemical toxins: Asbestos and mercury and perhaps dioxins have been implicated in autoimmunity. Asbestos is associated with systemic lupus erythematosus (SLE), scleroderma and rheumatoid arthritis.

Drugs: More than ninety medications from over 10 drug classes ranging from antibiotics to statins and anticonvulsants have been implicated in autoimmune diseases.

Low vitamin D: Having enough vitamin D helps keep the immune system in check, stopping it from attacking the body. If vitamin D levels are low, it can lead to too much inflammation, which is often seen in autoimmune diseases. Low vitamin D levels are linked to a higher chance of getting diseases like multiple sclerosis, rheumatoid arthritis, lupus, and type 1 diabetes. Sometimes, low vitamin D levels come before the symptoms of autoimmune diseases start.

Altered gut function: Gut microbiota play a crucial role in regulating the immune responses. Diets low in protective nutrients found in fruits, vegetables, and whole grains, such as vitamins A, C, and E, antioxidants and phytochemicals help to reduce inflammation. Their absence can contribute to autoimmune risk.

Food allergies or food sensitivities: Gluten from wheat, barley and rye as well dairy foods are common problems.

Emotional and physical stressors: About 80% of those with autoimmune disease report problems with emotional stress before the onset of their autoimmune disease. Severe childhood stress increases the risk of autoimmune disease in later life.

Hormonal triggers: Generally, oestrogen enhances immunity, but on the flip side it predisposes genetically susceptible females to more autoimmunity compared with their male counterparts. Prolonged oestrogenic stimulation has been reported in patients with SLE. Hormonal changes during pregnancy affect several autoimmune disease. Androgens, and perhaps progestogens, are somewhat protective, although androgens have also been shown to promote rheumatoid arthritis.

Reducing the antibody load: You can test for antibodies – they can identify many diseases and tell us about the inflammatory process in many autoimmune disorders. They can be very specific for the organs targeted by diseases of the thyroid, type 1 diabetes mellitus and coeliac disease.

Managing the symptoms and progress of these disease may be relatively simple with thyroid hormones, insulin in the case of diabetes and a gluten free diet for coeliac disease. But where the antibodies are less specific, like systemic lupus erythematosus (SLE), and if more than one organ is affected at the same time, the cause is often unclear. Medical practitioners need to be vigilant for signs and symptoms of autoimmune diseases in patients taking medications. As mentioned previously, many drugs commonly used to treat autoimmune diseases such as rheumatoid arthritis, psoriasis, and inflammatory bowel disease can paradoxically induce autoimmune diseases or exacerbate existing ones, such as lupus-like syndromes or demyelinating disorders such as multiple sclerosis or Guillain-Barré Syndrome (GBS).

Explore These Options for a Better Outcome

- Check allergy load via blood tests and skin prick tests. Check for gluten sensitivity.
- Antibody tests can often pinpoint out specific autoantibodies associated with different autoimmune diseases.
- Inflammatory markers and blood count provide clues on inflammation.
- Check hormone levels.
- Low vitamin D levels are often prevalent in autoimmune diseases. Anyone with a hint of an autoimmune disease should have vitamin D status checked.
- Genetic markers are associated with certain autoimmune diseases, such as HLA-B27 in ankylosing spondylitis or HLA-DR4 in rheumatoid arthritis.
- Do a hair analysis if there is concern re toxic metals such as mercury or lead as these can thereby be measured in the cells rather than in the blood. Blood levels may also be measured.
- Add probiotics and fibre to enhance the gut bacterial diversity.
- Manage weight as obesity is a driver of inflammation.
- Reduce stress with exercise, meditation, professional help, friends and family – see Chapters 12 and 31.
- Keep joints mobile with prescribed exercising: When times are tough and pain is high, it's not always easy to exercise. An exercise physiologist can help.
- Reduce inflammation via diet: reduce red meat, alcohol, lower allergens, lower sugar and avoid junk food and vegetable oils. Add fish and omega-3 fats and fresh fruit and vegetables.
- Supplement any deficiencies.

Reduce Inflammation and Pain

Start by supporting the immune system. Natural remedies can be helpful, the problem being that they take longer to work, so patience is a required part of the process!

- Always include vitamin D (See Chapter 35)
- Add the herb turmeric (*Curcuma longa*) is useful, inexpensive and safe with few side effects; it is better absorbed when taken with piperine (black pepper). It's traditionally used for inflammation, pain and wound healing, it also has anti-tumour necrosis factor (anti-TNFα) ability which also lessens the symptoms of multiple sclerosis, rheumatoid arthritis, psoriasis, and inflammatory bowel disease.
- Zinc, magnesium and B6 have anti-inflammatory properties, as have fish oils.
- N-acetylcysteine (NAC) is very useful as an antioxidant and has anti-inflammatory and detoxification properties.
- Copper has an anti-inflammatory effect, and the anti-inflammatory drugs compete with copper absorption and may render copper stores depleted. Copper may be checked by a hair mineral analysis at a cost of about $130. Blood is basically a transport medium and we need to assess the copper *within* the cells.

Why you Might Use Naltrexone

Naltrexone, known for its role in blocking opiate/endorphin receptors, typically serving those grappling with opioid addiction at doses ranging from 50–100 mg daily. However, a lesser-known application emerges in the form of low-dose naltrexone (3–4.5 mg), which has demonstrated efficacy in managing conditions such as multiple sclerosis, fibromyalgia, Crohn's disease, and inflammatory bowel disease and more recently long-COVID and fibromyalgia.

When low-dose naltrexone (LDN) is administered, it displaces the body's own endorphins. The cells then busily 'rebound' by increasing their receptor numbers and becoming more sensitive. This rebound compensates for the previous shortage and results in a greater production and greater utilisation of the endorphins with better pain relief. LDN only blocks these receptors for a few hours before it is naturally excreted, so the timing of the medication is important.

Low dose naltrexone treatment does not work for everybody. The *subjective* improvement is a decrease in pain and an increase in vitality. The *objective* measure is a decrease in antibodies – but these are very often not identifiable enough to measure.

Why Pregnenolone is Another Option

Pregnenolone, often called the 'Mother Hormone' or the 'Master Anti-inflammatory', shares similarities with the synthetic drug cortisone (prednisone), both discovered in the 1940s. While both offer anti-inflammatory advantages, prednisone is much stronger, being a hundred times more potent than pregnenolone.

Despite being a natural substance, pregnenolone lost popularity because it's less powerful, and there's less profit in natural, unpatentable substances. Prednisone, on the other hand, can cause various side effects at high doses or with prolonged use, including fluid retention, weight gain, high blood pressure, sleep issues, immune suppression, and bone loss. However, pregnenolone, though slower to act, causes minimal side effects even at high doses. Balancing these factors is important when considering treatment options.

Acupuncture May Be Helpful

A trial of three to four treatments of acupuncture at weekly intervals may be useful in painful conditions.

Navigating Treatment Options for Autoimmune Diseases

Autoimmune diseases pose formidable challenges, often necessitating specialised interventions to mitigate inflammation. Drugs like methotrexate serve as potent immune system suppressors, albeit with associated risks such as hepatic and hematologic toxicity, necessitating vigilant monitoring through regular blood tests.

Glucocorticoids, (e.g. prednisone) exert anti-inflammatory albeit with a propensity for adverse effects like fluid retention and immune suppression.

Disease-modifying antirheumatic drugs (DMARDs) suppress the spread of the inflammatory chemicals and have the capacity to reduce tissue and organ damage.

Non-steroidal anti-inflammatory drugs (NSAIDs) round out the arsenal against inflammation, offering relief from pain fever and inflammation albeit with a spectrum of potential side effects.

Aspirin: Is an old fashioned and cheap anti-inflammatory (NSAID) drug commonly used to reduce inflammation, relieve pain, and lower fever. It can be safe for adults long-term,. It can be effective in use in managing chronic inflammation but there are potential risks and side effects such as gastric and renal effects. It is nor recommended long term for children suffering from recovering from chickenpox or flu-like symptoms due to the risk of Reye's syndrome that affects the liver and brain.

FAECAL TRANSPLANT: ARE WE THERE YET?

Innovative therapies such as faecal transplant hold promise in addressing a spectrum of ailments. By transferring fecal matter from a healthy donor—ideally a healthy relative—to a recipient, this procedure has shown efficacy in treating recurrent Clostridium difficile infection and other conditions including Parkinson's disease, chronic fatigue syndrome, fibromyalgia, multiple sclerosis, obesity, and autism.

Despite its therapeutic potential, faecal transplant remains outside the Medicare rebate system, presenting a cost barrier with expenses typically exceeding $10,000. However, for immune-compromised individuals it represents a viable option warranting consideration.

AUTOIMMUNE DISEASE
ACTION PLAN – CHECKLIST

- Identify physical and neurological symptoms.
- Obtain a diagnosis via history, examination and tests.
- Seek specialist appointments with rheumatologists or neurologists.
- Identify/manage allergies or hormonal and nutrient deficiencies.
- Identify other triggers: foods, stress and poor sleep, toxins and climate.
- Improve nutrition.

References:

Choi, H. H., & Cho, Y. S. (2016). Fecal Microbiota Transplantation: Current Applications, Effectiveness, and Future Perspectives. *Clinical endoscopy*, *49*(3), 257–265. https://doi.org/10.5946/ce.2015.117

Toljan, K., & Vrooman, B. (2018). Low-Dose Naltrexone (LDN)-Review of Therapeutic Utilization. *Medical sciences (Basel, Switzerland)*, *6*(4), 82. https://doi.org/10.3390/medsci6040082

Chapter 4

COELIAC DISEASE AND GLUTEN SENSITIVITY

"Progress is not possible without change, and those who cannot change their mind cannot change anything."

GEORGE BERNARD SHAW

Coeliac disease is an autoimmune condition that affect many different organs. It is thought to have emerged thousands of years ago as societies transitioned from hunting and gathering to farming. New foods such as grains, milk, and eggs triggering reactions in some people unused to such a diet.

Affecting around 1% of the population, coeliac disease arises when the immune system reacts to gluten found in wheat, barley, and rye. Oats do not contain gluten, but crops may be contaminated with gluten containing grains. The reaction from gluten produce antibodies that attack the lining of the gut, causing inflammation of the villi and hindering the absorption of nutrients. If left untreated coeliac disease can cause serious health problems including headaches, thyroid disorders, diabetes, multiple sclerosis, osteoporosis, infertility, skin and neurological disorders.

Non-coeliac gluten sensitivity affects up to about 13% of the population. It occurs when gut and other symptoms develop in response to gluten. About half of those with gluten sensitivity have the genes that code for coeliac disease. Unlike coeliac disease however, gluten sensitivity in this population does not cause lifelong autoimmune disease. It doesn't trigger the production of the same antibodies nor do the same damage to the gut lining, but it can cause many other symptoms similar to coeliac disease.

Wheat allergies affect about 1% of the population. It occurs when the immune system produces antibodies in response to wheat. In rare cases, wheat allergies can trigger life-threatening reactions.

People with coeliac disease and those with non-coeliac gluten intolerance need to avoid gluten from wheat, rye, barley (and perhaps oats). Sometimes people with coeliac disease (or a non-coeliac gluten sensitivity) react to other grains, such as corn or rice, too. If that's you, it's worth consulting a dietitian with specific interest in grain sensitivities to help you work out your allergies.

HOW TO TEST FOR COELIAC DISEASE

Coeliac testing requires both genetic blood tests and a biopsy of the gut to confirm the disease. One must have wheat, bread and other gluten-containing foods for at least six weeks prior to testing – otherwise the tests may be inconclusive! A positive test indicates the need for a gluten-free diet for life. Sometimes the characteristics of coeliac disease don't differ much from that of non-coeliac gluten sensitivity or wheat allergy. The similarities and differences are outlined below:

IS IT NON-COELIAC GLUTEN DISEASE OR WHEAT ALLERGY?

Characteristics	Non-coeliac Sensitivity	Wheat Allergy
Rate in population	Unknown. Estimated at 0.6%.	1%
Genetic Link	50% carry the variant HLA-DQ2 or HLA-DQ8.	100% have inherited hyper-sensitivity
How it develops	Unknown. Probably occurs at first encounter, prompting the immune memory of gluten.	Immune system responds when wheat allergen comes into contact with IgE antibodies.
Symptoms	Intestinal: abdominal pain, diarrhoea, nausea, bloating and flatulence. Possible Other: chronic tiredness, headaches, muscle cramps, anaemia, depression, numbness of hands and feet, bone and joint pain.	Intestinal: diarrhoea, cramps, indigestion, nausea and vomiting. Other: skin rash, irritation of the mouth or throat, wheezing or asthma, stuffy/running nose and headache. Wheat allergies can (rarely) trigger anaphylaxis.
Effect on gut lining	None	May cause degeneration.
Effect on lifespan	Unknown	Decreased if anaphylaxis.
Time to eliminate trigger from the diet	Unknown	6 years average, it varies, ? off wheat for life.

If you are *not* coeliac but still think you may be sensitive to gluten, you need to eliminate all gluten from the diet for 4–6 weeks to reduce the gluten load in the system and see if you can alleviate symptoms. We often see improvements in stages: first, the bowel may become less irritable; then the brain starts thinking more clearly; then energy starts to return; then aches and pain diminish; and so on. If symptoms resolve by the end of the trial, you may have your diagnosis: non-coeliac gluten sensitivity. It's a new name for an old problem. It's much easier these days to go gluten-free, but you must be strict – no cheating!

Going Gluten Foods: Source:https://www.betterhealth.vic.gov.au/health/healthyliving/gluten-free-diet#gluten-free-foods

Type of Food	Free of Gluten	Contains Gluten
Meat products	Unprocessed meat, fish, chicken, bacon, ham off the bone. Meats that are frozen or canned, but with no sauce.	Products prepared with breadcrumbs or batter, sausages and other processed meats or small goods (unless labelled gluten-free), thickened soups, meat pies and frozen meals.
Dairy products	Eggs, full-cream milk, low-fat milk, evaporated milk, condensed milk, fresh cream, yoghurt, block cheese, and some custards, ice creams and soy milks.	Malted milk, ice cream cones, some ice creams and some soy milks.

Fruits and vegetables	Fresh, canned or frozen (but not sauced) fruit juices.	Textured vegetable protein (found in some vegetarian products) and fruit-pie filling.
Cereals and baking products	Corn (maize) flour, soya flour, lentil flour, rice flour and rice bran, potato flour, sorghum, buckwheat, millet, amaranth. Cereals made from corn and rice (without malt extract from barley), polenta and psyllium.	Wheat, wheat flour, wheaten cornflour, freekeh, spelt, semolina, couscous, wheat bran, barley, oats, porridge. Breakfast cereals containing wheat, rye, oats or barley, cereals made from corn or rice that also contain malt extract from barley. Some icing-sugar mixtures and some baking powders.
Breads, pizza, pastry, cakes and biscuits	Most rice crackers, corn cakes, rice crispbreads, corn tortillas and taco shells.	All bread, pizza, pastry, cakes and biscuits prepared with flours from a gluten source.
Pasta and noodles	Rice noodles, rice or bean vermicelli, and buckwheat noodles.	Spaghetti, pasta, lasagne, gnocchi, Hokkien noodles, soba noodles and two-minute noodles (read label).

Condiments	Tahini, jam, honey, maple syrup, cocoa, all vinegars (except malt vinegar), most tomato pastes, some sauces and salad dressings.	Malt vinegar, some mustards, relishes, pickles, salad dressings, stock, sauces, gravy and yeast extract from barley (for example, in Vegemite).
Snacks	Plain chips, plain corn chips and unflavoured popcorn.	Liquorice, lollies and chocolates, packet savoury snacks and some flavoured potato and corn chips.
Drinks	Water, full-cream and low-fat milk, fruit and vegetable juices, tea, coffee, mineral water, wine and spirits.	Coffee substitutes, cereal, and some milk-drink powders (Milo, Ovaltine, and malted milk powder), beer, lager, ale and stout (Guinness).
Other	Seeds, nuts and nut butters.	N/A
Specially made gluten-free foods	Packaged breads, biscuits, cakes, pasta, and beer labelled as 'gluten-free'.	N/A

In Australia, foods that are labelled 'gluten-free' must have a gluten content of less than three parts per million. There's now a wide choice of gluten-free foods available in supermarkets, although they're still slightly more expensive than comparable foods that contain gluten.

REBUILDING YOUR NUTRIENT STORES

If you've recently been diagnosed with coeliac disease, you might not have felt well for a long time. But you'll be amazed at how much better you can feel after a few months on a gluten-free diet and replenishing your deficient nutrients.

Your inflammed gut may have struggled to absorb nutrients properly for years, leaving you tired, moody, and troubled by various symptoms like headaches and joint pains. Diarrhoea from malabsorption might have worsened these deficiencies. You're likely deficient in minerals like iron, zinc, and magnesium, as well as vitamins D, K, and B12.

Getting injections of these vitamins and minerals can quickly restore optimal levels, bypassing the gut entirely. You may need to find a doctor with a focus on nutrition to help with this.

Remember, it can take time for gluten antibody levels to decrease, so another biopsy may be needed for confirmation. If antibodies remain high, a dietitian can help ensure your diet is truly gluten-free. Not everyone responds immediately to a gluten-free diet, especially with other medical conditions present.

COELIAC DISEASE & GLUTEN SENSITIVITY

ACTION PLAN – CHECKLIST

- Confirm coeliac disease with blood tests and a gut biopsy.
- Seek dietetic advice to maintain a gluten-free diet for life.
- Re-check gluten antibodies in six months, to confirm diet is on track.
- Add probiotics.
- Check the levels of the B vitamins especially B12.
- Check for deficiencies in zinc, iron, magnesium, and copper.
- Supplement vitamins D and K and the B vitamins as required.

References:

Czaja-Bulsa G. (2015). Non coeliac gluten sensitivity - A new disease with gluten intolerance. *Clinical nutrition (Edinburgh, Scotland)*, *34*(2), 189–194. https://doi.org/10.1016/j.clnu.2014.08.012

Biesiekierski, J.R., Iven, J. (2015). Non-coeliac gluten sensitivity: piecing the puzzle together. *United European Gastroenterol J.* 3(2):160–165. Doi:10.1177/2050640615578388.

Czaja-Bulsa G. (2015). Non coeliac gluten sensitivity - A new disease with gluten intolerance. *Clinical nutrition (Edinburgh, Scotland)*, *34*(2), 189–194. https://doi.org/10.1016/j.clnu.2014.08.012

Chapter 5

ECZEMA

"God is in the details."

LUDWIG MILES VAN DER ROHE

People with eczema have skin that dries out very easily, leaving it more open to allergens and prone to itchiness and redness. Rates of eczema peak in infancy, affecting about one in five children under two years but of course it can occur older children and adults too. It is a common condition, but sometimes it's not well managed. Allergy testing is important in eczema.

Eczema often has a genetic basis, afflicting people with family histories of asthma, hay fever and other allergies. But it also needs a trigger, which usually comes in the form of an irritant, an infection, stress, sweating, or nutritional deficiency.

GENETICS AND ENVIRONMENT COME TOGETHER

Questions for Eczema Sufferers

1. Are family members sensitive to gluten in food, drugs, moulds, animals, pollens or chemicals?
2. Is there a sensitivity to foods, additives or colours (e.g. MSG/chicken salt in flavoured packaged foods)?
3. Does eczema develop at a certain location (e.g. school, home, relative's house, picnics)?
4. Are laundry detergents, soaps or make-up aggravating the problem?
5. Do you have a sensitivity to chlorine or fluoride in the water supply?
6. Is there enough zinc or vitamin D in the diet?
7. Are you using moisturiser several times a day?
8. Is there a gut issue with poor diet and lack microbe diversity?

Common Causes of Eczema

- **Dust mite allergy** can affect people with eczema. The skin is often worse at night. Dust mites live in humid environments in bedding and carpets. Treat by soaking affected fabrics in a mix of pure tea tree oil and hot water (one capful of tea tree oil per litre of hot water) and detergent for one hour. Rinse and then wash as normal in hot water in the washing machine. Allow three weeks to see a difference.
- **Grass and pollen allergy:** Noticeable after sitting on the grass and on windy days. This commonly occurs when grass is pollenating and often affects the respiratory system, but skin and eyes can be irritated as well. Some plants cause problems, especially if the skin is dry and pollen sits in the skin folds.

- **Foods may cause problems with some people:** Check for food allergies. Sometimes foods with high salicylate content may cause problems for some people. Avoid stone fruit, citrus fruit, berries, herbs and spices.
- **Check if some drugs may cause skin irritation.** Commonly Aspirin and Ibuprofen or other non-steroidal anti-inflammatories, penicillins and other drugs.
- **Food colours, preservatives and flavour enhancers:** Avoid those labelled as tartrazine (102 and 124), monosodium glutamate or MSG (621), ribonucleotides (627, 631 and 635), sulphur dioxide (220), benzoates (210 and 211), potassium metabisulphite (224) and metabisulphite (223). Avoid the lot and then bring back one at a time for a few days.
- **Laundry detergents** many cause problems. Avoid powders, use small amounts of unscented liquid detergent and avoid fabric softener.
- **Formaldehyde:** Found in hand-cleaning products, shampoos and wrinkle-free textiles.
- **Rosin or colophony:** Found in cosmetics, toiletries, and shoe and car polish.
- **Wool and other prickly fabric:** Found in clothes and carpets.
- **Sodium lauryl sulphate (SLS):** Found in shampoos and soaps.
- **Chlorine:** Added to our water to kill off any bad bacteria. If you are suspicious, eliminate chlorine with a trial of bottled water. It's harder to remove chlorine from water used in the shower so tank water may be the best option if possible.
- **Fluoride:** Found in water supply and toothpaste. Some people who drink fluoridated water develop skin conditions as a result. Drinking water can be treated by reverse osmosis to remove fluoride; however, tank water is the best option for showering.
- **Nutrient deficiencies:** If your skin lacks certain fats (fatty acids), it'll become dry and sensitive. These fats can only come from the diet, so make sure you eat enough oily fish, nuts and seeds. Lowering vitamin D, zinc, magnesium and iodine tends to make the eczema symptoms worse. Supplementing with vitamin D 600–800 IU (International Units)/day and 30 mg of zinc per day for about three months may assist improvement.

· **Probiotics:** Our opinion is that anyone suffering from eczema should consider taking probiotics regularly. See Chapter 20, for more information.

TREATMENTS FOR ECZEMA

The conventional treatment for eczema is to focus on the use of antihistamines or steroid medications. These drugs are essential when skin flares are severe, but they only treat the symptoms, nor the cause of the eczema. It is worth trying to find the trigger and cause of the problem. Sometimes a skin biopsy is necessary when things don't improve.

Reducing the Triggers

1. Test for allergies and avoid/reduce allergens, additives, and maybe salicylates (see Chapter 2 on Allergies).
2. Avoid irritants – perfumes, soaps, and scented laundry powders.
3. Add half a cup of white vinegar at the end of the wash cycle or in the fabric softener dispenser.
4. Use dryer balls in place of fabric softeners in the washing machine.
5. Use non-allergenic cosmetics.
6. Assess if heat, cold and rapid temperature changes irritate the skin.

Care for the Skin

· Use non-soap body wash when showering or washing.
· Moisturiser should be applied after the shower and several times per day.

- Epsom salt baths to relieve the itch. Add two cups of Epsom salts per bathtub and soak for about half an hour about 2-3 times per week. Rinse off and apply skin creams and emollients straight away.
- Use a 5% solution of Dead Sea salt and soak the affected area for fifteen minutes daily for about six weeks. It can improve the skin barrier, hydration, and reduce skin roughness and inflammation.
- Reduce stress – stress can make the skin worse.
- Enhance the diversity of the gut. A mixture of different bacterial species or of *Lactobacillus* species showed greater benefit than did treatment with *Bifidobacterium* species alone.
- Add quercetin. It decreases inflammation in eczema. Usual dose: 1000 mg/day.

WHEN ECZEMA IS SEVERE

- **Adding bleach to bathwater**: This practice, known as bleach baths, is sometimes recommended for certain skin conditions like eczema to reduce bacterial colonisation on the skin. However, the concentration of bleach needs to be precise, typically around half a cup for a *full* bathtub. Ten minutes up to three times a week is a common recommendation for bleach baths. It's crucial to rinse thoroughly after a bleach bath to remove any residual bleach, as it can irritate the skin if left on. Moisturising immediately after bathing is also essential to lock in moisture.
- **Use of cortisone orally or topically**: Cortisone, whether oral or topical, can help reduce inflammation and itching associated with certain skin conditions. However, long-term use of oral cortisone should be under the supervision of a healthcare professional due to potential side effects.
- **Antihistamines**: These can indeed help alleviate itching and are commonly used for various skin conditions.

· **Applying wet wraps** to the affected areas will help rehydrate and calm the itch while delivering topical creams. The wraps are applied after bathing, and moisturising creams and medication are applied at this time. Wet cotton gloves or socks can be used on the hands and feet for the wet layer, with plastic/cling wrap applied on top as the dry layer. Gauze wraps (from chemists/shops) are moistened in warm water and applied to the affected skin with normal clean clothing for the top dry layer. The wraps can be left overnight, but don't allow them to dry out. Moisten them again before taking them off. The clinic nurse can demonstrate how and when these wraps are applied.

ECZEMA

ACTION PLAN – CHECKLIST

- Identify the triggers and avoid where possible.
- Use antihistamines and cortisone when necessary.
- Check for deficiencies especially vitamin D, zinc and essential fatty acids.
- Use cortisone and wet wraps when the symptom is severe.
- Moisturise heavily.
- Add probiotics, vitamin D, E, zinc and quercetin for immune support.

References:
Andreozzi, L., Giannetti, A., Cipriani, F., Caffarelli, C., Mastrorilli, C., & Ricci, G. (2019). Hypersensitivity reactions to food and drug additives: problem or myth? *Acta bio-medica: Atenei Parmensis*, *90*(3-S), 80–90. https://doi.org/10.23750/abm.v90i3-S.8168

Schlichte, M. J., Vandersall, A., & Katta, R. (2016). Diet and eczema: a review of dietary supplements for the treatment of atopic dermatitis. *Dermatology Practical & Conceptual, 6*(3), 23–29. https://doi.org/10.5826/dpc.0603a06

Kim, S. O., Ah, Y. M., Yu, Y. M., Choi, K. H., Shin, W. G., & Lee, J. Y. (2014). Effects of probiotics for the treatment of atopic dermatitis: a meta-analysis of randomized controlled trials. *Annals of allergy, asthma & immunology : official publication of the American College of Allergy, Asthma, & Immunology, 113*(2), 217–226. https://doi.org/10.1016/j.anai.2014.05.021

Chapter 6

ASTHMA

"Life isn't measured by the number of breaths we take, but by the moments that take our breath away."

AUTHOR UNKNOWN

If you have asthma, you find it hard to move air in and out of your lungs as you breathe. The difficulty is greater when you try to breathe out. You can feel wheezy and feel tight in the chest and suffer coughing fits that bring up mucous. As symptoms develop, the inflamed airways from your lungs will narrow. The lining of the bronchial tubes swell, making the circular muscles around them tight, twitchy and prone to spasms, triggering the production of mucous that interferes with your breathing.

Around 11% of Australians have asthma compared to the UK with 12%. In the USA just over 7% have an asthma diagnosis. We know that genetics, allergies, environment, infections, emotions and overuse of antibiotics in early childhood all play a part in this complex medical condition.

GENES VERSUS ENVIRONMENT

The cause of asthma can be divided into two categories:

1. **The first category is hereditary.** This first type comes from your parents. Scientists are studying the chromosomes that carry asthma traits, aiming to find treatments and maybe even a cure. They might find groups more likely to get asthma now that they've found the Bpifb1 gene, which controls mucus in the lungs.
2. **The second category is environmental.** The food you eat, the air particles you inhale, the chemicals you work with and the climate you live in can all trigger or exacerbate asthma.

Understanding the balance between genetics and environment in asthma development can be tricky. Kids with allergic parents face a higher risk, while babies born to smoking moms have double the chance. But even with a genetic predisposition, asthma might not show up unless environmental triggers come into play. Common triggers include dust mites, pollen, pets, and certain foods. Don't worry; Chapter 2 has tips on handling these irritants.

Certain foods high in salicylates or additives can worsen symptoms. Other triggers include smoke, infections, chemicals, medications, and stress. Around 5% of folks may react to food additives, especially if they've had issues with different foods or processed ones. Watch out for sulphites in wine, prawns, and dried apricots. Check out the list of risk factors for more details.

Risk Factors for Asthma

Genetics:

Family history of asthma or allergy

History of respiratory conditions and infections

High-risk occupations:

Baking

Woodworking

Farming

Laboratory assistants

Painters using paints containing isocyanates.

Cleaners using chemical cleaning agents

Work chemicals:

Chlorine gas

Sulphur dioxide

Paints

Adhesives that contain acrylate

Laminates

Soldering resins

Insulation packaging

Foam mattresses

Latex

Persulphate in hair chemicals

Farm sprays

Tobacco smoke

Dust mites

Animal fur

Pollen

Moulds

Common food allergens:

Milk and all dairy

Eggs

Nuts and peanuts

Wheat

Soy

Seafood

Food chemicals:

Naturally occurring salicylates and amines

Foods additives such as:

monosodium glutamate MSG (620-625),

ribonucleotides (627-635),

tartrazine (102),

sulphites (220-228),

nitrites (249-252),

benzoates (220-229),

butylated hydroxytoluene (BHT) 321

butylated hydroxyanisole (BHA) 320

Medicines:	Other:
	Exercise
Aspirin	Cold, dry air
Beta blockers for blood high pressure	Stress
ACE inhibitors heart disease	Thunderstorms
Eye drops for glaucoma	Laughter
	Sex

WHAT A DOCTOR CAN DO FOR YOU

The three main goals of asthma management are control of the symptoms, re-duction in risk of exacerbations, and minimisation of adverse effects of medications. A spirometry test measures the amount of air you breathe in and out within a certain period, can tell you how narrow your airways are and how well your lungs are working. You can also review your inhaler technique, medications, coexisting conditions and exposures to environmental triggers. For example, a runny nose may point to a pollen allergy worsening your asthma. If allergies are believed to be behind your asthma, your doctor may order skin prick tests or RadioAllergoSorbent (RAST) blood tests.

Preventer inhalers contain corticosteroids to reduce inflammation and may include long-acting medications to keep airways open. **Tiotropium (Spiriva)** relaxes airway muscles for up to 24 hours, mainly for severe asthma, with significant side effects.

Bronchodilators like **Ventolin** provide quick relief. **Ipratropium (Atrovent HFA)** is for emphysema or chronic bronchitis but can treat asthma attacks. **Trimbow**, a new pre-venter for severe asthma, reduces swelling and relaxes airway muscles.

Intravenous corticosteroids and **EpiPen** are for emergencies; EpiPen contains sodium metabisulfite but is still used in severe allergic reactions.

Immune system therapies like **Singulair and Omalizumab (Xolair)** target immune chemicals or IgE response, respectively, to alleviate asthma symptoms.

Asthma Action
Asthma Australia

Every asthmatic should have an Asthma Action Plan, available from organisations like the Australian National Asthma Council. This plan, completed by a doctor, should be understood by family, school, or work members in case of emergencies.

It's common for asthmatics to have low levels of zinc, selenium, and vitamin D. Boosting these nutrients can support your immune system, along with adding fatty fish and a nutrient-rich diet. Magnesium helps relax bronchial muscles, so it's worth checking blood levels and considering a trial of 400 mg per day for three weeks and see if the symptoms have improved. Quercetin is another helpful supplement, but it's high in salicylates, so be cautious if sensitive. It has antihistamine and antiallergy properties and can help break down mucus.

WHAT ELSE CAN YOU DO?

Medical treatment is key to keeping asthma under control. Other therapies may help as well.

- Acupuncture: It's not a replacement for modern asthma drugs, but it can help alongside them. Around 60% of kids with asthma experience side effects from their daily medications. The World Health Organization approves acupuncture for asthma, sinus issues, hay fever, bronchitis, and colds

· **Gentle thoracic spine manipulation**: If chest symptoms come from the spine, gentle adjustments might help. Sometimes, a misaligned spine could result from breathing problems, not the other way around.

· **Stress and Anxiety**: Stress and anxiety can make asthma worse, and asthma can make stress worse. Relaxation techniques like tai chi and yoga and mindfulness which focus on breathing, can help calm both body and mind.

· **Check for nutritional deficiencies**: Vitamin D, along with the minerals zinc, selenium and magnesium are important.

· **Herbal medicines**: Use with more caution. Many are high in salicylates that trigger allergic reactions or sensitivities in some asthmatics.

· **Mould** thrives in humid environments and can be harmful, especially for those with weakened immunity. Chapter 2 (Allergy) and Chapter 27 (When All Else Fails) provide comprehensive information on dealing with mould.

ASTHMA

ACTION PLAN

- Determine your Asthma Action Plan with your doctor.
- Have an EpiPen always available for emergencies.
- Ensure medications are available at home, work or school.
- Check allergies via skin prick tests and blood tests.
- Be aware of triggers – foods, chemicals and environmental pollutants.
- Avoid moulds and fungi.
- Supplement any nutritional deficiencies, especially vitamin D and zinc.
- Enjoy a Mediterranean diet (more in Chapter 30).
- Manage stress and include exercise within limitations.

References:

Allan, K., & Devereux, G. (2011). Diet and asthma: nutrition implications from prevention to treatment. *Journal of the American Dietetic Association*, *111*(2), 258–268. https://doi.org/10.1016/j.jada.2010.10.048

Asthma Australia. (2020). *Asthma Statistics & Facts*. Asthma Australia. https://www.asthmaaustralia.org.au/national/about-asthma/what-is-asthma/statistics

National Asthma Council Australia. (2024) Asthma Action Plan: https://www.nationalasthma.org.au/living-with-asthma/resources/health-professionals/asthma-action-plans/hp-asthma-action-plans-by-national-asthma-council-australia

Dubus, J. C., Marguet, C., Deschildre, A., Mely, L., Le Roux, P., Brouard, J., Huiart, L., & Réseau de Recherche Clinique en Pneumonologie Pédiatrique. (2001). Local side-effects of inhaled corticosteroids in asthmatic children: influence of drug, dose, age, and device. *Allergy*, *56*(10), 944–948. https://doi.org/10.1034/j.1398-9995.2001.00100.x

Miraglia Del Giudice, M., Indolfi, C., Capasso, M., Maiello, N., Decimo, F., & Ciprandi, G. (2017). Bifidobacterium mixture (B longum BB536, B infantis M-63, B breve M-16V) treatment in children with seasonal allergic rhinitis and intermittent asthma. *Italian journal of pediatrics*, *43*(1), 25. https://doi.org/10.1186/s13052-017-0340-5

Chapter 7

MIGRAINE

"And I have learned now to live with it, learned when to expect it, how to outwit it, even how to regard it, when it does come, as more friend than lodger. We have reached an understanding, my migraine and I."

JOAN DIDION

Migraines can be tough to pin down. They often start with a pounding, one-sided headache, sometimes with eye pain, and come with sensitivity to light and sound, plus nausea. They can stick around for hours or days. Although they can start in youth, they become more common in adulthood, affecting about 1 in 5 women and 1 in 10 men.

We're still figuring them out. They might involve changes in brain blood flow and chemicals. Too much glutamate can make the brain overreact to pain, while too little GABA can make it worse. Low serotonin levels can play a role too.

Hormones also play a part. Just before a period, dropping oestrogen levels can mess with serotonin, leading to menstrual migraines. Pregnancy, birth control pills, and hormone therapy can also trigger them. Keeping a migraine calendar can help track patterns over time.

Diagnosis: The first step in managing migraines is getting the right diagnosis. There are three hundred different types of headaches, so a doctor may order tests such as MRI (Magnetic Resonance Imaging) and scans to rule out other possible conditions such as strokes and tumours if the evidence is not clear.

Prevention: The second step in managing migraines is preventing them. If you can identify the causes or the triggers for your migraines, you'll be much better placed to prevent the next one.

Hit them hard, hit them early: The third step is intervening early if migraines occur. Take your migraine medication as soon as you feel one coming on. Don't wait until your migraine intensifies. Specialists will often tell you to 'hit it hard and hit it early' with painkillers and anti-inflammatory medicines.

THE MANY MIGRAINE TRIGGERS

Migraines can begin with your genes. Within the labyrinth of our DNA lies the methylentetrahydrofolatereductase gene, best known (for obvious reason) as the MTHFR gene. Its the main character in the realm of headaches and ethereal 'auras'.

Numerous genetic pathways intertwine and these predispositions shape our migraine experiences.

While these genetic mutations may not wield the power to summon migraines alone, they join with physical, mental, and environmental stressors to produce the migraine. It is well understood that headache frequency is increased by emotional factors and while 75% of sufferers recognise a range of triggers for their migraines, only about 2% consider food as *not* being a trigger. The major triggers seem to be stress, hormones, fasting and food. All triggers are additive and attacks happen when an individual's stress/environmental threshold is exceeded.

Super-sensitive 'migraine brains' do not adapt quickly to change. And yes, migraines are more common in a Hypersensitive Person (HSP) – see Chapter 26. Here are some of the recognised triggers:

- Stress-related changes, which play a role in around 70% of chronic daily migraines.
- Neck pain.
- Fluctuations in hormones and neurotransmitters.
- Weather, heat and changes in barometric pressure.
- Sleep – too little or too much.
- Alcohol – that extra glass of red wine or beer.
- Strong light, smells, smoke or sounds cause more acute attacks.
- Exercise and sexual activity.
- Fatigue (over-exertion and lack of sleep).
- Allergies – check out wheat or other allergies mentioned in the previous chapters.
- MSG or other additives in packaged chips or takeaway foods.
- Nutritional deficiencies.

PREVENTION RATHER THAN CURE

By the time you pop a pill for a migraine, you already have one. There are other strategies to prevent migraines:

1. **Gentle physical therapies** such as acupuncture, simple massage and gentle manipulation can have a remarkable effect on migraines caused by tense, tender muscles around the head and neck.
2. **Botox injections** have also been used effectively when all else fails. Referral to a neurologist is required. About 31 injections (across the neck and head) every 12 weeks may be required.
3. **Changes to your diet** can also help, especially if migraines occur after you consume certain foods or additives. When migraines happen, it's worth recording what you ate or drank beforehand. A tailored diet can also go a long way towards addressing some of the nutritional, blood sugar and neurotransmitter imbalances behind migraines.
4. **Low-glycaemic foods:** Avoid the high and low blood sugars that trigger symptoms.
5. **Food allergies and sensitivities** are common among migraine sufferers. If you can see a pattern, ask your doctor for a skin prick test and/or RadioAllergoSorbent test (RAST) blood test to check for allergies. Regarding sensitivities to foods, a study (Lance, 2012) of more than 500 adults with a history of migraines found many had sensitivities (not allergy) to alcohol (17%), cheese (17%) and chocolate (17%). Another study found 11% were sensitive to citrus. Among children, a study of 100 children found that the foods which caused the most problems were caffeine (28%), cocoa (22%), cheese (13%), citrus (10%) and tomato (one patient), as well as the additives monosodium glutamate or MSG (25%), aspartame (13%)

and nitrates (6%). The trigger food generally had to be consumed more than once to cause a headache, so the cumulative effect made all the difference.

6. **A ketogenic diet** (low in carbs and high in protein and fat) may be useful for some people. Studies suggest this very low carbohydrate diet may decrease the frequency of migraines but consult a doctor before making such a change.

7. **Eating lots of foods rich in folate** has been beneficial for migraine sufferers, especially those with a connection to the MTHFR gene. These individuals, who often experience migraines with auras, struggle to process folate properly. They also tend to have high levels of homocysteine, an amino acid linked to migraines and other health issues. Taking folate and other B vitamins as supplements can lower these homocysteine levels and potentially ease migraine symptoms.

8. **Supplement with fish oils.** Fish oils with omega-3 fats have been shown to reduce inflammation and migraines.

9. **High-dose vitamin B2 (riboflavin).** 400 mg of B2 daily often reduces the frequency of migraines.

10. **Keep a diary of what you eat.** Don't be caught by surprise.

11. **Manipulation/chiropractic/osteopathy/physiotherapy/massage** can all play a therapeutic role, especially if the migraine is a result of referred pain from the neck.

12. **Biofeedback** is where electrical sensors are attached to the head to measure brain waves, breathing, heart rate and muscle contraction. A computer graphic feedback assists changes necessary for managing anxiety and stress and many associated conditions.

13. **Practice deep-breathing exercises** which increase oxygen supplies to the brain.

MIGRAINE

ACTION PLAN – CHECKLIST

- Confirm the diagnosis. There are many causes of headaches.
- Use modern drugs in the prevention and treatment of migraine.
- Consider other pain management options.
- Check hormones, gluten sensitivity and other foods or chemical triggers.
- Try a low amine diet for three weeks.
- Try weekly acupuncture.
- Keep a diary for two weeks re: pain intensity and frequency.
- Try vitamin B2 and fish oil supplements.
- Keep well hydrated.
- Manage stress effectively.
- Avoid low blood sugar swings.
- Get enough sleep.
- Use tinted glasses on sunny days.
- Stay indoors if affected by the weather conditions.

References:

Alpay, K., Ertas, M., Orhan, E. K., Ustay, D. K., Lieners, C., & Baykan, B. (2010). Diet restriction in migraine, based on IgG against foods: a clinical double-blind, randomised, cross-over trial. *Cephalalgia: An International Journal of Headache*, *30*(7), 829–837. https://doi.org/10.1177/0333102410361404

Lance, J. W. (2012). Impact commentaries: Observations on 500 cases of migraine and allied vascular headache. *Journal of Neurology, Neurosurgery & Psychiatry*, *83*(7), 673–674. https://doi.org/10.1136/jnnp-2011-301630

Taheri, S. (2017). Effect of exclusion of frequently consumed dietary triggers in a cohort of children with chronic primary headache. *Nutrition and Health*, *23*(1), 47–50. https://doi.org/10.1177/0260106016688699

Woolhouse, M. (2005). Migraine and tension headache – a complementary and alternative medicine approach. *Australian Family Physician*, *34*(8), 647–651.

Chapter 8

ARTHRITIS

"Success is a journey – not a destination."

BEN SWEETLAND

Arthritis is the most common disease in the Western world and a leading cause of disability in old age. There are more than one hundred different types of arthritis, including the two most common (osteoarthritis and rheumatoid arthritis). They all have all the characteristics of inflammation – redness, swelling, heat, pain and loss of function. Infections, hormonal imbalances, obesity, trauma, infection and stress can play a role in the inflammatory processes, particularly among people genetically predisposed to arthritis.

Inflammation can start in specific joints. Over time, the smooth, shock-absorbing cartilage tissue that protects the joints wears away and, in some cases, bone spurs develop. Arthritic symptoms can take decades to develop but can affect many joints in your body – from your hips, knees and lower back to your fingers and toes. As you age, the pain can become chronic, creating a whole new set of problems.

No single lab test can definitively diagnose the disease. Generally it can be classified as bilateral, peripheral and symmetrical. There are many useful markers characteristic of rheumatoid arthritis:

- **Anti-CCP antibody test.** A positive anti-CCP test is considered diagnostic of rheumatoid arthritis. Around 60–70% of people with rheumatoid arthritis test positive for anti-CCP antibodies. The CCP (cyclic citrullinated peptide) antibodies are made by the immune system and mistakenly attack healthy tissues.
- **Rheumatoid factor** is also an antibody (protein) found in the blood. Raised levels and joint pain on both sides of the body is an indicator for rheumatoid arthritis. In 30% of cases, however, the test is not always positive in early stages of the disease, while around 80% test positive when the disease is established.
- **C-reactive protein (CRP).** CRP is considered the best general inflammatory marker. It is not specific for arthritis but it is often used to monitor a person's response to treatment.
- **Erythrocyte sedimentation rate test (ESR).** Similar to CRP, this test also screens for inflammation.

We strongly advocate for the Mediterranean diet (Chapter 30) with the reduction of refined grains and sugar products typical of a pro-inflammatory diet. The vegan diet has also been shown to improved pain and stiffness. The usual suspects of the allergy world – gluten, dairy and food additives – can also trigger arthritic symptoms. Nightshade vegetables, such as tomatoes, potatoes, eggplants, and peppers, contain a group of compounds called alkaloids. Some people believe that these alkaloids may contribute to inflammation and exacerbate arthritis symptoms. However, scientific evidence on this relationship is conflicting.

Nutrients for Pain: There is a myriad of nutrients that help alleviate pain and/or inflammation: The components of cartilage glucosamine and chondroitin are commonly used supplements for arthritis. S-adenosyl-methionine (SAM-e) has anti-inflammatory, cartilage-protecting and pain-relieving effects. Other anti-inflammatory nutrients include fish oil, turmeric with black pepper (piperine), ginger, magnesium and vitamin B 12.

Herbs for Pain Management: Commonly used are devil's claw (*Harpagopytum*) and perhaps *Boswellia serrata*. Most natural anti-inflammatory preparations contain multiple nutrients, so there's no need for lots of tablets or needing to remember the names of all the herbs.

Exercise, like a good diet, has multiple benefits. It keeps the blood pumping to deliver nutrients, eliminate waste and lubricate stiff, inflamed joints so they're better able to move. It reduces weight, builds muscle, restores energy, and improves fitness, balance and flexibility. Crucially, it releases endorphins that can lift your mood, relieve pain and relax your body. An exercise physiologist can develop a personalised training program to get you started safely, especially since exercise can hurt at first. Some forms of exercise such as stretching or hydrotherapy hurt less because they have less impact on joints. Swimming and water aerobics are ideal when non-weight-bearing exercise is necessary.

CONVENTIONAL MANAGEMENT

Early aggressive treatment reduces the risk of severe joint damage and disability. If you achieve remission, the drug dose is reduced. The non-steroidal anti-inflammatory drugs, e.g. Celebrex, Mobic and Naproxen (Naprosyn), are useful starters, but where inflammation is severe, prednisone is prescribed for a short time to suppress the immune system.

Rheumatologists are more likely to prescribe the disease-modifying antirheumatic drugs (DMARDs) such as methotrexate (e.g. Rheumatrex and Trexall), which also suppress the immune system and are very effective. There are side effects, which include folate deficiency causing mouth ulcers, gastrointestinal problems and liver toxicity. Janus kinase (JAK) inhibitor drugs can only be accessed after meeting certain criteria, but like all medications they have both benefits and side effects, and they don't help everyone. All require close monitoring.

Lifestyle factors play a huge role, so weight management, exercise and diet are crucial to management.

ARTHRITIS

ACTION PLAN – CHECKLIST

- Diagnose early – for example, with blood tests and X-rays.
- Check for allergies, gluten sensitivity and chemical irritants.
- Manage pain with pharmaceuticals, natural medicines or acupuncture.
- Keep joints supple with activity, good fats and hydration.
- Keep weight under control.
- Use a vegan or Mediterranean diet. Add fish oil and turmeric.
- Recognise triggers for flares – for example, gluten and sugary foods.
- For pain, try glucosamine sulphate and chondroitin for six weeks.

References:

Alwarith, J., Kahleova, H., Rembert, E., Yonas, W., Dort, S., Calcagno, M., Burgess, N., Crosby, L., & Barnard, N. D. (2019). Nutrition Interventions in Rheumatoid Arthritis: The Potential Use of Plant-Based Diets. A Review. *Frontiers in nutrition*, 6, 141. https://doi.org/10.3389/fnut.2019.00141

Khanna, S., Jaiswal, K. S., & Gupta, B. (2017). Managing Rheumatoid Arthritis with Dietary Interventions. *Frontiers in Nutrition*, 4, 52. https://doi.org/10.3389/fnut.2017.00052

van de Laar, M. A., & van der Korst, J. K. (1992). Food intolerance in rheumatoid arthritis. I. A double blind, controlled trial of the clinical effects of elimination of milk allergens and azo dyes. *Annals of the Rheumatic Diseases*, 51(3), 298–302. https://doi.org/10.1136/ard.51.3.298

Wilsdon, T. D., & Hill, C. L (2017). Managing the drug treatment of rheumatoid arthritis. *Australian Prescriber*, 40(2), 51–58. https://doi.org/10.18773/austprescr.2017.012

Chapter 9

CHRONIC PAIN

*"He has the right to criticise who
has the heart to help."*

ABRAHAM LINCOLN

Chronic pain is when discomfort sticks around for six months or more, shifting from temporary to long-lasting. Pain is a personal experience, shaped by lots of things like how you're feeling emotionally, what society expects, and cultural influences. Your ability to handle pain changes depending on how you're feeling, how well you've slept, and what you're up to. Since pain is tricky to pin down, explaining it well to your healthcare provider—like describing how it feels, when it happens, where it hurts, how bad it is, and what it stops you from doing—really helps in figuring out your best treatment.

4 MAJOR TYPES OF PAIN

Pain can be categorised into several types based on various factors such as its duration, underlying cause, and location.

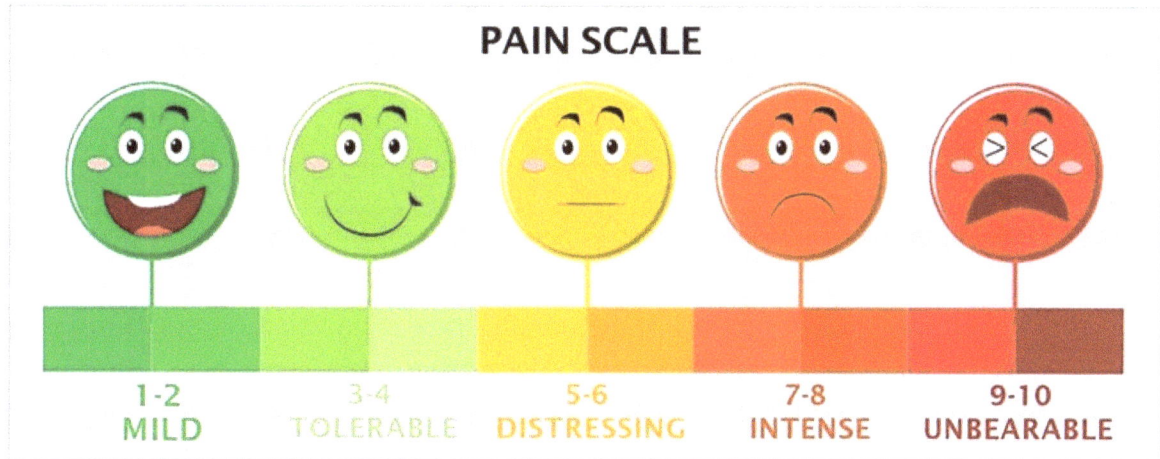

PAIN SCALE

| 1-2 MILD | 3-4 TOLERABLE | 5-6 DISTRESSING | 7-8 INTENSE | 9-10 UNBEARABLE |

Emojis are fun; while pain ... not so much. The tolerance for pain depends on personality traits and attitudes, your previous experience of pain, financial status and even gender (women are more sensitive to pain).

DIFFERENT TYPES OF PAIN

1. **Acute pain** that occurs with accidents, illnesses and surgery is different from chronic pain. It is generally self-limiting and settles as the healing process occurs. Drugs and physical therapy are helpful in these situations, with full function and healing being restored in a timely manner. But pain can persist well beyond the time of the original tissue damage, and the site of the pain location can change and be quite different from the site of the original injury.

2. **Chronic pain** affects every part of your body, intertwining with inflammation and challenging your immune system. Even without injury, hypersensitive nerves can send pain signals to the brain. Managing it requires a holistic approach, including simple remedies like ice and heat, as well as pain management programs. These programs, led by specialists like doctors, physiotherapists, and psychologists, take a whole-person approach to address the complexities of chronic pain. Stress, prior pain experiences, and fear of movement can make chronic pain worse. Long-term opioid use is then less than ideal.

3. **Neuropathic pain or nerve pain** is often described as a 'shooting' or burning pain, and sometimes pins and needles. Common causes include nerve injuries, diabetes, and conditions like sciatica. Nerve pain is the most difficult to treat, and the opioids and anti-inflammatory drugs are often unsatisfactory. Drugs such as antidepressants (e.g., amitriptyline, nortriptyline) and selective serotonin and norepinephrine reuptake inhibitors (SNRIs) are often prescribed. Anticonvulsants such as gabapentin and pregabalin (Lyrica), help stabilise abnormal nerve activity. Stretching and strengthening exercises and manual therapies can help improve mobility, reduce muscle tension, and alleviate pain. Transcutaneous Electrical Nerve Stimulation (TENS) uses a battery-operated device that delivers mild electrical impulses to the affected area, which can help disrupt pain signals and provide relief. Techniques such as cognitive-behavioral therapy (CBT), mindfulness-based stress reduction and relaxation techniques can help individuals cope with neuropathic pain and reduce its impact on daily life (see Chapter 12).

4. **Complex regional pain syndrome** can occur after an injury, such as a fracture of an arm, hand, leg or foot. Nobody knows why it occurs, and it can be very debilitating. It happens more in females than males, and it can occur in children. The pain can be mild to really severe and vary in intensity, lasting years after the injury. The limb may be hot or cold, with changes in colour and restricted blood flow or muscle spasm. Management includes a combination of medications

(such as pain relievers, antidepressants, anticonvulsants, and anti-inflammatory drugs), physical therapy, occupational therapy, sympathetic nerve blocks, spinal cord stimulation, and psychological therapy. A surgical nerve block can work by destroying particular nerve cells.

MANAGING CHRONIC PAIN

About 70% of patient visits to a GP for chronic pain result in a medication script, with fewer than 15% of these patients being referred to a pain specialist. Suicidal behaviour is 2–3 times higher in people with chronic pain. There is much that can be done, but there are broader issues always at play and lifestyle factors are an added factor in pain management.

Self Management

· **Assessing lifestyle factors** such as diet, hydration, stress levels, and work-life balance as part of routine evaluations to identify areas for improvement.

· **Regular exercise is important** in managing pain, improving mobility, and maintaining overall health.

· **Psychological support** and coping strategies help manage stress, mood swings, and other emotional factors that may exacerbate pain.

· **Individualised Care**: Customising the pain management plan based on the individual's goals, lifestyle, and specific needs, whether focussed on pain relief, prevention, or both.

Pain Medications

· **There is a plethora of natural medicines available.** This usually means that one type is not the answer. It also reflects the fact that different people respond to different products. Fish oil is the go-to nutrient to treat inflammation, then curcumin and ginger. Arnica can be rubbed on the skin for joint pain and inflammation. While there is debate about the effectiveness of glucosamine and chondroitin, our experience is that combinations of glucosamine (approx. 600 mg) with chondroitin (approx. 300 mg) plus MSM (approx. 400 mg) twice a day for a trial of six weeks is a good start for joint pain. MSM can be very helpful on its own. These things take time – and they don't work when left in the bottle!

· **Common drugs used for pain:** Panadol, non-steroidal anti-inflammatory drugs (NSAIDs), opioids, muscle relaxants and sometimes anticonvulsants are useful. There are side effects, and opioids are probably considered the most dangerous because of cognitive deficiency, motor impairment and respiratory depression, among other problems. They also represent a significant addiction risk in certain groups of patients.

· **PEA (palmitoylethanolamide)** offers a promising option for managing pain and inflammation while also enhancing mood. Particularly effective for nerve pain, it's naturally produced in the body after injury and can also be found in certain foods like soy, peanuts, and eggs. With minimal side effects, it's considered safe for pain relief, inflammation, and possibly conditions like eczema and dementia. Studies have shown it to be as effective than non-steroidal anti-inflammatory drugs in relieving pain after two weeks. The typical dose for chronic pain is 400–500 mg taken three times a day, either in capsule or powder form. Despite its short half-life, PEA stands out for its excellent tolerability and safety compared to other medications.

· **Vitamin B12** is beneficial for regeneration of nerves and inhibiting pain-signalling pathways in people with diabetic neuropathy and feet pain. The dose with oral methylcobalamin is 1500 μg daily for three months.

· **Trigger point injections.** In this treatment, a doctor first finds your 'hot spots' – usually taut knots of muscles – by using pressure or ultrasound. Medication (usually cortisone and/or local anaesthetic) is injected into these areas. Cortisone injections affect the tissue, so it's worth consulting an exercise physiologist to help rehabilitation.

· **Spinal drug pumps.** In this treatment, a neurosurgeon inserts a small pump under the skin to deliver drugs (usually morphine or clonidine). They insert this into the fluid around the spinal cord to alleviate symptoms from the deep, painful areas along the spine. While a spinal drug pump can dramatically reduce pain, it doesn't seem to improve function or mood.

Common Procedures for Pain Management

· An orthopaedic and neurosurgical surgeon can operate to relieve pain – for example, by taking the pressure from a disc lesion off a nerve root, cutting nerves or using heat to destroy those that transmit pain from worn-out joints. If it's clear what's causing the pain, you'll generally get better results, but surgery may not be 100% successful.

· **Transcutaneous electrical nerve stimulation (TENS) and dorsal column stimulation.** Both treatments electrically stimulate the nerves to block the normal pathways that carry messages of pain to the brain. They adopt a similar approach to the 'gate theory' where pain signals can be let through or restricted at the spinal cord. The stimulators are placed on the skin with TENS or they're implanted within the body with dorsal column stimulation.

· **Shockwave therapy.** Radiologists have recently introduced this non-invasive procedure that uses high-energy sound waves, similar to those used in a common ultrasound, to break down existing scar tissue, encourage new, healthy blood vessels, and stimulate a new process of repair. Take care afterwards as shockwave therapy, like cortisone injections, affects the tissue.

· **Biofeedback** makes use of electrical sensors to monitor muscle tension, body temperature and brain wave activity over time. Once you're aware of those reactions, you can intervene and alleviate the pain response by making subtle changes such as slowing your breathing and relaxing certain muscles.

· **Acupuncture.** Another traditional practice with proven benefits for pain relief is acupuncture. It uses needles to fire electrical signals up the spinal cord to the brain, 'shutting the gate' so troubling pain signals can't make it through. Usually, you'll know after about three treatments if acupuncture will help. If there is no response, it's probably not worth continuing.

· **Alternative treatments.** You may want to ask about cannabis and low-dose naltrexone (discussed earlier in Chapter 2) as an alternative to conventional anti-inflammatory drugs, especially if you can't tolerate their side effects.

We'd recommend other less invasive therapies, too. They can be as simple as exercise, relaxation and counselling, and include massage and acupuncture. Don't leave home without your hot or cold pack

Stress management. Pain can be isolating. It can help to talk to a trusted friend or someone outside your immediate circle about specific problems. We'd urge you to consider the range of available support out there, from counselling and group therapy to behavioural therapy or psychotherapy.

CANNABIS: WHAT YOU NEED TO KNOW IN A NUTSHELL

Let us give you a little background information to shed light on why cannabis is such a hot topic for such an ancient herb. There has been uncertainty and caution towards the use of medical cannabis.

Firstly, we have the **endocannabinoid system (ECS)**, which is basically a signalling system in the central and peripheral nervous system and in the endocrine and immune systems. In the 80s and 90s, cannabinoid receptors type 1 (CB1) and type 2 (CB2) were discovered:

- CB1 receptors are involved in pain relief and present in several tissues and organs, including the gastrointestinal tract, the spinal cord, adrenal and thyroid glands, liver, and reproductive organs.
- CB2 receptors are in some nervous tissues but mostly in the immune cells, which support the anti-inflammatory effects of cannabis.

Secondly, we have the cannabis plant (Cannabis sativa), otherwise known as marijuana, which contains a host of chemical components. Over a hundred of these are phytocannabinoids, which are the main active chemical components of the cannabis plant. They exert their pharmacological effects via the nervous system and the immune cells. The two main extracts of interest are tetrahydrocannabinol (THC) and cannabidiol (CBD), which are produced from the buds, flowers and leaves of the plant. Hydroponically grown cannabis typically contains between 6% and 8% THC, and the CBD content is between 1% and 4%.

Hashish/hash is made from the more potent sticky resins on the stalk of the cannabis plant, which has a much higher THC content (30–90% depending on the strain).

Hemp, on the other hand, is still the same cannabis plant, but a different variety with a THC content of less than 0.3%. However, extraction methods are the same from hemp as marijuana, so there is a small amount of THC in hemp extractions – about 5%. Hemp seed oil has little or no CBD (75 mg/kg) and even less THC (50 mg/kg) and is legally sourced without prescription.

Tetrahydrocannabinol (THC) provides pain relief, affects cognition and motor function, and has the psychotropic effects that give you a 'high'. It works mainly on the CB1 receptors. The side effects are mostly sleepiness, dizziness and impaired memory, confusion, anxiety, and immune suppression and dry mouth. THC affects people soon after smoking cannabis, with psychotropic effects after 15–30 minutes and declining within three hours.

Cannabidiol (CBD) is nonintoxicating and does not alter mood and cognition, but has significant analgesic, anti-inflammatory, anti-convulsant and anti-anxiety effects that counteract some of the negative effects of THC. It is the second most prevalent active ingredient of the cannabis/marijuana plant. CBD has anti-inflammatory properties and may be applied on the skin to help lower pain and inflammation in arthritis. Side effects include nausea, fatigue and irritability. Patented CBD oil for pharmaceutical use has a purity of at least 98%. There many types of CBD oils are defined by the cannabinoid content in the oil.

There are various delivery forms of cannabis products – either orally, via sprays or inhalation, smoking (or vaporisation) and absorption. Oral or sublingual delivery is common. Pain trials use 4% THC. Patches and lozenges are also available. CBD is not recommended if you are on blood thinners.

CHRONIC PAIN

ACTION PLAN – CHECKLIST

- Identify the cause of the pain.
- Use anti-inflammatory foods, drugs and natural medicines.
- Try PEA or cannabis if other methods fail.
- Use the Mediterranean diet long-term.
- Use trigger-point therapy and acupuncture to increase endorphins.
- Try TENS stimulation to block severe pain.
- Use heat packs for chronic pain and muscle soreness
- Use ice packs on bruising and to numb pain.
- Use meditation, yoga and exercise several times a week.

References:

Marini, I., Bartolucci, M. L., Bortolotti, F., Gatto, M. R., & Bonetti, G. A. (2012). Palmitoylethanolamide versus a nonsteroidal anti-inflammatory drug in the treatment of temporomandibular joint inflammatory pain. *Journal of orofacial pain*, *26*(2), 99–104.

Mücke, M., Phillips, T., Radbruch, L., Petzke, F., & Häuser, W. (2018). Cannabis-based medicines for chronic neuropathic pain in adults. *The Cochrane Database of Systematic Reviews, 3*(3), CD012182. https://doi.org/10.1002/14651858.CD012182.pub2

Gabrielsson, L., Mattsson, S., & Fowler, C. J. (2016). Palmitoylethanolamide for the treatment of pain: pharmacokinetics, safety and efficacy. *British journal of clinical pharmacology*, *82*(4), 932–942. https://doi.org/10.1111/bcp.13020

Chapter 10

KEY NUTRIENTS IN INFLAMMATION

"Where all men think alike, no one thinks very much."

WALTER LIPPMAN

DIETARY SOURCES

DIETARY NUTRIENTS	FUNCTION
Essential fatty acids - Omega-3 (mostly from fish) and omega-6 (mostly plant based).	Omega-3 fatty acids reduce inflammation; included are skin conditions, asthma and lung function. Source: Fish, especially salmon, tuna, mackerel. Supplement: for rheumatoid arthritis - 2.7 g/day.
Pomegranate	Pomegranate has high antioxidant and weak anti-inflammatory effects. Fresh fruit is best.
VITAMINS	FUNCTION
Vitamin A	Vitamin A supports immunity but is toxic in excess. Source: liver, fish, eggs, milk, Amount: 25,000 IU/day.
B vitamins	Found in many foods, B vitamins are water-soluble and have a role in metabolism and cognition.
Vitamin C	Vitamin C supports cardiac and respiratory function (asthma). Source: citrus fruit, kiwi fruit, berries, tomatoes. Amount: 600–1000 mg/day.

Vitamin D	Vitamin D supports the immune system. Helpful in asthma and migraines. Source: oily fish such as mackerel, salmon, eggs. Amount: For migraines: 1500 IU/day of vitamin D.
Vitamin E	Clinical trials have shown vitamin E to be helpful in treating skin conditions. Taken for 3 months. Source: wheat germ oils, nuts, pumpkin. Amount: 400 IU/day.
MINERALS	FUNCTION
Magnesium	Magnesium relaxes muscles, alleviates pain and stiffness, and reduces inflammation. Source: pumpkin seeds, spinach, yoghurt, grains. Amount: 400 mg/day.
Selenium	Selenium supports the immune system and cardiovascular function. Sources: nuts, seeds, eggs, liver, oily fish, poultry. Amount: 200–250 µg/day.
Zinc	Zinc boosts the immune system, aids the healing process and helps process. Source: oysters, fish, meat, eggs, dairy products, sunflower seeds. Amount: 10 - 30 mg/day.
Boron	This trace mineral helps with pain relief. Amount: 6 mg/day.
HERBS	FUNCTION

Turmeric (curcumin)	Used to heal wounds and relieve pain; anti-inflammatory. Better absorbed if complexed with other nutrients. Amount: 400 mg/twice a day is the usual dose.
Ginger	This herb root has anti-inflammatory and antioxidant effects. Amount: 500–4000 mg/ day.
Garlic	Helps clear up mucous and works well with horseradish. Amount: 750 mgs/ per day.
Boswellia serrata	An Indian plant with anti-inflammatory effect. Dose for rheumatoid arthritis: 1200 - 3600 mg/ day.
Devil's claw (*Harpagophytum*)	An African plant for pain, it has anti-inflammatory properties. Nil in pregnancy. 150 –1500 mg twice per day.
Aloe vera	Can help alleviate inflammation, particularly in the gut. Useful for sunburns and eczema. Dose: 200 mg/day if taking a capsule (equal to 20 ml of cream).
Arnica	Creams applied to the skin for swelling and pain relief. Amount: Rub gel into joints three times per day.

Feverfew (*Tanacetum parthenium*)	For classical migraine and cluster headaches, but also for premenstrual, menstrual, and other headaches. Amount: 100–300 mg, 4 times daily with 0.2–0.4% parthenolides.
OTHER SUPPLEMENTS	FUNCTION
Quercetin	Counters the inflammatory effects of histamine that can trigger allergic reactions. Source: onion, apple, grapes, berries, red wine and cocoa. Amount: 500 mg twice/day.
Glucosamine	Naturally found in cartilage, helps repair cartilage and alleviate joint pain. Harvested from shellfish. Amount: 1500 mg/day. Avoid if allergic to shellfish.
Chondroitin sulphate	Keeps cartilage healthy and prevents swelling, used for arthritis. Amount: 1200 mg/day.
Methylsulfonylmethane (MSM)	An anti-inflammatory compound used for joint and muscle pain and arthritis. Amount: 600–750 mg twice per day.
Probiotics	*Lactobacillus casei, Lactobacillus rhamnosus GG, Bifidobacterium lactis*, and *Streptococcus thermophiles* all improve gut health. Fermented foods.

Chapter 11

THE MIND AND ITS MESSENGERS

"I not only use all the brains that I have, but all that I can borrow."

WOODROW WILSON

This is the story of two 'messenger' systems that link the brain and the body – the nervous system and the endocrine system. It's a cautionary tale about what happens when either system malfunctions or the two systems stop working together. The nervous and endocrine systems are called organ systems for a reason – they affect every organ in the body, from the brain and the gut to the reproductive organs. Thus, the fallout from a failing nervous system or endocrine system is far-reaching. If you struggle through the day feeling tired, moody, unmotivated or forgetful, with brain fog and little interest in sex or other pleasures, then read on.

Stay with us as we explain more about your nervous system, your endocrine system and their interactions. If you know more about what ails you, you can best understand what treatment options you have. Some of the signs that indicate these two systems are in trouble can take the form of hormonal imbalances, depression and other mood disorders, adrenal fatigue, hypothyroidism, low libido, prostate problems and diabetes.

THE NERVOUS SYSTEM

The nervous system is always active, regulating body functions such as breathing, blood pressure and digestion without conscious effort on your part. But it also coordinates your body's response to your thoughts and moods, so your muscles contract when you want to move, your attention focuses when you're working to a deadline, and tears fall when you're feeling sad. Nerve cells transmit the impulses from one to the other via long, thin fibres that almost – but not quite – connect them. Chemicals called neurotransmitters bridge the 'synaptic gap' between nerve cells so that transmission of the electrical impulse continues until it reaches its target cells in the body.

THE ENDOCRINE SYSTEM

The endocrine system is a separate but related part of the brain's command structure. It acts as both messenger and regulator, providing information to and from the brain. It's made up of a collection of glands that profoundly influence your growth, metabolism and digestion. The endocrine glands are throughout the body – in the brain (pituitary and pineal glands), neck (thyroid and parathyroid glands), chest (thymus), abdomen (adrenal glands and pancreas) and gonads (ovaries and testes).

But, unlike the nervous system, the endocrine system doesn't communicate with fast-acting electrical signals, but via hormones produced by the glands and released into the bloodstream, often needing to travel a significant distance to reach their target cells. Some chemicals, such as acetylcholine and norepinephrine (a form of adrenaline), are both hormones and neurotransmitters, and are produced by the glands in the endocrine system as well as by the nerve cells in the nervous system. They're the same chemicals, but they just act in a different way.

HOW TWO SYSTEMS WORK TOGETHER – THE HPA

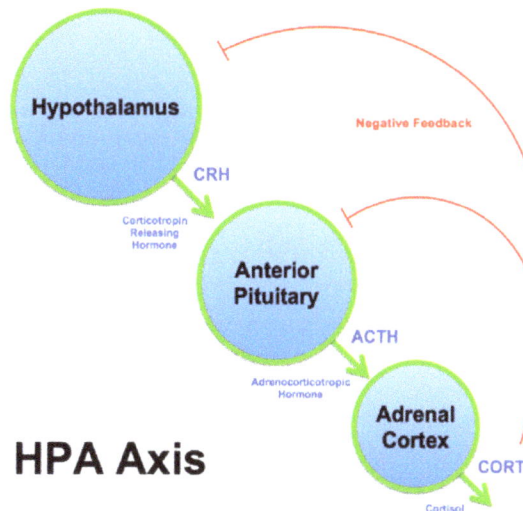

Image courtesy of Brian Sweis (2012) under Wikimedia Commons

The nervous and endocrine systems coordinate via the hypothalamic pituitary axis (HPA) during stress.

1. The nervous system reacts first, releasing adrenaline and norepinephrine. The hypothalamus then prepares the body for 'fight or flight', enhancing blood flow, energy release, and potentially engaging the endocrine system.

2. The hypothalamus starts the 'chain reaction' in the endocrine system, triggering the release of a hormone that acts on the nearby pituitary gland. This action causes the pituitary gland to release of a number of hormones, prompting the adrenal glands to flood the bloodstream with stress hormones such as cortisol.

3. Cortisol is released in a pulse motion that lasts about fifteen minutes. It then circulates in the blood for another one hundred minutes.

That's fine if you have a near miss in traffic or are sitting an exam. But if you're getting the same hormonal response to everyday stressors such as a work deadline or family argument, it can overload your threshold for stress. Repeated and prolonged release of stress hormones may result in 'burn-out', affecting hormonal and neurological functions but may also compromise the immune, cardiovascular and metabolic systems. Your body may stay on alert, your blood pressure and blood sugars remain elevated, your sleep be disrupted, your mood disturbed, your digestion compromised, and your effective responses to allergies compromised. For example, your genetics, early life experiences, any past traumas and current life stressors can collectively affect how much cortisol you'll be exposed to as an adult. So, if you think stress is just short term, think again. Over the long term, stress can actually change the areas in the brain that control the whole chain reaction (the HPA) making the problem more intractable.

CHEMICAL MESSENGERS – HORMONES AND NEUROTRANSMITTERS

1. Hormones travel through the bloodstream to affect distant organs.

· Adrenal glands produce cortisol, adrenaline, and DHEA, regulating stress response and energy levels.
· Thyroid gland releases T3 and T4, controlling baseline energy and metabolism.

· **Ovaries and testes produce sex hormones** (oestrogen, progesterone, testosterone) for reproductive development.

When the hormones are out of whack, it's akin to signals getting mixed up in the body's communication system, the HPA axis. Amino acids (think adrenaline) or cholesterol (think oestrogen) and dietary factors influence hormone functions (e.g fish oils affect metabolism, fibre impacts the gut microbiome and neurotransmitter production). So, stress isn't the only thing that affects hormones.

2. Neurotransmitters, from proteins, aid cell growth and repair.

· **Inhibitory neurotransmitters** calm the brain and slow down the flow of information. The neurotransmitters serotonin and GABA (gamma-aminobutyric acid) are important in generating this sense of peace and stability.
· **Excitatory neurotransmitters** stimulate the brain. Glutamate, adrenaline (epinephrine) and norepinephrine are the main excitatory neurotransmitters.
· **Some can be both excitatory and inhibitory.** For example, acetylcholine can excite the muscular system, signalling muscles to contract, but may also inhibit the cardiovascular system, signalling the heart to slow down. Since all bodily functions are linked to the nervous system, depleted neurotransmitters chemicals affect everything, including the hormonal system.

Dealing with these imbalances often involves a multifaceted approach, including lifestyle modifications, adjusting your diet, psychotherapy, managing medications, and getting to the bottom of any health issues lurking underneath. Healthcare professionals are crucial for proper evaluation and treatment. Here are some of the reasons why your neurotransmitters may be out of whack;
· Genetics: Genetic variations can influence the synthesis, release, reuptake, and degradation of neurotransmitters, affecting their levels and function in the brain.

· **Environmental Factors:** Exposure to environmental toxins, pollutants, drugs, or chemicals can disrupt neurotransmitter function. For example, heavy metal exposure or pesticide exposure may interfere with neurotransmitter manufacture or signalling.

· **Stress:** Chronic stress can negatively affect the hypothalamic-pituitary-adrenal (HPA) axis, leading to alterations in neurotransmitter levels. Cortisol levels impact neurotransmitter manufacture and receptor sensitivity, affecting mood and cognition.

· **Diet and Nutrition:** Inadequate intake of essential nutrients such as amino acids, vitamins, and minerals, can impair neurotransmitter production and function. Additionally, excessive intake of alcohol or caffeine can disrupt neurotransmitter balance.

· **Medical Conditions:** Neurological disorders, such as Parkinson's disease, Alzheimer's disease, multiple sclerosis, and epilepsy, can involve dysfunction of specific neurotransmitter systems. Additionally, psychiatric disorders like depression, anxiety disorders, bipolar disorder, and schizophrenia are associated with alterations in neurotransmitter levels and signalling.

· **Trauma and Injury:** Head injuries, concussions, or traumatic brain injuries can disrupt neurotransmitter function and lead to cognitive and emotional changes.

· **Medications:** Certain medications, including antidepressants, antipsychotics, stimulants, and drugs of abuse, can directly influence neurotransmitter levels or receptor activity, leading to imbalances.

· **Hormonal Changes:** Fluctuations in hormone levels, such as those occurring during puberty, menstruation, pregnancy, or menopause, can affect neurotransmitter function and contribute to mood swings or emotional changes.

NUTRIENTS ARE KEY TO NEUROTRANSMITTER HEALTH

GABA (Gamma Amino Butyric Acid)	Inhibitory neurotransmitter derived from the amino acid glutamate requiring vitamin B6. GABA and glutamate work together to balance brain activity.
Function	GABA relaxes and sedates your mind and body. It helps to relieve stress and nervous tension
Imbalance	Too little GABA causes muscle tension, racing mind, poor sleep, lack of focus, anxiety and stress- related disorders.
Food Source	Fermented foods – kimchi, miso, kefir, tempeh, sauerkraut and *Lactobacillus* in yoghurt – produce GABA.
SEROTONIN	Inhibitory neurotransmitter (5-hydroxytryptamine or 5-HT for short) derived from the amino acid tryptophan.
Function	Stabilises mood and behaviour, sleep, learning and memory. 90% of serotonin production occurs in the gastrointestinal tract.

Imbalance	Low serotonin can result in depression, anxiety, anger and other emotional disorders. It can disrupt sleep, appetite and sexual behaviour, and cause bowel and skin conditions
Food Source	Serotonin is derived from tryptophan. Food high in tryptophan include meat, fish, dairy products, nuts, seeds, oats, beans, lentils, tofu and eggs.
DOPAMINE	**Both an excitatory and inhibitory neurotransmitter. Dopamine can convert into the 'arousal' hormones – adrenaline (epinephrine) and norepinephrine. Dopamine is derived from tyrosine (with help from vitamin B6).**
Function	Critical to movement and motivation, it has an inhibitory effect. It also plays a role in the reward system for behaviour, focus, learning, attention, arousal and sleep.
Imbalance	Too little dopamine results in rigidity, tremors, restless legs, ADD/ADHD and Parkinson's disease. Excessive dopamine is linked to schizophrenia and mania.

Food Source	Derived from tyrosine occurs in highest concentrations in meat, fish, dairy, eggs, nuts, seeds and wholegrains
ACETYLCHOLINE	**Acetylcholine is both excitatory and inhibitory. It is made from choline as well as acetyl-coenzyme A and vitamin B5.**
Function	Responsible for muscle contraction, it has a role in memory and cognition, sleep, behaviour and arousal.
Imbalance	Reduces in ageing. Deficiencies are seen in Alzheimer's disease, poor focus and muscle weakness.
Food Source	Choline is found in high-fat dairy products, fish, meat, eggs (yolks) and poultry.
GLYCINE	**Considered an inhibitory neurotransmitter but does promote the action of the excitatory neurotransmitter glutamate.**
Function	It's involved in motor control, pain perception and processing information. Used to treat schizophrenia and cancer, and build muscle.

Imbalance	Problems are rare, but mental retardation can result if glycine levels are too high in the cerebrospinal fluid
Food Sources	Highest in meat, fish, dairy products and eggs, but also occurs in banana, cauliflower, kiwi and beans.
GLUTAMATE	**Glutamate is the principle excitatory neurotransmitter and the most abundant, occurring in more than half the brain.**
Function	Central to brain development and metabolism. It is involved with learning, memory, digestion and DNA formation.
Imbalance	High levels are toxic. Associated with seizures, epilepsy, Parkinson's disease, Alzheimer's, stroke, schizophrenia and addiction.
Food Sources	Sourced from matured cheeses, cured meats, fish, oysters, tomatoes, mushrooms, broccoli, walnuts and peas.

HISTAMINE	An excitatory neurotransmitter derived from the amino acid histidine
Function	Histamine plays a role in the sleep/wake cycle. Histamine keeps you awake and alert. It is also involved in immunity, inflammation and allergies.
Imbalance	High levels of histamine may cause skin rashes, sneezing, gut pain, headaches or migraines in some people.
Food Sources	High histamine levels are found in tuna, mackerel, anchovy, spinach, wine, cheese and fermented foods.
ADRENALINE AND NORADRENALINE	Adrenaline/epinephrine and noradrenaline (also called norepinephrine) are excitatory neurotransmitters. Both are made from dopamine and secreted by the endocrine and the nervous system.
Function	Both are involved in the 'fight or flight' response to stress that increases arousal, focus, blood sugar, heart rate and blood flow to the muscles.

Imbalance	Excessive levels cause anxiety, panic attacks, mania, sweating and poor sleep cycles. Low levels are associated with fatigue, inability to focus, poor attention span and poor sleep. Adrenaline is given to people in cardiac or ana- phylactic shock or other emergency situations to increase blood pressure and blood flow.
Food Sources	Derived from dopamine via tyrosine and occurs in highest concentrations in meat, fish, dairy, eggs, nuts, seeds and wholegrains.

References:

Briguglio, M., Dell'Osso, B., Panzica, G., Malgaroli, A., Banfi, G., Zanaboni Dina, C., Galentino, R., & Porta, M. (2018). Dietary Neurotransmitters: A Narrative Review on Current Knowledge. *Nutrients*, *10*(5), 591. https://doi.org/10.3390/nu10050591

Gómez-Pinilla, F. (2008). Brain foods: the effects of nutrients on brain function. *Nature reviews. Neuroscience*, *9*(7), 568–578. https://doi.org/10.1038/nrn2421

Smith, S. M., & Vale, W. W. (2006). The role of the hypothalamic-pituitary-adrenal axis in neuroendocrine responses to stress. *Dialogues in clinical neuroscience*, *8*(4), 383–395.

Chapter 12

EMBRACING MINDFULNESS FOR HOLISTIC HEALTH

"Training your mind to be in the present moment is the number one key to making healthier choices."

SUSAN ALBERS

What is Mindfulness?

Mindfulness is a practice steeped in ancient wisdom, dating back around 2,500 years to its origins in Buddhist meditation. Yet, it resonates profoundly with our contemporary lives, offering a moment-by-moment awareness that encompasses our thoughts, feelings, bodily sensations, and environment—all approached with a non-judgmental attitude. This timeless practice provides a vital connection to managing the complexities of modern living with grace and composure.

Mindfulness and Managing Pain, Stress, and Chronic Illnesses

The transformative journey of mindfulness from ancient practice to modern therapeutic intervention was significantly advanced by Dr. Jon Kabat-Zinn. In the late 1970s, he founded the Mindfulness-Based Stress Reduction (MBSR) program at the University of Massachusetts Medical School. This pioneering program married Eastern meditation techniques with Western scientific methods, offering a revolutionary non-pharmaceutical approach to managing pain, stress, and chronic illnesses. Since its inception, mindfulness principles have been increasingly embraced by hospitals and wellness centres globally, highlighting its growing importance and efficacy in contemporary medical practices.

Mindfulness in Hospitals and Wellness Centres

As mindfulness has integrated into the fabric of Western medicine, it has transformed many aspects of patient care. Hospitals and wellness centres around the world now utilise mindfulness techniques to significantly improve health outcomes. This approach has proven especially effective in managing conditions ranging from chronic pain to mental health disorders, enhancing both physical and mental well-being.

The Functions of Mindfulness

This table details the diverse functions of mindfulness, underscoring its broad applicability and effectiveness in our fast-paced modern world:

Function	Description
Pain Management	Mindfulness helps patients manage chronic pain, reducing the need for pharmaceutical interventions by focusing on coping mechanisms through meditation and awareness.
Stress Reduction	Clinical studies and meta-analyses show that mindfulness-based therapies significantly alleviate stress, enhancing overall mental health.
Mental Health Disorders	Employed in treating anxiety, depression, and other mental health disorders, mindfulness meditation can significantly reduce symptoms, improving emotional and psychological resilience.
Immune System Support	Regular mindfulness practice has been linked to better immune system responses, crucial for overall health and disease prevention.
Heart Health	Techniques in mindfulness can contribute to cardiovascular health by reducing stress and improving heart rate variability.
Emotional Regulation	By cultivating a moment-by-moment awareness of emotions without judgment, mindfulness assists in better emotional control and resilience.

Function	Description
Enhanced Mental Functions	Includes improvements in working memory, cognitive flexibility, and focus, essential for both personal and professional development.
Decreased Emotional Reactivity	Mindfulness enables individuals to disengage effectively from negative stimuli, fostering a calmer and more composed demeanour.
Improved Relationship Satisfaction	Practicing mindfulness can enhance communication skills and relationship satisfaction, fostering deeper connections and understanding between individuals.

By integrating these functions of mindfulness into daily routines, individuals and healthcare providers can harness its full potential, fostering a healthier, more balanced lifestyle amidst the complexities of modern living. This holistic approach is not limited to adults; it extends significantly to younger populations as well.

When to Begin Mindfulness

"The best time to plant a tree was 20 years ago. The second best time is now." This proverbial wisdom holds true for beginning mindfulness, especially when considering its profound impact on our lives. If the journey into mindfulness didn't begin in the past, the next best moment is undoubtedly the present.

In educational environments, mindfulness has emerged as a powerful tool for fostering emotional and cognitive development in children. A landmark study, known for its extensive duration and comprehensive analysis, conducted by researchers from the University of British Columbia, provides compelling evidence on the long-term benefits of mindfulness training initiated in early childhood.

Mindfulness Study over a Ten-Year Period

The study followed several hundred students who began mindfulness training in elementary school and were tracked over a ten-year period. These students participated in a structured program that incorporated daily mindfulness practices, focusing on awareness of their internal and external experiences without judgment.

Key Findings

1. **Improved Academic Performance:** The children who consistently engaged in mindfulness practices demonstrated significant improvements in their academic performance. This was attributed to enhanced concentration, better memory recall, and a greater ability to engage in complex cognitive processes.
2. **Enhanced Emotional Regulation:** One of the most significant findings was the marked improvement in emotional regulation. Students trained in mindfulness showed decreased reactivity to negative stimuli and an increased ability to manage stress and anxiety effectively.
3. **Reduced Behavioural Issues:** The study noted a decrease in incidents of disruptive behaviour and disciplinary actions among students who practiced mindfulness. This change was linked to better emotional control and increased patience and empathy towards others.
4. **Social Benefits:** Mindfulness-trained students displayed better social skills, such as improved communication with peers and adults, and a higher level of empathy. They were more adept at resolving conflicts and more frequently engaged in pro-social behaviours.
5. **Long-term Mental Health Benefits:** Remarkably, the benefits of early mindfulness training appeared to extend into adolescence. Participants reported lower levels of depression and anxiety compared to their peers who had not received such training.

This long-term study underscores the profound impact that mindfulness education can have on a child's development. By integrating mindfulness into school curricula, educators can equip children with essential skills to manage their mental, emotional, and social health. These skills not only enhance academic success but also contribute to building a foundation for well-being that supports children through their schooling years and beyond.

Mindfulness and the Greatest Olympian

Michael Phelps, the most decorated Olympian of all time, has been a vocal advocate for the power of mindfulness in achieving peak performance and overcoming personal challenges. Phelps's use of mindfulness techniques provided him with a psychological edge over his competitors, contributing to his record-breaking 28 Olympic medals.

Diagnosed with ADHD as a child, Phelps was introduced to breathing exercises and meditation techniques by his mother at a young age to help him focus. These early mindfulness practices laid the foundation for what would become an integral part of his training regimen, profoundly impacting his approach to competition and life. His commitment to mindfulness techniques helped him manage stress and maintain concentration, contributing significantly to his Olympic successes.

What We Can Learn from Mindfulness Techniques Used by Phelps

Michael Phelps's application of mindfulness techniques provides valuable insights into how these practices can be adapted to enhance performance and personal growth. Here's what we can learn from the techniques he used:

1. **Visualisation:** Phelps used visualisation not just as a preparatory tool but as a way to build confidence and take control over his mental state. By visualising every detail of the race, he prepared himself to face any scenario, enhancing his focus and reducing performance anxiety. This teaches us that mental rehearsal can prepare us for challenges, helping to manifest desired outcomes in high-pressure situations.

2. **Breathing Exercises:** Regular incorporation of breathing exercises helped Phelps manage stress and maintain clarity of mind. This practice regulated his heart rate and calmed his nerves, essential for peak performance. From this, we learn that controlled breathing is a powerful tool for managing physiological responses to stress, making it applicable not only in sports but in any stressful situation.

3. **Routine Meditation:** By engaging in regular meditation, Phelps developed a heightened awareness of his thoughts and emotions, which allowed him to remain focused and present during competitions. This practice underlines the importance of consistent mental training to cultivate concentration, resilience, and mindfulness, which are beneficial across all areas of life.

Impact on Performance

Michael Phelps's journey with mindfulness demonstrates its transformative power, not just in sports but in personal recovery and growth. His story highlights the critical role mindfulness can play in high-pressure environments, showcasing its benefits for focus, emotional regulation, and overall mental health. Through his advocacy, Phelps continues to inspire others to embrace mindfulness, whether they are athletes, professionals, or individuals facing personal challenges.

How to Build Mindfulness into your Life

Mindfulness involves engaging actively with the present moment in a non-judgmental way. It is a valuable tool for enhancing well-being and managing the stresses of daily life. Below is a guide on how to incorporate mindfulness into everyday routines to cultivate mental, emotional, and physical health.

Introduction to Daily Mindfulness Routine

Incorporating mindfulness into your daily routine is a transformative practice that can enhance your overall well-being and provide a peaceful break from the hustle and bustle of everyday life. Mindfulness involves being fully present and engaged in the moment, aware of your thoughts and feelings without distraction or judgment. Here's a structured approach to integrating mindful moments throughout your day, helping you cultivate a deeper sense of peace and focused awareness.

Common Mindfulness Techniques and Their Benefits

Technique	Description	Benefits
Body Scan Meditation	Involves mentally scanning your body for areas of tension.	Increases bodily awareness and helps release stress.
Sitting Meditation	Practiced by sitting quietly and paying attention to thoughts, sounds, the sensations of breathing, or parts of the body.	Enhances focus and calms the mind.
Walking Meditation	Focuses on the experience of walking, being aware of the sensations of standing and the subtle movements that keep your balance.	Integrates mindfulness into physical activity, enhances physical and mental balance.
Mindful Eating	Eating slowly and savouring each bite.	Improves digestion and promotes enjoyment of food, reduces overeating.
Loving-kindness Meditation	Sending wishes of loving-kindness to the world.	Boosts compassion towards oneself and others, fosters a positive mindset.
Guided Imagery	Using visualisation to improve mood and calm the mind.	Enhances relaxation and reduces anxiety.

5 Tips for Enhancing Your Mindfulness Practice

1. **Set Reminders:** Use phone alerts or sticky notes as reminders to engage in mindfulness activities until they become a habitual part of your routine.
2. **Be Patient:** Mindfulness is a skill that develops with practice. Start with short sessions and gradually increase the duration as you become more comfortable.
3. **Create a Mindful Space:** Establish a designated quiet area in your home for mindfulness exercises, particularly for breathing and meditation, to enhance focus and minimise distractions.
4. **Use Guided Sessions:** If you're new to mindfulness, guided sessions via apps or online platforms can provide structure. Explore 10-minute mindfulness videos on platforms like YouTube to find guided exercises that fit into a busy schedule.
5. **Reflect and Adjust:** Regularly assess what aspects of your mindfulness practice are effective and what might need adjustment. Tailor the activities to better fit your daily schedule and personal preferences.

Daily Mindfulness Action Plan Table

Time	Activity	Description
Morning	Mindful Breathing	Begin the day with 10 minutes of focused breathing. Sit in a quiet place, close your eyes, and tune into the natural rhythm of your breath.

Time	Activity	Description
Midday	Mindful Walk	Take a 15-minute mindful walk. Pay attention to the sensations of your feet touching the ground, the sounds around you, and the temperature of the air.
Evening	Mindful Eating	Eat dinner mindfully, concentrating on the tastes and textures of your food. Chew slowly and savour each bite.
Night	Reflective Meditation	End the day with a 10-minute meditation, reflecting on the day's experiences and contemplating what went well and what could be improved.
Anytime	Mindful Movement	Engage in physical activities like yoga or tai chi, focusing on each movement and the sensations in your body.
Anytime	Mindful Listening	Actively listen during conversations. Focus on the words, tone, and emotions being expressed.

Time	Activity	Description
Anytime	Mindful Seeing	Practice mindful observation of your surroundings. Notice colors, shapes, and movements that are usually overlooked.

Conclusion: Embracing Mindfulness as a Way of Life

Mindfulness transcends being merely a practice; it embodies a philosophy for living deeply rooted in ancient wisdom, fostering a balanced and mindful approach to life. By integrating mindfulness into our daily routines, individuals of all ages not only enhance their own mental and physical health but also contribute positively to the broader community. As mindfulness continues to permeate modern medicine and everyday living, its role in promoting healthier, happier societies becomes increasingly vital. Through mindfulness, we have the opportunity to transform our lives and the lives of those around us, making each moment more meaningful and enriched.

Join Our Mindful Community at Think2Be Healthy

Think2Be Healthy, an initiative inspired by entrepreneur and philanthropist Hilton Misso, is at the forefront of building a global community that values holistic and balanced approaches to health. Our platform is dedicated to reviving and enhancing the ancient philosophies of natural health and wellness. We invite both individuals and health professionals to connect with us, sharing in the journey of embracing traditional wisdom that has nurtured human well-being for centuries.

Our community is a dynamic network of individuals and holistic medical professionals dedicated to integrating these profound health practices into modern healthcare. By joining Think2Be Healthy, members gain access to a supportive environment where they can learn, share, and grow in their mindfulness practices, ensuring a comprehensive approach to health.

We encourage everyone interested to connect with us and receive our newsletter for regular updates. Visit us at www.think2behealthy.com.au to learn more and become part of a movement towards a more mindful, health-conscious world. Together, we can inspire and catalyse a broader movement towards well-being and mindfulness.

References

Kabat-Zinn, J. (1990). *Full Catastrophe Living: Using the Wisdom of Your Body and Mind to Face Stress, Pain, and Illness*. Delta. This seminal book introduces the Mindfulness-Based Stress Reduction (MBSR) program and its applications in medical settings.

Benson, H. (2015). *The Relaxation Response*. This work explores the physiological mechanisms behind mindfulness and its capacity to reduce stress.

Phelps, M. (2017). *No Limits: The Will to Succeed*. An autobiography that includes insights into how mindfulness and mental training contributed to Phelps's Olympic success.

Hofmann, S. G., et al. (2010). "The effect of mindfulness-based therapy on anxiety and depression: A meta-analytic review." *Journal of Consulting and Clinical Psychology*. This study provides a comprehensive review of how mindfulness-based interventions affect mental health outcomes.

Morone, N. E., et al. (2008). "Mindfulness meditation for the treatment of chronic low back pain in older adults: A randomized controlled pilot study." *Pain*. This article details a study on the effectiveness of mindfulness meditation in managing chronic pain.

Grossman, P., et al. (2004). "Mindfulness-based stress reduction and health benefits: A meta-analysis." *Journal of Psychosomatic Research*. A key study that aggregates the health benefits of mindfulness across various clinical settings.

Ong, J. C., et al. (2014). "A randomized controlled trial of mindfulness meditation for chronic insomnia." *Sleep*. Research highlighting the effectiveness of mindfulness meditation in improving sleep quality.

Beach, M. C., et al. (2013). "Mindfulness training for clinician well-being." *The New England Journal of Medicine*. Discusses the impact of mindfulness on healthcare providers' stress and burnout.

Chapman, A. L., et al. (2016). "The cost-effectiveness of mindfulness-based stress reduction for the management of anxiety and depression." *Journal of Affective Disorders*. This article evaluates the economic benefits of using mindfulness to treat anxiety and depression.

Tatter, G. (2019). "Making Time for Mindfulness." *Harvard Graduate School of Education*. Provides insights into the practical applications of mindfulness in educational settings.

Meisner, J., et al. (2020). "Effectiveness of a mindfulness-oriented substance use prevention program for boys with mild to borderline intellectual disabilities: study protocol for a randomized controlled trial." *BMC Public Health*. A study protocol examining mindfulness interventions for preventing substance use.

Merkes, M. (2010). "Mindfulness-based stress reduction for people with chronic diseases." *Australian Journal of Primary Health*. Reviews the effectiveness of MBSR programs in treating chronic conditions.

Chapter 13

UNDERACTIVE THYROID

*"Every great advance in natural
knowledge has involved the
absolute rejection of authority."*

THOMAS HUXLEY

Your thyroid, nestled in your neck, is the mastermind behind your metabolism, heart rate, and body tempreature. But for women, it can sometimes go awry because of genetics, immune issues, or just random disruptions. Getting older or catching an infection can throw it off too. By the time you reach your 80s, your thyroid might be functioning about 40% less than it did in your 30s.

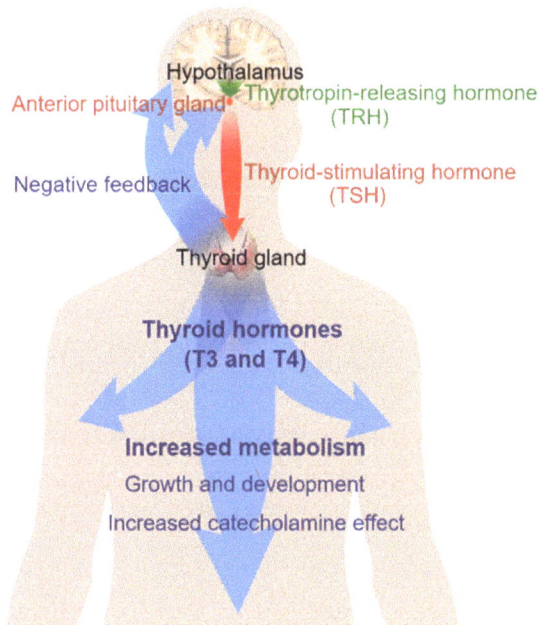

THYROID SYSTEM
Mikael Häggström, Public domain, via Wikimedia Commons
https://commons.wikimedia.org/wiki/File:Thyroid_system.svg

Thyroid Gland: This gland is located in the front of your neck, below your Adam's apple. Its primary function is to produce hormones that regulate various bodily functions, including metabolism, growth, and energy expenditure.

Thyroxine (T4) and Triiodothyronine (T3): These are the two main hormones produced by the thyroid gland. They are synthesised from the amino acid tyrosine, along with iodine. T4 is less potent but more abundant, while T3 is more potent but less abundant. Both hormones play crucial roles in regulating metabolism, growth, and development.

Thyrotropin-Releasing Hormone (TRH): TRH is produced by the hypothalamus, a region of the brain located above the brain stem. It acts by stimulating the release of thyroid-stimulating hormone (TSH) from the anterior pituitary gland.

Thyroid-Stimulating Hormone (TSH): TSH is produced by the anterior pituitary gland, located at the base of the brain. To put the story simply - it tells your thyroid gland to make and release hormones called T4 and T3. The amount of TSH your body makes is controlled by how much T4 and T3 are already in your bloodstream. When these two (T4 and T3) levels are low, the hypothalamus (in the brain) releases TRH (Thyrotropin-Releasing Hormone), which in turn tells the pituitary gland to make more TSH. This mechanism boosts thyroid hormone production. When T4 and T3 levels are high, TRH and TSH production slows down, which means less thyroid hormone is made. This system helps keep your thyroid hormone levels steady.

Underactive thyroid, also known as hypothyroidism, is more common than overactive thyroid, known as hyperthyroidism. Hypothyroidism occurs when the thyroid gland does not produce enough thyroid hormones, leading to a slowing down of bodily functions. The main causes are autoimmune diseases, iodine deficiency, or thyroid surgery. Hypothyroidism can be either *primary* - the thyroid gland just produces insufficient hormones - or *secondary* - which is rare, due to malfunction of the hypothalamus or pituitary gland.

On the other hand, **hyperthyroidism happens when the thyroid gland produces an excess of thyroid hormones**, causing an acceleration of bodily functions. It can be caused by conditions like Graves' Disease, thyroid nodules, or thyroiditis. Here we will consider hyperthyroidism first.

SYMPTOMS OF AN OVERACTIVE THYROID

1. Increase in metabolism with unintended weight loss.
2. Loss of appetite.
3. Increased heart rate and palpitations.
4. Tremors.
5. Insomnia - very poor sleep.
6. Nervousness and irritability.
7. Increased sweating.
8. Increased bowel movements and diarrhoea.
9. Bulging eyes and eye irritation.
10. Thyroid gland enlargement.
11. Thinning of the skin and brittle nails.
12. Brittle nails.

13. Menstrual irregularities.

Causes of Hyperactive Thyroid: Excess secretions is a serious condition. Autoimmune disease, inflammation, excess iodine, cancerous nodules and medications are some of the common causes.

Managing the Condition: An overactive thyroid requires specialist consultation and usually antithyroid medicines are added to radioactive iodine to destroy the thyroid cells. Beta blockers can alleviate symptoms of a rapid heart beat. However, sometimes surgical removal of a part or all of the thyroid gland may be necessary. Close monitoring and underlying causes need to be addressed by the clinician, and follow up to check if some thyroid medication is warranted.

SYMPTOMS OF AN UNDERACTIVE THYROID

Symptoms can vary and develop gradually over time but if you have a significant number of the following it is time to have your thyroid hormone levels checked:

1. Tired and sluggish - more than normal.
2. Slow pulse.
3. Dry skin.
4. Weight gain.
5. Cold intolerance.
6. Constipation.
7. Joint aches and pains.
8. Muscle weakness and cramping.
9. Unsteady gait.
10. Puffy hands and feet
11. Heavy periods in women of reproductive age.

Hashimoto's thyroiditis is an autoimmune condition and the leading cause of low thyroid hormone secretions. The immune system mistakenly attacks the thyroid gland instead of defending it and inflammation reduces thyroid output. However, once Hashimoto's thyroiditis is diagnosed, there's often very little follow-up testing or management of the antibodies attacking the thyroid. Conventional remedies for an underactive thyroid tend to focus on synthetic hormone replacement therapy of T4 alone, which may offer some relief of symptoms, but neglects to manage the cause – the antibodies which initially trigger thyroid gland damage. We argue that it's an error to neglect the progressive damage done by untreated Hashimoto's thyroiditis, as antibodies will then inflame and further disable the hormone-producing cells of the thyroid.

MANAGEMENT OF AN UNDERACTIVE THYROID

This comprehensive approach aims to address the underlying causes, symptoms, and complications associated with Hashimoto's Thyroiditis to optimize thyroid function and overall well-being.

Testing and Diagnosis: Monitoring thyroid function and antibodies in well people over time can help diagnose the condition. A rising trend in TSH levels, along with symptoms, suggests underactive thyroid. Subclinical hypothyroidism with TSH > 10 mIU/L warrants treatment.

Hormone Replacement: If thyroid hormone levels are low, replacement therapy may be necessary. Testing T3 levels can help determine if synthetic T3 medication is needed in addition to T4.

Symptom Management: Addressing symptoms like depression, which often coexist with hypothyroidism, is important. Thyroid hormones influence stress hormones and neurotransmitters, impacting mood and emotions.

Identifying Triggers: Eliminating potential triggers like gluten, which can provoke an immune response, may help reduce antibody levels and alleviate thyroid inflammation. Genetic testing may help identify gluten as a culprit.

Reducing Antibodies: Low-dose naltrexone (LDN) therapy may help reduce thyroid antibodies over time, potentially minimising thyroid damage.

Checking Nutrient Levels: Ensuring adequate levels of nutrients such as iodine, selenium, iron, zinc, and vitamins A and C is crucial for proper thyroid function.

Supplementation: While synthetic T4 medication is commonly prescribed, some individuals may not effectively convert it to T3. Exploring alternative treatments or supplementation options may be necessary for better management. The natural form of T3 is readily absorbed by cells, reducing the reliance on converting T4 to T3, a process that can be inconsistent for many. Supplements like Thyroid Extract, Armour Thyroid, or Natural Desiccated Thyroid, made from dried pig thyroid extract, were commonly used for hypothyroidism until the 1950s.

Associate Professor Christopher Strakosch, an expert in thyroid disease, highlighted in a review in the medical magazine Australian Doctor (2016) that many hypothyroid patients felt better with natural desiccated thyroid (combining T4 and T3) rather than synthetic T4 alone. He suggested that the concerns about natural desiccated thyroid's risks, especially for younger women, might be overstated and advocated for clinical trials if patients remain unwell despite synthetic T4 treatment.

If combination products like natural desiccated thyroid don't work, it may be due to insufficient dosage or other factors like iron and selenium deficiencies or cortisol imbalances. Selenium deficiency exacerbates hypothyroid symptoms. Foods rich in selenium include pork, beef, turkey, chicken, fish, shellfish, and Brazil nuts.

Persistence may be necessary until symptoms resolve. Some individuals with early-stage hypothyroidism might only receive help in their fifties, despite experiencing symptoms since their thirties, due to rigid diagnostic criteria. A study from northeast England found that more than one in ten women over fifty-five had 'subclinical hypothyroidism,' surpassing the number of undiagnosed type 2 diabetes cases.

UNDERACTIVE THYROID

ACTION PLAN – CHECKLIST

- Check for symptoms and clinical signs of underactive thyroid
- Do comprehensive blood tests if signs are positive
- Test hormones – TSH, T3, T4, thyroid antibodies,.
- Check for gluten sensitivity, allergies and blood sugar control.
- Check levels of iodine, selenium, iron, zinc, and vitamins A and C.
- Supplement effectively – hormones (natural T4 Plus T3 preferred)
- Supplement important nutrients if necessary.
- Check regularly for improvements in symptoms and thyroid hormone levels.

References:

Hoang, T. D., Olsen, C. H., Mai, V. Q., Clyde, P. W., & Shakir, M. K. (2013). Desiccated thyroid extract compared with levothyroxine in the treatment of hypothyroidism: a randomized, double-blind, crossover study. *The Journal of clinical endocrinology and metabolism*, *98*(5), 1982–1990. https://doi.org/10.1210/jc.2012-4107

Koulouri, O., Moran, C., Halsall, D., Chatterjee, K., & Gurnell, M. (2013). Pitfalls in the measurement and interpretation of thyroid function tests. *Best practice & research. Clinical endocrinology & metabolism, 27*(6), 745–762. https://doi.org/10.1016/j.beem.2013.10.003

Strackosh, C (2016). A "natural" thyroid therapy still finds favour in patients. *Australian Doctor.*

Teixeira, P. F. D. S., Dos Santos, P. B., & Pazos-Moura, C. C. (2020). The role of thyroid hormone in metabolism and metabolic syndrome. *Therapeutic advances in endocrinology and metabolism, 11*, 2042018820917869. https://doi.org/10.1177/2042018820917869

Vadiveloo, T., Donnan, P. T., Murphy, M. J., & Leese, G. P. (2013). Age- and gender-specific TSH reference intervals in people with no obvious thyroid disease in Tayside, Scotland: the Thyroid Epidemiology, Audit, and Research Study (TEARS). *The Journal of Clinical Endocrinology and Metabolism, 98*(3), 1147–1153. https://doi.org/10.1210/jc.2012-3191

Chapter 14

WOMEN'S HORMONAL HEALTH

"Sometimes the questions are complicated and the answers are simple."

DR SEUSS

If life begins at forty and you've gained valuable life experience and self-awareness, it's worth noting that, for women especially, hormonal changes can present challenges. As with many things, hormone production decreases with age.

Unfortunately, different hormones decline at different ages and hormonal imbalances become prominent challenges. Deficiencies in progesterone around forty, testosterone in their forties, and oestrogen nearing fifty, disrupt both the endocrine and nervous systems, affecting mood-regulating neurotransmitters like serotonin and GABA.

Produced mainly by the ovaries, oestrogen and progesterone are crucial for development, fertility, menstrual cycle regulation, libido and successful sexual function.

OESTROGEN

Oestrogen dominates the first half of the menstrual cycle, aiding in endometrial buildup. During this time, mood is pretty good because of increased serotonin. With high oestrogen and low progesterone around the ages of the 30s and 40s, conditions like endometriosis, ovarian cysts, and fibroids can affect fertility, causing difficulties in conception and risks of miscarriage. Levels decline during menopause, often causing sleep disturbances, concentration issues, and digestive and thyroid problems.

Oestrogen Deficiency and Excess

	1.	Hot flushes, night sweats
	2.	Poor sleep
	3.	Painful intercourse
	4.	Vaginal dryness and low libido
Oestrogen Deficiency	5.	Dry skin
	6.	Heart palpitations
	7.	Headaches and fuzzy thinking
	8.	Depression
	9.	Bone loss

Oestrogen Excess	1.	Water retention
	2.	Breast swelling and tenderness
	3.	Cravings for sweets
	4.	Fibrocystic breasts
	5.	Uterine fibroids
	6.	Nervousness/anxiety/irritability
	7.	Heavy irregular menses
	8.	Fatigue
	9.	Weight gain
	10.	Mood swings
	11.	Underactive thyroid
	12.	Yeast infections

Treating Oestrogen Deficiency: Apply an oestrogen cream, such as Biest (containing 20% oestradiol and 80% oestriol), to a hairless area of the forearm to prevent the cream from optimal absorption. Biest offers two safe compounds to alleviate deficiency.

Treating Oestrogen Excess: Incorporate natural progesterone to rebalance elevated oestrogen levels. DIM (Diindolylmethane), derived from cruciferous vegetables, reduces excessive oestrogen activity. Administer during the first half of the menstrual cycle if excess oestrogen is detected. Maintain supplementation throughout the month if symptoms like sore breasts and fluid retention persist. Include phytoestrogen-rich foods (such as soy, mung beans, and tofu) which help regulate hormonal balance by competitively occupying oestrogen receptors, potentially reducing the overall oestrogenic effect.

PROGESTERONE

Progesterone: Progesterone is mainly produced after ovulation until the next period; it balances oestrogen. When all's well, each hormone keeps the other in check. But as progesterone levels fall in women over thirty, oestrogen starts to dominate since it doesn't fall until near menopause. Without progesterone's counterbalancing effect, excessive oestrogen can contribute to mood swings and weight gain. Progesterone boosts GABA, calming the mind and body. Deficiency may contribute to anxiety, which may explain why women aged forty suffer from anxiety, at a time when they often have their lives worked out pretty well.

Progesterone Deficiency and Excess Symptoms

Progesterone Deficiency	1. Swollen breasts 2. Headaches 3. Mood swings, depression and anxiety 4. Irregular menses and cramping 5. Low libido 6. Acne 7. Weight gain 8. Joint pain

Progesterone Excess	1.	Mild depression
	2.	Sleepy during the day
	3.	Yeast infections
	4.	Tummy bloating
	5.	Weight gain
	6.	Brain fog
	7.	Shortness of breath
	8.	Dizziness

Treating Progesterone Deficiency: Take natural progesterone via a cream or troche (lozenge) to bypass the gut and liver. Take it in the latter half of the menstrual cycle, from the twelfth to twenty-sixth day of the cycle (day one is the first day of bleeding), since that's when progesterone is needed most. Natural progesterone works better with fewer side effects than the synthetic version.

Treating Progesterone Excess: Test hormonal levels before supplementing. Progesterone supplementation is commonly recommended to balance oestrogen. Cease or reduce progesterone supplementation when levels are too high.

TESTOSTERONE

Testosterone: The ovaries and adrenal glands produce small amounts of testosterone in women. The testes, and to a lesser extent the adrenal glands, secrete far more in men. Testosterone helps build bone and muscle mass, boosts sex drive and energy levels, and supports brain function in both sexes. When levels fall too far, women can experience muscle loss, develop osteoporosis and feel general aches and pains. Testosterone, like oestrogen, enhances the effects of serotonin, and also affects the neurotransmitter dopamine, which also gives the body a bit of an energy boost.

Testosterone Deficiency and Excess Symptoms

Testosterone Deficiency	1. Prolonged fatigue
	2. Depression
	3. Loss of mental sharpness
	4. Blunted motivation and wellbeing
	5. Muscle weakness and muscle loss
	6. General aches and pains
	7. Vaginal dryness
	8. Decreased libido
	9. Heart palpitations
	10. Bone loss
	11. Incontinence
	12. Fibromyalgia
	13. Thinning skin
	14. Increased fat mass
Testosterone Excess	1. Aggression
	2. Irritability
	3. Acne and oily skin
	4. Increased muscle mass

Treating Testosterone Deficiency: Apply testosterone cream on the hairless forearm. Oral forms of testosterone don't work as well as the creams. Methyl testosterone taken orally has many side effects. Testosterone cream can be mixed with either or both oestrogen or progesterone creams, often with better results than when used alone.

If using intra-muscular injections for men, monitor the levels as excessive levels of testosterone or abrupt fluctuations can sometimes lead to increased irritability and aggression in susceptible individuals. Women do not appreciate the side effects of excess testosterone: being angry and hairy!

THE ROLE OF DHEA

DHEA, a hormone made by the adrenal gland, helps produce testosterone and oestrogen. If you boost DHEA you're likely to produce more of these two sex hormones and address deficiencies that may be affecting your quality of life.

DHEA can be added to natural progesterone cream or lozenges. Maintaining the right balance is crucial. Healthy DHEA levels can enhance well-being, cognition, immunity, and bone health, while reducing abdominal fat and insulin resistance. Low DHEA levels can cause fatigue, weakness, low libido, poor sleep, and can also increase the risk of various health issues. However, excessive DHEA can raise cancer risk and cause masculine traits in women. Using 7-keto-DHEA, which does not convert to testosterone or oestrogen, may be a safer option.

NATURAL HORMONE REPLACEMENT

"Natural" progesterone, commonly sourced from wild Mexican yam (Dioscorea uillosa), involves extracting the active substance diosgenin and converting it into progesterone in a laboratory. This conversion is necessary because the body cannot convert diosgenin into progesterone on its own. The resulting progesterone's chemical structure is identical to the one produced by the human body. Each batch of natural progesterone undergoes purity testing, confirmed by a Certificate of Analysis.

Similarly, oestrogen can also be extracted from yam through a similar laboratory process. This method contrasts with synthetic progestins, which are commonly used in birth control pills and hormone replacement therapy. Natural forms of hormones are reported to have fewer side effects compared to synthetic progestins, such as reduced breast tenderness, bloating, and irritability.

Prescribing Natural Hormone Replacement

· **For pre-menopausal symptoms**, progesterone is typically taken daily from the 12th to the 26th day of the menstrual cycle. Prescription of a natural cream or troche (a type of lozenge) depends on age, symptoms, and hormone levels in blood or saliva. A common HRT cream contains progesterone (2.0%), testosterone (0.5%), DHEA (2.0%), and Biest (0.125%). Instructions for skin cream application usually entail daily use from Monday to Saturday. Both skin cream and oral troche forms offer reliable absorption and overcome gut or liver absorption issues.
· **Pregnenolone** is often referred to as "the mother of all hormones" because it serves as a precursor for the synthesis of various hormones, including oestrogen, testosterone, progesterone, and cortisol. Supplementation, typically 25–50 mg at bedtime, can benefit emotional and cognitive issues, with higher doses used in some studies for depression, schizophrenia, and bipolar symptoms. Pregnenolone also enhances deep sleep duration.
· **Long-term use of testosterone and oestrogen** together may hinder the conversion of cholesterol to pregnenolone, affecting hormone regulation and various bodily functions, including cognition and mood.

Hormone replacement therapy, while beneficial, carries a heightened risk of breast cancer. It should be used at the lowest effective dose and for the shortest duration possible. Some evidence suggests that bioidentical oestrogen *may* have a lower risk of certain health concerns compared to synthetic forms.

WOMEN'S HORMONAL

HEALTH ACTION PLAN – CHECKLIST

- Identify symptoms re: deficiencies or excesses of various hormones.
- Test hormonal levels: oestrogen, progesterone, testosterone and DHEA.
- Treat with natural hormones if necessary – via the skin or buccal troches.
- Review symptoms monthly initially.
- Retest hormonal levels second monthly.

References:

Amin, Z., Gueorguieva, R., Cappiello, A., Czarkowski, K. A., Stiklus, S., Anderson, G. M., Naftolin, F., & Epperson, C. N. (2006). Estradiol and tryptophan depletion interact to modulate cognition in menopausal women. *Neuropsychopharmacology : official publication of the American College of Neuropsychopharmacology*, *31*(11), 2489–2497. https://doi.org/10.1038/sj.npp.1301114

Klinge, C. M., Clark, B. J., & Prough, R. A. (2018). Dehydroepiandrosterone Research: Past, Current, and Future. *Vitamins and hormones*, *108*, 1–28. https://doi.org/10.1016/bs.vh.2018.02.002

Navarro-Pardo, E., Holland, C. A., & Cano, A. (2018). Sex Hormones and Healthy Psychological Aging in Women. *Frontiers in aging neuroscience*, *9*, 439. https://doi.org/10.3389/fnagi.2017.004

Warren, M. P., & Shantha, S. (1999). Uses of progesterone in clinical practice. International Journal of Fertility and Women's Medicine, 44(2), 96–103.

Chapter 15

MOOD DISORDERS

*"What mental health needs is
more sunlight, more candour, and
more unashamed conversation."*

GLENN CLOSE

Did you know that according to the World Health Organization about 1 in 4 people worldwide will experience a mental disorder at some point in their lives? That's a lot of people, but it also means you're not alone if you're going through something!

In Australia, about one in every five Aussies deals with some form of mental illness. That's a significant number, but it's also a reminder that there's support and understanding out there. Anxiety seems to be the most common, affecting 17% of the population. Depression affects about 8%, while substance abuse issues affect 3%. Bipolar disorder affects around 3.5% of males and 4% of females, and schizophrenia, though less common, impacts 2.4 in every 1000 people.

ANXIETY DISORDERS

Anxiety can stem from a combination of biological, psychological, and environmental factors. The range of disorders include generalized anxiety disorder, panic disorder, social anxiety disorder, and specific phobias. Then there are medical conditions such as thyroid disorders, cardiovascular and respiratory problems, chronic pain, epilepsy and Alzheimer's disease that produce anxiety symptoms. Overall, the environment plays a crucial role in shaping brain function and influencing anxiety levels, to date there are no definitive tests for a diagnosis.

Genetics: People with a family history of anxiety disorders may be more likely to experience anxiety themselves.

Personality: Certain personality traits - perfectionism, neuroticism, and those with a tendency to worry have increased risk of developing anxiety disorders.

Stressful Life Events: Things like trauma, abuse, accidents, and major life changes can trigger anxiety disorders. Stressors from work, relationships, finances, or school can also exacerbate anxiety. Chronic illness or pain can add even more stress, making anxiety symptoms worse.

Substance Use or Withdrawal: Alcohol, caffeine, nicotine, and certain drugs or medications can worsen or trigger anxiety symptoms.

Brain Chemistry: Imbalances of serotonin, dopamine, and gamma-aminobutyric acid (GABA) regulate mood and stress responses and can contribute to anxiety. There is no 'one size fits all' because the effects of neurotransmission depend on how much neurotransmitter is released, any defects in processing or delivery, and its mode of action, be it excitatory (increasing activity) or inhibitory (decreasing activity).

Causes of Anxiety:

Serotonin: Low levels of serotonin have been linked to depression and anxiety. Serotonin plays a role in regulating sleep, appetite, and digestion, which can be disrupted in individuals with anxiety disorders.

Gamma-Aminobutyric Acid (GABA): GABA is an inhibitory neurotransmitter that helps calm and reduce the activity of neurons. Low levels have been implicated in a heightened arousal and increased anxiety symptoms.

Norepinephrine: Also known as noradrenaline, it is involved in the body's "fight or flight" response to stress. Poor regulation contributes to racing thoughts, restlessness, and hypervigilance.

Dopamine: Dopamine levels can influence mood, motivation, and pleasure. Poor regulation contributes to anxiety and other mood disorders.

Glutamate: Excess glutamate with overstimulation of neurons may lead to heightened anxiety symptoms. Monosodium glutamate (MSG) should be avoided.

Treatment of Anxiety: Anxiety typically involves a combination of the approaches tailored to the individual's needs.

1. **Lifestyle Changes:** Regular exercise, adequate sleep, and a healthy diet can help reduce anxiety symptoms. Avoiding caffeine, alcohol, MSG, and nicotine, which can exacerbate anxiety, may also be beneficial.

2. **Stress Management Techniques:** Mindfulness (Chapter 12), deep breathing, progressive muscle relaxation, meditation, and yoga can help reduce stress and promote relaxation.

3. **Support Groups**: Support groups or online communities can offer a sense of belonging and reduce feelings of isolation. Any activity that brings joy and relaxation can help improve mood and reduce anxiety.

4. **Professional Support**: Therapists, counsellors, or psychiatrists can provide guidance and support. They provide treatment options tailored to the individual. Cognitive-behavioral therapy (CBT) is often effective. Therapy helps individuals identify and challenge negative thought patterns and develop coping strategies to manage anxiety symptoms.

5. **Medication**: Selective serotonin reuptake inhibitors (SSRIs) or serotonin-norepinephrine reuptake inhibitors (SNRIs), are drugs commonly prescribed to treat anxiety disorders. Benzodiazepines (e.g. valium) may be used for short-term relief of severe anxiety symptoms, but they are generally not recommended for long-term use due to the risk of dependence and tolerance with repeated use. Some people with anxiety disorders may use medical cannabis as a treatment option.

DEPRESSION

Depression is also a multifaceted condition, and individual experiences may vary. Some 75% of people with clinical depression experience more than one episode within ten years and about 10% develop chronic depression. Mood disorders (including depression) are the most common factors associated with suicide, accounting for 43% of all suicides. Not everyone with these risk factors experience depression, and not all cases of depression can be attributed to these causes.

Depression is common in women who are transitioning to menopause. In fact, females aged forty to forty-four years experience higher rates of suicidal thoughts compared to other age groups. That said, the overall rate of suicide among males is much greater than that for females. Several different factors that come into play when diagnosing depression and mental health disorders.

1. **Biological Factors**: Changes in neurotransmitter levels (such as serotonin, dopamine, and norepinephrine) and alterations in brain structure and function can contribute to depression. Genetic factors may also play a role, as depression tends to run in families.
2. **Psychological Factors**: Again, as with anxiety, personality traits, such as low self-esteem, pessimism, or a tendency toward perfectionism, can increase the risk. Additionally, unresolved trauma, stressful life events, and ongoing stressors can contribute to the onset of depression. Social factors such as loneliness, social isolation, or a lack of supportive relationships can also contribute.
3. **Medical Conditions**: Chronic illnesses such as cancer, diabetes, heart disease and neurological disorders are factors. Similarly, hormonal changes associated with conditions like thyroid disorders, menopause, or pregnancy can contribute to mood disturbances.
4. **Medications and Substance Abuse**: Some medications, including certain types of birth control, corticosteroids, and beta-blockers, may increase the risk of depression as a side effect. Substance abuse, including alcohol, drugs, and prescription medications, can also contribute to or exacerbate depression.

Symptoms of Depression

- Feeling down
- Tired all the time
- Listless and unable to concentrate
- Lacking enjoyment or interest in once pleasurable activities
- Lacking in confidence
- Feeling worthless
- Feeling guilty

· Poor sleep
· Poor appetite
· Low sex drive
· Recurrent thoughts of death or suicide

There are other conditions that can mimic depressive symptoms and it is important to rule out these conditions through careful assessment to avoid misdiagnosis. There are no specific blood tests to diagnose depression.

Exclude the Following Before Diagnosing Depression

· Personality and eating disorders.
· Latent bipolar disorder.
· Substance abuse – alcohol, ice, cocaine.
· Decreased blood flow to the brain.
· Subclinical hypothyroidism.
· Sleep apnoea.
· Narcolepsy – excessive sleepiness in daytime.
· Early dementia.

BRAIN SERENITY, STABILITY AND FIREPOWER

Let's have a look at how serotonin, GABA, and dopamine impact mental health. Serotonin and GABA, often referred to as the "happy" chemicals, are two key inhibitory neurotransmitters. They help calm the nervous system, particularly when it's overstimulated by stress hormones like adrenaline.

Serotonin: Serotonin plays an important role in mood regulation, behavior, sleep and learning. It's also involved in digestion, since 90% of serotonin actively occurs in the gastrointestinal tract. Because serotonin is derived from the amino acid tryptophan, adequate dietary protein is essential.

GABA: GABA (gamma-aminobutyric acid) promotes restfulness and reduces nervous tension. It is primarily produced in the brain from glutamate, not commonly found in significant amounts in food sources. However, fermented foods such as *Lactobacillus* and *Bifidobacterium* have small amounts. Supplements may indirectly influence GABA levels in the brain. Low GABA levels can go hand in hand with irritable bowel syndrome and fibromyalgia. We recommend you try it for yourself if you have poor sleep and a '"busy" brain with high anxiety.

Dopamine: Dopamine is known as the "great motivator." Dopamine can act as both an excitatory and inhibitory neurotransmitter. It's renowned for its role in the brain's reward system, influencing feelings of pleasure and motivation. However, dopamine also affects blood pressure, digestion, and voluntary movements. Certain behaviours like eating chocolate, engaging in sexual activity, or consuming addictive substances trigger dopamine release. However, prolonged substance abuse can lead to decreased sensitivity to dopamine, contributing to mental health issues like anxiety and depression. While dopamine is primarily sourced from protein-rich foods, the natural opioids/ endorphins released during exercise and pleasurable activities can also has a positive influence mood, pain perception, and immunity.

As mentioned previously, neurotransmission depends on how much neurotransmitter is released, any defects in processing or delivery, or mode of action may cause an imbalance. So it's not surprising people with major depressive disorder are prescribed antidepressant drug therapy – and reasonably in many cases. Some don't find them useful or stop because of side effects. And not everyone who has symptoms of mild to moderate depression has a significant risk of progressing to a major depressive disorder.

DRUGS AND MOOD DISORDERS

Let's explain how drugs can affect the levels neurotransmitters in the brain. Normally, serotonin is relayed across a microscopic cleft/space to other neurons and then is reabsorbed back into the original neuron through a process called reuptake. Importantly, you can inhibit that reuptake, so the neurotransmitters are then increased in the synapse. The increased concentration leads to more prolonged and enhanced serotonin signaling between neurons.

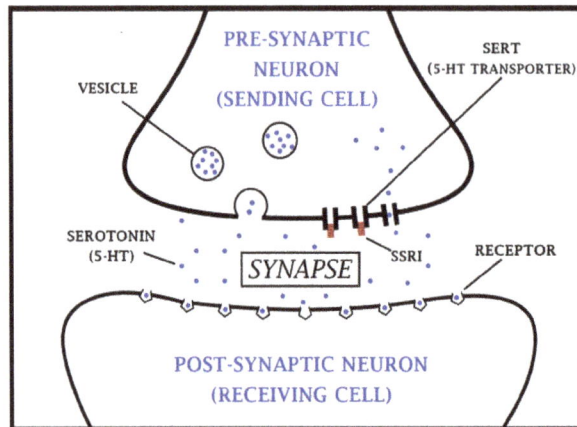

HOW SSRIs WORK
https://creativecommons.org/licenses/by-sa/4.0/

Selective serotonin reuptake inhibitors, or SSRIs increase the concentration of serotonin leading to enhanced neurotransmission. Their use is recommended for moderate to severe depression, and not all patients benefit from the treatment. The most common side effects experienced are nausea, dry mouth and insomnia. Some cause weight gain.

Similarly, **Norepinephrine-dopamine reuptake inhibitor (NDRI)** blocks the reuptake of norepinephrine and dopamine. NDRI drugs effect mood, cognition, and behavior.

So, if the aim is to increase the levels of serotonin, why not add the foods and the precursors 5-HTP (5-hydroxytryptophan) that raise the levels naturally (turkey, salmon, nuts and dairy)? After all, 90% of serotonin resides in the gut.

FEEL-GOOD FOODS FOR A BETTER MOOD

What you eat affects how you feel, emotionally as well as physically. 'Comfort food' is called that for a reason – it can offer you solace when you're feeling down and raise your blood sugar. Western-type diets have been found to be a risk factor for anxiety and depression, because of the deficiencies in nutrients like omega-3 fatty acids, B vitamins, and magnesium. Traditional diets like those found in the Mediterranean, Norwegian, or Japanese cultures emphasise abundant intake of fruits, vegetables, legumes, whole-grain cereals, nuts, and seeds, all rich sources of omega-3 fatty acids. They tend to minimise processed foods, fast foods, commercial baked goods, and sugary treats. Additionally, these diets often prioritise the cultivation of probiotic gut bacteria for overall health.

The Mediterranean Diet: In this diet you will find nutrients that improve depressive symptoms. These are the protein foods, with fish, meats, lentils, leafy greens, lettuces, peppers and cruciferous vegetables. Inherent within these foods are the nutrients considered essential to balance our mood via the omega-3 fatty acids in fish as well the B vitamin plus zinc, magnesium, iron, potassium, selenium, and vitamins A, B12, C and D.

Diets High in Sugar Don't Help: There's a strong relationship between the gut and brain: microbes stimulate cells in the intestines to produce serotonin. If the microbes are out of balance, you can develop problems such as uncontrolled yeast infections that depress mood. Conversely, you can restore their balance and lift your mood; high fibre foods and probiotics such as *Lactobacillus* and *Bifidobacterium* strains have shown to be the most beneficial, but a mix is usually best.

Specific Nutrients: There is convincing evidence that, fish oils, S-adenosyl-methionine (SAMe regulates hormones), N-acetyl cysteine (anti-inflammatory), the B vitamins and vitamin D are beneficial for mental health disorders. Magnesium, selenium and zinc also support neurochemical activities. We would add the herb St John's Wort which helps increase mood to your list. The importance of nutrient based supplements in combination or in isolation have been acknowledged in mainstream psychiatry (Sarris, 2015).

A Few Words of Caution: If you are already on antidepressant drugs, taking St John's Wort, SAMe or any other products that induce excess serotonin may be a problem - also known as serotonin syndrome. Feeling drunk or dizzy, agitated, confused with twitching and low-grade fever are some signs of excessive serotonin.

Pyrroles and Neurological Disorders

Some studies have identified elevated levels of pyrroles in the urine (called hydroxyhemepyrrolin-2-one (HPL)). These raised pyrroles were hypothesised to result in a range of psychiatric disorders. Pyrroles are molecules that have the potential to bind irreversibly to zinc and vitamin B6 in the body and lead to the excretion of these essential nutrients. Many practitioners believe that elevated pyrrole levels may be linked to conditions such as anxiety, depression, ADHD and schizophrenia, but more robust scientific evidence is needed to establish these connections definitively. Refer to Chapter 16 on ADHD.

POST TRAUMATIC STRESS DISORDER

Eye movement desensitisation and reprocessing (EMDR) may be helpful where depression results from past traumatic events. A therapist will ask you to think about a distressing image while moving your eyes from side to side, following the movement of the therapist's finger. This side-to-side movement establishes connections between the right and left brain so that the experience is then processed as a past event, rather than being continually relived in the present. An improvement is often achieved in three to five treatments. See more on EMDR in Chapter 31 (Stress Less).

TIPS FOR TACKLING MOOD DISORDERS

- Have a general health check, check hormone and nutrient levels.
- Supplement hormones, neurotransmitters and nutrients if deficient.
- Identify the type of depression for best treatment options.
- Manage diabetes or heart disease, which can make depression worse.
- Discuss major life changes/ traumatic events with a therapist.
- Avoid alcohol, foods with MSG, nicotine and other drugs of dependence.
- Rule out sleep apnoea. Aim for restful sleep.
- Get more sunlight and vitamin D.
- Increase serotonin with exercise, mindfulness, yoga, or tai chi. .
- Add probiotics, adequate protein and a Mediterranean diet.
- Consider rapid eye movement desensitisation reprocessing (EMDR) if your depression may stem from a past trauma.

References:

Australian Institute of Health and Welfare. (2022). https://www.aihw.gov.au/mental-health/overview/prevalence-and-impact-of-mental-illness

Briguglio, M., Dell'Osso, B., Panzica, G., Malgaroli, A., Banfi, G., Zanaboni Dina, C., Galentino, R., & Porta, M. (2018). Dietary Neurotransmitters: A Narrative Review on Current Knowledge. *Nutrients*, *10*(5), 591. https://doi.org/10.3390/nu10050591

Chopra, C., Mandalika, S., & Kinger, N. (2021). Does diet play a role in the prevention and management of depression among adolescents? A narrative review. *Nutrition and health*, *27*(2), 243–263. https://doi.org/10.1177/0260106020980532

Sánchez-Villegas A, Delgado-Rodríguez M, Alonso A, et al. (2009). Association of the Mediterranean Dietary Pattern With the Incidence of Depression: The Seguimiento Universidad de Navarra/University of Navarra Follow-up (SUN) Cohort. *Arch Gen Psychiatry*. 2009;66(10):1090–1098. doi:10.1001/archgenpsychiatry.2009.129

Sarris, J., Logan, A. C., Akbaraly, T. N., Amminger, G. P., Balanzá-Martínez, V., Freeman, M. P., Hibbeln, J., Matsuoka, Y., Mischoulon, D., Mizoue, T., Nanri, A., Nishi, D., Ramsey, D., Rucklidge, J. J., Sanchez-Villegas, A., Scholey, A., Su, K. P., Jacka, F. N., & International Society for Nutritional Psychiatry Research (2015). Nutritional medicine as mainstream in psychiatry. *The lancet. Psychiatry*, *2*(3), 271–274. https://doi.org/10.1016/S2215-0366(14)00051-0

Chapter 16

ATTENTION DEFICIT HYPERACTIVITY DISORDER AND AUTISM SPECTRUM DISORDER

"Common sense is a genius in working clothes."

RALPH WALDO EMERSON

Attention Deficit Hyperactivity Disorder (ADHD) and Autism Spectrum Disorder (ASD) are common conditions. Both are generally diagnosed by developmental/behavioural paediatricians or behavioural neurologists in early to mid-childhood, and both are complex disorders that require a range of assistance from health professionals. ADHD may be accompanied by autism spectrum disorder (ASD) in 20–50% of cases.

However, if the primary diagnosis is ASD, many symptoms of ADHD are present in 30–80% of cases, with genetic factors overlapping.

ATTENTION DEFICIT HYPERACTIVE DISORDER (ADHD)

The main problems in ADHD relate to behavioural symptoms where the child or adult shows lack of attention, hyperactivity and impulsiveness, which make the dynamics at home and at school very difficult. Depending on their severity, these core symptoms impact on academic performance, as well as social development. Globally, around 7% of children and adults have ADHD symptoms. Where the father is hyperactive, the number of siblings with the disorder is around 34%, indicating a highly genetic association. Without the problem of hyperactivity, problems of attention deficit disorder (ADD) may also exert some cognitive challenges.

In making the diagnosis, the behaviours must be obvious both at home and at school and interfere with the normal function of the child. The problems are multiplied when there are other related behaviours, such as obsessive-compulsive disorder and conduct disorder (due to similar sets of genes). Other related disorders are more obvious in later years such as the likelihood of developing depression or anxiety, bipolar disorders, substance abuse, alcoholism and drug addiction. Apart from psychological disorders, allergies, eczema, dermatitis, sinusitis and asthma are more common in those with ADHD.

Challenges for Development and Education

Coping with the inattentive hyperactive child in the home and at school is tricky. The resilience of the parents and teachers has been shown to be a key factor in decreasing the symptoms. Patience and tolerance may wear thin, especially when children are disruptive and fail to follow directions, but especially when children/adults are non-compliant and experience poor sleep, mood swings, aggression, temper tantrums and clumsiness.

Literacy, immature language and other learning problems are often part of the disorder, making school a very unhappy place. Many children with ADHD are quite intelligent, but they tend to become frustrated and underachieve because of their inability to finish their tasks, leaving them – and their parents – frustrated, and teachers impatient. A teacher, counsellor and friend of many years' experience expressed the view that there is a misconception that ADHD kids/people have trouble focusing. They don't. Their ability to focus can be awesome if they're interested. The child will see things very broadly and so can get easily distracted by what others see as trivial – to them it isn't.

The course of ADHD from school age to adulthood may present differently. People with ADHD tend to be disorganised, having lots of projects on the go that remain unfinished. They can be difficult to live with due to clutter and the flight of ideas.

The extreme activity seen in early years may change to excessive fidgetiness and restlessness towards their teenage years. Excessive use of digital media such as Facebook, YouTube and Instagram may be observed. Teenagers commonly avoid treatment, employ risky behaviours leading to injury, and may at times seek illicit drugs and alcohol to cope.

However, attention span can improve with age, as will many of the other symptoms. By age twenty-five, only 15% of those with ADHD will meet the criteria for the ADHD diagnosis, but only about 10% will seek treatment.

ADHD DIAGNOSIS

Many psychologists utilise the Conners questionnaire to gather insights into the behaviors and habits of children with ADHD. By inputting specific scores into a computer program, comprehensive feedback is generated, providing a clear snapshot of the child's current state. This tool is invaluable as ADHD symptoms can fluctuate over time, making it essential to track attention and behavior patterns consistently.

CAUSES OF ADHD

ADHD has genetic and biological causes that influence activity in certain parts of the brain. There is no one cause – there are the inherited risks, environmental risks, and risks associated with low birth weight and prematurity or birth injury. Toxins such as cigarette smoke in pregnancy, lead and pesticides, chemicals (food additives/MSG) and nutrient deficiencies – low iron and zinc – often precipitate symptoms of ADHD. Then there are additional problems if a parent or carer suffers from a mood disorder and needs antidepressants or anxiolytics.

Although there is a high genetic influence in ADHD, it is not all about the genes. Variations in the ability of the neurons to fire normally depend on the nutrients and precursors in the blood plasma arising from the diet. Changes in dietary proteins and B vitamins affect these precursors and regulate not only the rate at which we make neurotransmitters, but also the concentration in the nerve terminals and the quantity released when the neurons fire. Dietary considerations are a major factor in the treatment of ADHD; it is not all about drugs.

Genetic factors	Up to 35% of family members are also likely to have ADHD. Around 42 different genes are involved.
Neurotransmitters: excitatory and inhibitory, with altered levels	Altered dopamine and serotonin pathways. Reduced inhibition and altered glutamate and GABA.

Nutrient deficiencies	Zinc, iron, magnesium, vitamin B6.
Food sensitivities, chemicals and additives	Food additives and some natural food chemicals.
Exposure to environmental toxins	Lead, mercury, pesticides, fluoride, cigarette smoke and BPA.
Brain injury	Postnatal injury to the prefrontal regions of the brain.
Low-birth-weight and premature births	Multiple causes: placenta abnormalities, mother's ill-health and infection.
Exposure to antidepressants in pregnancy	In women with mood disorders.
Alcohol, heroin and tobacco in pregnancy	Smoking by parents, grandparents and carers.
Pyrrole disorder	Biochemical abnormality with low vitamin B6 and zinc.

NEUROTRANSMITTERS AND ADHD

ADHD has a strong genetic component, but nutrients and substances in the diet play a major role too. Changes in proteins and B vitamins in our diet affect how neurons work, impacting neurotransmitter production, concentration, and release. Diet is a crucial part of ADHD treatment, not just medication.

Both low and high levels of norepinephrine and epinephrine are found in children with ADHD. These neurotransmitters help regulate attention. Too little when bored, and too much when stressed, and this will affect planning and organising thoughts and behaviours– otherwise known as executive function.

Stimulant medications like Ritalin inhibit the epinephrine and norepinephrine transporters or pathways, as well as the dopamine pathways to increase focus. Nutrients or medications that optimise these neurotransmitters often assist with dampening down the hyperactivity and impulsive behaviours.

Dopamine for Attention and Motivation: Dopamine transporters are the target of the medications for hyperactivity (Concerta and Ritalin). Dopamine levels really depend on the intake of protein foods. Volkow (2009) found lower dopamine receptors in two key areas of the brain in dealing with reward and motivation in adults with ADHD. The authors suggested that this could be a reason why those with ADHD prefer small immediate rewards over larger delayed rewards – in other words, they want things now! To boost dopamine, consider protein-rich foods, iron, zinc, exercise, B vitamins, and ginseng.

Serotonin for Mood and Impulse Control: Serotonin, our mood-enhancing neurotransmitter, also comes from tryptophan in proteins. Long-term protein deficiency might worsen ADHD symptoms. Boost serotonin with protein, vitamin B6, sunlight, exercise and zinc-rich foods (red meat).

Glutamate for Aggression and Impulse: Glutamate, an excitatory neurotransmitter, is often high in ADHD kids. Avoid foods with monosodium glutamate (MSG or additive number E 621) to manage impulsive, aggressive and anxious behaviors.

GABA for Calming: Many ADHD kids have low GABA levels. GABA is made from glutamate but needs vitamin B6 and zinc as well. While it's hard to increase GABA through diet alone, GABA supporting supplements might help.

CONSIDERATIONS BEFORE TREATMENT

- Get a diagnosis early; start behavioural training or other programs as soon as possible.
- Are there other issues like anxiety or obsessive-compulsive disorder (OCD) – making management more complex?
- Are there nutrient deficiencies due to poor diet?
- Who else in the house has ADHD or other psychological disorders?
- Assess the challenges for implementing treatment – diets, supplements or drugs – or any other interventions with parents and family.
- What are the support systems and the likelihood of success?

PARENT TRAINING AND BEHAVIOURAL INTERVENTION

There are many forms of behaviour therapy and counselling that are helpful for parents and children with ADHD. These are best when the children are young. Specialists in ADHD (or autism) are essential for the greater benefit – therapists who have seen it all and done it all and seen failures and success over years. Parents and carers should be taught skills to manage the behaviour and be consistent. They also need to be able to impose discipline on the child with agreed protocols. The child will need support at home and at school. They need to be taught to be able to control their behaviour, which leads to better relationships, improved schooling and a happier environment. In short, they need to feel better, happier and calmer.

DIET AND ADHD

The Elimination Diet from the Royal Prince Alfred Hospital in Sydney has been beneficial for many with ADHD. Spearheaded by Dr. Robert Loblay and dietitian Anne Swain in the 1980s, the hospital refined protocols for identifying food intolerances. Booklets are provided with helpful protocols and recipes. While caregivers are often willing to manage the diet, some specialists remain skeptical.

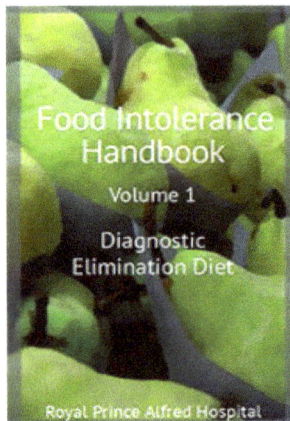

FOOD INTOLERANCE
HANDBOOK
Royal Prince Alfred Hospital

However, adverse reactions to food additives, colors, and flavors may be evident with hyperactivity or aggression linked to certain foods. Parents can decide whether to continue the dietary intervention and adjust for triggers as needed, (see Chapter 2). Here are some key nutrients in the management of ADHD symptoms;

1. **Iron**: Iron deficiency, even without anemia, can impact learning, behavior, and emotional well-being in children. Iron helps produce important brain chemicals like dopamine and GABA, which help regulate mood and excitability.

2. **Zinc**: Many children with ADHD may have low zinc levels, affecting their behavior and eating habits. Supplementing with 15 mg/day of zinc can help, especially if split and taken outside of mealtimes. Testing levels after ten weeks can guide further supplementation.

3. **Magnesium**: Diets low in magnesium can make ADHD symptoms worse. Supplementing with 200 mg/day for six months has been shown to reduce symptoms of ADHD, anxiety, and improve sleep.

4. Essential Fatty Acids (EFAs): Omega-3 and omega-6 fatty acids from sources like fish, nuts, and seeds are crucial for nerve function and brain development. Combining EFAs with stimulant medications can enhance ADHD symptom management.

5. Melatonin: Many people with ADHD struggle with sleep issues. Around 3–6 mg taken before bedtime, can help improve sleep quality.

6. Probiotics: Gut health influences mood and cognition. Including high-fiber foods, fermented foods, and quality yogurt in the diet can support a healthy gut microbiome.

7. B Vitamins: B vitamins play a role in various brain functions and the production of neurotransmitters. Folinic acid is often preferred over folic acid, especially in individuals with a genetic influence like MTHFR.

DRUGS AND ADHD

In terms of efficacy, stimulant medications work in approximately 65–80% of children. Depending on the severity, the complexity and different complaints, doctors or psychiatrists may recommend versions of these drugs that reduce the core symptoms of ADHD. Complaints of insomnia, decreased appetite and perhaps growth, stomach aches, headaches and jitteriness can worry parents having to give these medicines to their children. That said, the challenges of parenting and teaching children with ADHD can be enormous, and when the case is severe, drugs are often the only option to maintain some level of normality within the home and at school. Here are some of the reasons why the drugs ae used:

Stimulant Medications: Ritalin and Adderall, work by increasing the levels of certain chemicals in the brain, namely dopamine and norepinephrine. These chemicals help regulate attention, focus, and impulse control and help those with ADHD concentrate better and manage their behavior more effectively.

Non-Stimulant Medications: Medications, such as Strattera, Intuniv, and Kapvay, work differently than stimulants. They target other neurotransmitters like norepinephrine, to help improve attention and impulse control. These medications may take longer to show effects compared to stimulants, but they can be helpful for those who don't respond well to stimulants or have certain medical conditions that prevent them from using stimulants.

Overall, both types of medications aim to balance brain chemicals to reduce ADHD symptoms and improve daily functioning.

PYRROLE DISORDER – IS IT AN ISSUE IN ADHD?

Sometimes, due to genetic factors or stress, our bodies can produce too many pyrroles. Pyrroles are chemical structure and part of an important molecules like heme (found in blood cells), vitamin B12 and bile pigments. These extra pyrroles get removed from our bodies via urinary output, but they also bind to zinc and vitamin B6, causing our levels of these nutrients to drop. This may lead to problems with brain chemicals like dopamine and GABA, which are important for mood and behavior.

The research is not conclusive but suggest some people with a pyrrole disorder might experience symptoms like depression, ADHD, autism, schizophrenia. Characteristics of the disorder include mood swings and anxiety, heightened sensory sensitivity and digestive problems, trouble sleeping, muscle weakness, tantrums and learning difficulties.

Pyrrole tests are done via a urine sample. If positive, supplementing with vitamins like B6 and zinc can help. However, it can be challenging to get children to take these supplements regularly! Parents often notice a difference when their child stops taking the supplements, as the symptoms can come back quickly without them.

ADHD

ACTION PLAN – CHECKLIST

- Check symptoms against the Conners' Parent Rating Scale.
- Ascertain the diagnosis. (Government assistance relies confirmation).
- Check for deficiencies, especially iron, zinc, magnesium and vitamin D.
- Check for allergies and chemical sensitivities that exacerbate ADHD.
- Ensure the diet is adequate in protein, supplement deficiencies.
- Supplement with melatonin to improve sleep, add fish oils and magnesium.
- Implement behavioural therapies.
- Keep the teachers informed so they know how to help.
- Review progress.
- If progress is poor, seek specialist review who may consider a trial of drugs.

References:

Volkow, N. D., Wang, G. J., Newcorn, J. H., Kollins, S. H., Wigal, T. L., Telang, F., Fowler, J. S., Goldstein, R. Z., Klein, N., Logan, J., Wong, C., & Swanson, J. M. (2011). Motivation deficit in ADHD is associated with dysfunction of the dopamine reward pathway. *Molecular psychiatry*, *16*(11), 1147–1154. https://doi.org/10.1038/mp.2010.97

Mikirova N (2015) Clinical Test of Pyrroles: Usefulness and Association with Other Biochemical Markers. Clin Med Rev Case Rep 2:027. 10.23937/2378-3656/1410027

Loblay, R. H., & Swain, A. R. (1986). Food Intolerance. *Recent Advances in Clinical Nutrition*, *2*,169–177.

AUTISM SPECTRUM DISORDER

Autism, or neurodiversity, is a common developmental difference in processing the world around you, characterised by different degrees of impaired social behaviour, communication and language. Individuals may have a narrow range of interests and repetitive behaviours, such as hand flapping or whole-body movement. Sensory issues are common: sensitivities to light, sound, taste and touch are features of ASD, to the extent that there may be a dislike for wearing clothes, covering ears to avoid noise or much preferring foods with a certain texture. Puberty transition can be difficult for some. For example, some may have seizures for the first time. Anxiety and depression are common associations.

There is a wide range of cognitive abilities – from severe retardation to quite high IQ. Over half receive special tuition and around 44% use a counsellor or disability support.

While the challenges are many, parents of children with autism generally cope well. On bad days, when routine must be changed for some reason, the meltdowns, upsets, and tantrums can be difficult for everyone involved. Specific phobias, obsessive compulsive disorder, social anxiety or separation anxiety all require some cognitive strategies for management.

Savant syndrome is relatively common in autism. From the French word savoir, meaning 'to know', around 10% of those with autism (mostly boys) can do the most intricate mathematical calculations and have incredible memory and musical ability. This compares with fewer than 1% of savants in the general population. Possibly one of the greatest challenges is the inability to communicate in a similar way to the general population by reading gestures and facial expressions.

The prevalence of Autism Spectrum Disorder (ASD) is estimated to be around 1 in 54 children, according to the Centers for Disease Control and Prevention (CDC) in the United States. However, prevalence rates may vary slightly depending on the region and methodology of data collection.

COMMON SUBTYPES OR PROFILES OF ASD

Classic Autism: This subtype is characterised by significant impairments in social interaction and communication, as well as restricted interests and repetitive behaviors.

Asperger's Syndrome: Previously considered a separate diagnosis, Asperger's syndrome is characterised by milder social and communication difficulties but often includes intense interests and adherence to routines.

Pervasive Developmental Disorder-Not Otherwise Specified (PDD-NOS): This subtype was previously used to describe individuals who did not fully meet the criteria for classic autism or Asperger's syndrome but still exhibited significant social and communication challenges.

Childhood Disintegrative Disorder (CDD): This rare subtype involves a significant loss of previously acquired skills, such as language, social, and motor skills, typically occurring after a period of normal development.

Rett Syndrome: Another rare subtype, Rett syndrome primarily affects females and is characterised by a loss of motor and language skills, repetitive hand movements, and other neurological symptoms.

Autism with Intellectual Disability: Some individuals with ASD also have intellectual disability, characterised by significant limitations in intellectual functioning and adaptive behaviors.

EARLY INDICATORS

Restrictive and Repetitive Behaviours Relating to Autism

- Avoids or does not keep eye contact.
- Does not respond to name by 9 months of age.
- Does not show facial expressions like happy, sad, angry, and surprised by 9 months of age.
- Does not play simple interactive games like pat-a-cake by 12 months of age.
- Uses few or no gestures by 12 months of age (for example, does not wave goodbye)
- Does not share interests with others by 15 months of age (for example, shows you an object that they like).
- Does not point to show you something interesting by 18 months of age.
- Does not notice when others are hurt or upset by 24 months of age.
- Does not notice other children and join them in play by 36 months of age.
- Does not pretend to be something else, like a teacher or superhero, during play by 48 months of age.
- Does not sing, dance, or act for you by 60 months of age.

Source: CDC (2024); Autism Spectrum Disorder. *https://www.cdc.gov/ncbddd/autism/signs.html*

Autism varies widely among individuals, with unique genetic and environmental influences. We're still learning how DNA reactions affect brain development and conditions like ASD. Genetic testing can be helpful, as treatments may involve nutrients like folate, choline, and B vitamins for those with methylation issues. Both nutrition and genetics play a role in treatment.

Neurological Abnormalities: Some children show signs early on, with rapid brain growth until age two, followed by slower growth. **Choline, important for brain function,** is lower in those with autism, and the severity may be linked to this deficiency. Acetylcholine, which choline helps produce, affects muscle movement, sleep, pain, and learning. **Eggs are a good source of choline.** GABA issues can lead to constipation in half of those with autism. Both autism and ADHD can involve GABA and glutamate imbalances, leading to irritability, anxiety, and other issues. ASD is often associated with high inflammation levels and antibodies related to seizure disorders in childhood. Avoid MSG (additive number E621).

Immunity and ASD: Core ASD features are high inflammatory markers. Antibodies against glutamate receptors have been implicated in childhood seizure disorders.

Detoxication of Heavy Metals: First, guard against continuing uptake of the toxic metals and check out the nutrients that may be affected. Any decrease in essential nutrients such as magnesium, zinc and iron will put those who are malnourished at greater risk. The aim is to enhance the body's natural detoxification pathways, and where necessary pharmaceutical chelators create a bond with a toxic metal to make it water soluble for excretion in the urine.

ENVIRONMENTAL TOXINS TO BE AVOIDED

TOXINS	EFFECTS
Lead Air, soil, dust in mining areas. Solders used to copper pipes in houses and brass in taps still contain about 4% lead. Some PVC contains lead carbonate. Lead leaching is increased in copper pipes and brass fixtures where water is fluoridated.	Effects on intellect, behavioural disturbance, and ADHD. Children absorb more lead than adults because of their exposure from crawling around floors and hand-to-mouth activity. There is no safe amount of lead exposure.
Mercury Amalgam teeth fillings, large fish: shark, marlin, swordfish, ray, barramundi, gemfish, orange roughy, ling and southern bluefin tuna. Medical waste, old clocks, barometers, mirrors. Electronics -some in laptops and LCD screens.	Toxic to the central and peripheral nervous system mostly through long term exposure. Amalgam fillings with mercury are banned in Europe. Mercury can be measured in blood, urine and hair.
Cadmium Mining, smelting, or engraving. Cigarette smoke.	High amounts may interfere with development in early life.
Organophosphates From pesticides used in agriculture, homes, gardens and veterinary products.	Chronic toxicity and neurological complications are well documented. Children have reduced amounts of detoxifying enzymes compared to adults; they are more at risk.

Bisphenol A (BPA)	
BPA is a chemical compound used in manufacturing plastics. It can be found in receipt paper, the lacquer lining of canned food, toys, water pipes, medical tubing and food-container linings.	Affects behaviour (ADHD). It also has links to the prostate gland, blood pressure, cardiovascular disease and diabetes.
Fluoridated Water	
High levels in naturally water sources. Water fluoridation levels above 1.5mg/L are toxic to humans and animals.	Moderate to high levels of fluoride (1.5mg/L) in drinking water have been shown to affect IQ in the developing brain.

Detoxication of Heavy Metals: First, guard against continuing uptake of the toxic metals and check out the nutrients that may be affected. Any decrease in essential nutrients such as magnesium, zinc and iron will put those who are malnourished at greater risk. The aim is to enhance the body's natural detoxification pathways, and where (if necessary) pharmaceutical chelators create a bond with a toxic metal to make it water soluble for excretion in the urine. Important nutrients required for detoxification include:

Iron: Counteracts the toxic effects of lead. Cadmium and lead exposure cause the loss of essential metals, which leads to iron-deficiency anaemia and osteoporosis.

Selenium: Counteracts the effects of heavy metals such as mercury.

Zinc: Helps binding proteins (metallothioneins) that improve excretion of lead and arsenic.

Lactobacilli probiotics: Can protect against the toxicity of lead, cadmium and other metals.

α-Lipoic acid: A sulphur containing fatty acid that assists urinary excretion for the metals arsenic, barium, manganese, mercury and nickel following oral application.

Glutathione: A sulphur-containing molecule and the body's primary means for excretion of toxic metals.

L-cysteine: Has high affinity for binding mercury, copper, lead and cadmium, allowing their excretion from the body. N-acetyl-cysteine (NAC) is the precursor to L-cysteine and consequently glutathione. Found in onions, meat, poultry, yoghurt, eggs and grains.

Taurine and methionine: Sulphur-containing amino acids which decrease oxidative stress resulting from heavy metal exposure.

Cilantro (leaves of coriandrum sativum): An alcohol extract of the common coriander herb lowers lead concentrations – found in studies with rats!

Pharmaceutical detoxification agents: Doctors/toxicologists will often favour one type of agent over another. Here are two of the more common agents in modern use:

1. **Dimercaptosuccinic acid (DMSA)** is the main pharmaceutical agent that increases urinary excretion of arsenic, cadmium, lead, methylmercury and inorganic mercury, tin and copper. DMSA can be administered via oral, intravenous, rectal and transdermal (skin) routes.
2. **Penicillamine** may be used for cadmium, copper, arsenic and lead excretion, but is not as popular as DMSA.

WHAT TO DO

An early autism diagnosis requires early interventions and education programs. Months matter – toddlers' brains develop very rapidly, and every month that goes by is a missed opportunity to make a difference. Behavioural or other therapies are aimed at developing new cells and synapses in the brain and minimising the deficits of ASD. Visual training, speech therapy and physical or occupational therapy are essential.

1. **Specialist assessment** will give a good overall picture of basic problems, and it might be useful to press for a comprehensive stool analysis and genetic testing, biochemistry and allergy profile, with referrals to a dietitian specialising in the area of autism. While genetic differences may be the root cause of the problem, biochemical abnormalities, infections, toxicities, inflammatory markers, nutritional deficiencies and allergies are common.

2. **Attend to the issues that are most pressing and observe any progress or increased symptoms.** Deal with the major problems first. From our experience, it can be confusing to try dealing with lots of issues at the same time, although some parents manage very well.

3. **Sleep deprivation usually makes ASD symptoms worse**, with less concentration and exacerbated ADHD symptoms. For children with ASD, typical starting doses of melatonin range from 0.5 mg to 3 mg, taken about 30 minutes to an hour before bedtime. Some children may require higher doses, up to 6 mg or even 9 mg. However, sleep disturbance may be caused by a number of factors, including night terrors, reflux, seizures and heightened sensory issues, and dislike of bedclothes, light or noise. Keep a diary so you can keep track of the patterns.

4. **Check the diet for adequacy, because nutritional deficiencies are common** due to sensitivities to taste and textures. Fussy eaters preferring either white or brown food can be tricky. Supplementing zinc where the levels are low will often help improve appetite. Those who have 'pica' (where the child eats non-food

items such as paper or dirt) are thought perhaps to have an associated nutrient deficiency and sensory issues. Having sufficient foods with protein, iron, zinc, fibre, B vitamins and essential fats all on the one day may be impossible for some, and supplements may be an easier option. If children like eating soft, mushy food, egg custards (homemade) and blended meats will increase the macronutrient content.

5. **Consider short-term restrictions for dairy and perhaps gluten to see if there is a difference,** but certainly get rid of additives like MSG in the high-flavoured junk foods that can trigger poor behaviour or meltdowns and poor sleep. Elimination diets low in dairy or chemicals can take just three to four weeks before you see improvements in communication. For gluten, changes may take up to six weeks. The gains in communication and speech or other ASD symptoms need to be worth the trouble of the dietary restrictions.

6. **Probiotics, anti-infectives and dietary changes all play a role, but one can't do everything at once** as the treatments can sometimes make the symptoms worse at the start. A case in point is the antifungal treatment for *Candida* infections. 'Die-off' of *Candida* can produce toxins which overwhelm the system, and you will find autistic behaviours increase.

7. **Limit toxic substances and improve detoxification:** Improve detoxification pathways with adequate zinc and the glutathione precursor N-acetyl-cysteine. Protect the cells with antioxidants and omega-3 fatty acids.

8. **Drug therapy:** Specialist physicians are absolutely necessary in autism. It's important to note that medication should not be the sole or primary approach to managing autism-related symptoms. Behavioral interventions, educational supports, speech therapy, occupational therapy, and other forms of support are **typically considered first-line treatments.** Medication should be made on an individual basis, taking into account the specific needs and circumstances of the person with autism.

AUTISM

ACTION PLAN

- ASD confirmation by a specialist is necessary for government assistance.
- Check for nutrient deficiencies and genetic abnormalities.
- Tend to the most pressing issues first.
- Test stool for pathogens.
- Try Movicol for constipation.
- Check pyrrole levels. Supplements can assist behaviour.
- Start behavioural and educational interventions as soon as possible.
- Sleep disturbance is common; melatonin is often helpful.
- Keep a diary and review regularly.

References:

Chang, Z., Ghirardi, L., Quinn, P. D., Asherson, P., D'Onofrio, B. M., & Larsson, H. (2019). Risks and Benefits of Attention-Deficit/Hyperactivity Disorder Medication on Behavioral and Neuropsychiatric Outcomes: A Qualitative Review of Pharmacoepidemiology Studies Using Linked Prescription Databases. *Biological psychiatry*, *86*(5), 335–343. https://doi.org/10.1016/j.biopsych.2019.04.009

Australian Family Physician. (2011). Autism Detection in Early Childhood Indicators. *Australian Family Physician*, *40*(9), 675

Bashash, M., Marchand, M., Hu, H., Till, C., Martinez-Mier, E. A., Sanchez, B. N., Basu, N., Peterson, K. E., Green, R., Schnaas, L., Mercado-García, A., Hernández-Avila, M., &

Téllez-Rojo, M. M. (2018). Prenatal fluoride exposure and attention deficit hyperactivity disorder (ADHD) symptoms in children at 6-12 years of age in Mexico City. *Environment international*, *121*(Pt 1), 658–666. https://doi.org/10.1016/j.envint.2018.09.017

Bidwell LC, McClernon FJ, Kollins SH. (2011). Cognitive enhancers for the treatment of ADHD. *Pharmacol Biochem Behav*. (2):262–274

Jurewicz, J., & Hanke, W. (2008). Prenatal and childhood exposure to pesticides and neurobehavioral development: review of epidemiological studies. *International journal of occupational medicine and environmental health*, *21*(2), 121–132. https://doi.org/10.2478/v10001-008-0014-z

Li, Y., Zhang, H., Kuang, H., Fa,n R., Cha, C., Li G, Luo, Z., Pang, Q. Relationship between bisphenol A exposure and attention-deficit/ hyperactivity disorder: A case-control study for primary school children in Guangzhou, China. Environ Pollut. 2018 Apr;235:141-149. doi: 10.1016/j.envpol.2017.

Reichelt, K. L., Hole, K., Hamberger, A., Saelid, G., Edminson, P. D., Braestrup, C. B., Lingjaerde, O., Ledaal, P., & Orbeck, H. (1981). Biologically active peptide-containing fractions in schizophrenia and childhood autism. *Advances in biochemical psychopharmacology*, *28*, 627–643.

Stuckey, R., Walsh, W., & Lambert, B. (2010). The Effectiveness of Targeted Nutrient Therapy in Treatment of Mental Illness. *ACNEM Journal*, *29*(3).

Wagner-Schuman, M., Richardson, J.R., Auinger, P. *et al*. Association of pyrethroid pesticide exposure with attention-deficit/hyperactivity disorder in a nationally representative sample of U.S. children. *Environ Health* **14**, 44 (2015). https://doi.org/10.1186/s12940-015-0030-y

Chapter 17

LOW LIBIDO, ERECTILE DYSFUNCTION AND TESTOSTERONE DEFICIENCY

*"And in the end, it's not the years
in your life that count.
It's the life in your years."*

ABRAHAM LINCOLN

Yes, it's true that sex is one of the many functions of the body that becomes less efficient with ageing. Obesity, ageing, high blood pressure, diabetes, smoking and stress levels all play a role when it comes to sex. But you don't have to give up on your sex life or rely solely on drugs to 'keep it up'.

Age, depression and stress or marital/partner differences may cause loss of libido. Deficiencies in oestrogen, testosterone and dehydroepiandrosterone (DHEA) can wreak havoc on sex drive. Both men and women produce all three sex hormones, but their quantity and importance differ by gender. Testosterone decreases in men, causing a decrease in sex drive after about thirty years, while women's hormones decrease in their premenopausal years, with subtle changes in their thirties becoming more established in their forties.

ERECTILE DYSFUNCTION (ED)

Erectile dysfunction (ED) or impotence is the inability for a male to have or maintain an erection hard enough for satisfactory sexual intercourse. If not related to obvious causes, for example prostate surgery, it is often related to narrowing of the small penile arteries delivering blood to the penis. If you are over fifty, poor sexual function becomes an emerging issue. In all age groups, and with both sexes, there are significant health benefits of a safe and active sex life. For both men and women, sex is usually a pleasurable event aside from the health benefits.

Benefits of Safe and Active Sex

1. Reduces risk of heart disease.
2. Helps your immune system.
3. Improves women's bladder control.
4. Lowers your blood pressure.
5. Improves confidence and relationships.
6. Increases endorphins and reduces chronic pain.

7. Reduces frequency and severity of headaches.
8. Lower risk of prostate cancer.
9. Reduces stress.
10. May reduce risk of dementia.

PROSTATE CANCER AND BENIGN PROSTATIC HYPERTROPHY

Benign prostatic hypertrophy (BPH) is a major cause for surgery. This is diagnosed in some 60% of men over sixty years, though not all of these cases lead to surgery. The other cause is prostatic cancer, where the likelihood of the loss of erectile function post-operatively is (controversially) anywhere up to 80% within two years of surgery. Many men require assistance to attain and maintain erections after surgery for both these conditions.

All the issues of BPH and prostate cancer are presented in Chapter 18. There we present details of a new non-surgical technique for BPH which is not associated with erectile dysfunction (ED). This procedure, undertaken by a radiologist rather than a urologist, is called prostatic artery embolisation (PAE).

YOUR OPTIONS FOR ERECTION DYSFUNCTION

Here we will initially give you all the orthodox managements which are somewhat invasive but more likely to be prescribed by doctors. The more natural options are presented at the end of the chapter.

The Cause of The Problem: The main causes of erectile dysfunction are poor circulation and poor blood flow through the penis. Constriction and hardening of the arteries may be related to diabetes, hormonal imbalance, thyroid dysfunction, adrenal disorders, nerve disorders, prostate disease and/or drug side effects. Drugs for blood pressure, antidepressants or relaxants may cause problems. Another problem is excess weight. Men who are obese are particularly prone to impotence.

If you're impotent, it's important to identify which of these causes applies to you and work with your doctor to better manage the underlying conditions. If you are deficient in key hormones and neurotransmitters, you may be physically less able to achieve an erection and psychologically less ready to attempt one. If you're impotent once, the resulting anxiety and loss of confidence can sabotage future attempts.

Narrowing of small arteries in the body may be a warning that a compromise of the diameter of the larger arteries may later occur, with risk of heart disease and stroke. The argument suggests that ED should be considered a risk factor for these conditions, just the same as other risk factors – hypertension, diabetes and smoking.

Treatment: There is concern and some contra-indication for use of phosphodiesterase (PDE) inhibitors like Viagra, which we will introduce in the next paragraph. In particular, PDE5 inhibitors should not be given if the patient is on nitrates and nitrate-like medications that dilate the blood vessels to prevent chest pain.

Oral medications: The PDE5 inhibitors include sildenafil (Viagra), tadalafil (Cialis), vardenafil (Levitra) and avanafil (Spedra). The latter is a recent addition with quick action within fifteen minutes to help attain and maintain an erection. They are taken orally, the first three being taken half an hour to an hour before sexual activity. The effects of assisting penile erection can last a few hours, with the duration depending on the drug. This is usually the first, and most common, medical intervention.

Our preference: Cialis over Viagra for the following reasons:

· You're less likely to get flushing of the skin and headaches at the standard dose of a 20 mg tablet.

- You're more likely to achieve spontaneous morning erections at a lower dose of 5 mg a day (i.e. 5 mg taken every day as a maintenance, rather than 20 mg at the time of intended intercourse).
- At the lower dose of 5 mg a day, Cialis can offer some relief from symptoms of prostatism or chronic bladder irritation (when there is an unexplained but recurrent and persistent need to pass urine).
- **Penile injections:** Caverject is injected into the side of the penis, promoting blood flow into the penis. The patient needs to be taught how to do this procedure. This is the next most common procedure for ED suggested by doctors.
- **Male penis pump or vacuum constrictive device (VCD):** A pump is placed over the penis. As air is pumped out of the cylinder, blood is drawn into the penis to produce an erection. A ring slides over the base of the penis to keep the blood in the tissues to maintain an erection for up to half an hour.
- **Suppository:** A suppository is placed in the opening of the penis using an applicator.
- **Penile prostheses (implants):** These are rods that are placed in the penis. Devices which can be inflated and deflated are more commonly used.
- **Therapy:** For about one in ten men with erectile dysfunction, the underlying condition is psychological rather than medical. Therapy focuses more on counselling and other non-drug approaches such as mindfulness (Chapter 12) and relaxation techniques. These therapies are best in anxiety-based erection problems with partners involved in the sessions. But there are other important factors to consider:
- **Lifestyle:** As with other forms of sexual dysfunction, exercise, smoking and weight loss are issues that need to be assessed.
- **Increase nitric oxide:** This molecule dilates blood vessels and it increases the blood flow to the penis, as it does for the heart. Antibacterial mouthwashes and, antacids reduce nitric oxide. L-citrulline supplement of 1.5 g per day helps generate nitric oxide.

· **Herbal medicines:** There are many herbs that have pharmacological effects as an aphrodisiac, but would you be likely to use them in your hour of need? Probably the best researched herbs are Ginseng (Panax ginseng) and Yohimbe. Both these herbs are also believed to be effective by dilating blood vessels and improving blood flow to the penis, as does Saw Palmetto. Only ripe Saw Plametto berries have active constituents. Dried stinging nettle is also reported to assist. Both saw palmetto and stinging nettle have additional benefits in decreasing the size of a benignly enlarged prostate (BPH) – this is discussed in Chapter 18).

LIBIDO IN WOMEN AND MEN AND HORMONE DEFICIENCY

Oestrogen shapes girls into women at puberty and makes menstruation possible. But as menopause approaches, natural levels of oestrogen fall. The decline can coincide with a fall in levels of the soothing neurotransmitter serotonin. At best, a sense of wellbeing can be undermined. At worst, the depletion of oestrogen and serotonin can trigger the onset of depression. Either way, libido and sexual responsiveness are likely to suffer.

There are the other hormonal symptoms that can arise with oestrogen deficiency, such as atrophy of the mucous membranes of the vagina and vulva and decreased natural lubrication of these sensitive areas. The result – an unresponsive clitoris – it is the nearest female equivalent to 'erectile dysfunction' and deserves as much attention and treatment. Testosterone, in combination with oestradiol, is more effective for increasing desire in women post-menopause.

Factors Other Than Age That Cause Oestrogen Deficiency

1. **Testosterone Deficiency, Men and Women:** Testosterone helps boys to develop into men and makes sperm production possible. It's made largely by the testes (in men) and in much smaller amounts by the ovaries (in women) and adrenal glands

(in both genders). Testosterone levels in both men and women start falling as they reach their forties. If levels fall too low, the result can be significant or absolute loss of libido. Fatigue, muscle weakness and blunted motivation also don't help sex drive.

2. **Excess weight and poor diet:** Since testosterone is converted into oestrogen in fat tissue, more fat tissue results in a higher rate of conversion. An ageing male who develops a 'pot belly' is asking for trouble if he eats a meal high in saturated fat, which reduces testosterone for up to four hours.

3. **Stress:** High stress with high cortisol levels decreases both testosterone and DHEA.

4. **Alcohol:** When alcohol is metabolised, it stimulates an enzyme called aromatase which converts testosterone to oestrogen. Men can develop fertility problems and may develop breast tissue, especially if they are heavy drinkers. Beer, wine and bourbon have plant oestrogens, which raise oestrogen levels and decrease testosterone.

Testing for Testosterone: A common inexpensive blood test by a medical practitioner can show you whether your testosterone is above or below the 'normal' level of 12 to 30 nmol/L for a male, or 0.5 to 3.2 nmol/L for a female. However, 'normal' levels may not help much. For example, one man may perform satisfactorily in libido and erectile function only when testosterone is at the higher end of the normal range, yet another man or woman might get the same result at the lower-middle levels.

The normal serum values for male testosterone have a wide range between 12 and 32 nmol/L. If a male in his mid or later years has the 'normal' range at a level of, say, 14 mmol/L, but spent most of his former life with successful sexual activity at higher levels over 20 nmol/L, the figure of 14 is probably not relevant to him.

When testosterone is not the answer: For many men, testosterone works up to a point. And some men need more options. Nitric oxide (NO) can help sustain an erection, but it's not the whole story either. Other general long-term issues that are worth considering facilitating a successful erection include:

1. α-lipoic acid, which stops the early breakdown of NO.
2. Vitamin D is favourable for arterial health.
3. Vitamin B12 and folic acid assist arterial wall health and help decrease homocysteine, a risk factor in NO supply.
4. Vitamin C, as a free radical scavenger, supports healthy blood pressure levels, arterial health and blood flows.
5. Doses of L-arginine of 1.7 g per day, pycnogenol (an antioxidant) 40 mg twice per day and ginseng (herb) 600 mg three times per day have been shown to assist in different studies. The herb Tribulus has shown a positive influence on testosterone. The dose of 250mg -500mgs per day.

Check for DHEA Deficiency: Dehydroepiandrosterone (DHEA) is the most abundant hormone in the body made by the adrenal glands, testes, ovaries and brain. It regulates the production of oestrogen, testosterone, cortisol and adrenaline, assists immunity and supports bone and muscle health. Deficiency may be associated with very significant fatigue/exhaustion, decreased sex drive, and loss of body hair. DHEA levels fall from our twenties onwards, dropping to 50% by our forties and a further 20% by our seventies.

Since DHEA is needed to make the sex hormones oestrogen and testosterone, any deficiency can have a major impact on your sex drive. We often prescribe it in a cream, as with the women's hormones. Skin creams bypasses any problems with gut (absorption) and liver (inappropriate breaking down) which may occur via the oral route It's often combined with testosterone in the same cream mixture.

The Prescription: Hormones can be prescribed for compounding pharmacists in creams to be rubbed on the skin, or as troches via the buccal (inside mouth) mucous membranes. A combined cream for men with 5% DHEA and testosterone 6–8%, applied daily to soft, hairless skin; or alternatively, DHEA capsules, usually in 50 mg doses for men and 25 mg for women.

Women should understand that adequate testosterone often makes them sensuous and physically powerful, but we also warn that excessive testosterone may make them 'angry and hairy,' and they'll need regular testing and clinical reviews to avoid this distressing scenario.

LOW LIBIDO, ERECTILE DYSFUNCTION (ED) AND TESTOSTERONE DEFICIENCY

ACTION PLAN – CHECKLIST

- Aim for an ideal body weight.
- Measure, then treat, for any testosterone or DHEA deficiencies.
- Look for other causes – diabetes, heart disease.
- Are psychological issues or drugs an issue?
- Consider natural vasodilators.
- Seek prescription medicines that assists achievement of erections.
- For women with low libido, use appropriate skin cream with hormone complexes.

References:

Borrelli, F., Colalto, C., Delfino, D. V., Iriti, M., & Izzo, A. A. (2018). Herbal Dietary Supplements for Erectile Dysfunction: A Systematic Review and Meta-Analysis. *Drugs, 78*(6), 643–673. https://doi.org/10.1007/s40265-018-0897-3

Carruthers M. (2009). Time for international action on treating testosterone deficiency syndrome. *The aging male : the official journal of the International Society for the Study of the Aging Male, 12*(1), 21–28. https://doi.org/10.1080/13685530802699067

Chapter 18

BENIGN PROSTATIC HYPERTROPHY (BPH) AND PROSTATE CANCER

"Unfortunately, with men's health, we don't talk about it enough, and prostate cancer gets lost in the conversation."

ERIC MCCORMACK

The prostate is a small gland that surrounds the neck of the bladder and the urethra (the tube passing down the middle of the penis, which facilitates the passage of urine from the bladder to the outside).

The prostate is about the size of a walnut, it encircles the bladder neck and urethra, aiding in semen production. By age sixty, it often enlarges to the size of a lemon, causing benign prostatic hypertrophy (BPH) and urinary difficulties. BPH affects around 50% of men at fifty and 80% at eighty.

When it comes to prostate cancer, symptoms often show up later and are less severe compared to benign prostatic hyperplasia (BPH). Prostate cancer is typically detected through rising PSA levels and abnormal lumps found during a rectal exam, confirmed by MRI.

On the other hand, BPH symptoms, like frequent urination, occur earlier. A rectal exam and ultrasound can confirm an enlarged prostate, which causes difficulties in urination but isn't associated with cancer.

Any ageing man who has to get up several times overnight to pass urine knows how disruptive a benignly enlarged prostate (BPH) can be. It's harder to pass urine and takes longer, ending with a dribble and a night of broken sleep. It can also contribute to urinary tract, bladder and bowel problems, but is not in any way linked to cancer of the prostate.

BPH AND THE HORMONE CONNECTION

In BPH there are multiple factors at play: hormonal imbalance, increasing cell numbers and inflammation all drive prostate disorders in ageing men. Over time, this excess cell growth can create fairly large, discrete nodules in the prostate, which in turn press against, restrict or block the urethral canal that eliminates urine from the bladder via the penis.

When the progesterone hormone levels decline, there is an increase of the oestrogen (oestradiol) hormone, plus another hormone called dihydrotestosterone (DHT). It's the DHT that causes the prostate to enlarge.

Progesterone has several important functions. It curbs excessive production of oestradiol (which can thus cause increased breast tissue in men) and reduces the conversion of testosterone to the more active DHT, which causes the prostate to enlarge. Hormonal balance is key if progesterone is low, a trans-dermal cream (2–5 mg /day) can help.

INTRODUCTION TO LOWER URINARY TRACT SYMPTOMS (LUTS)

BPH results in less control over the urinary process – so much so that there's now a special name for the condition: lower urinary tract symptoms (LUTS). Lower Urinary Tract Symptoms (LUTS) include:

- Weak urinary stream
- Intermittent flow and hesitation
- Urgency to empty the bladder
- Frequent urination during day and night.

One in five men are affected by LUTS. Urinary tract infections, diabetes, obstructive sleep apnoea, obesity, heart and renal problems plus alcohol and caffeine consumption at night can make those symptoms worse. A referral to a urologist will see you on your way if you have a urinary infection, incontinence, retention symptoms or if you have a raised PSA. You may require:

1. **Ultrasound:** An ultrasound of the kidney, bladder and prostate will usually settle the diagnosis of BPH. This test, which involves an ultrasound of the lower abdomen region, is non-invasive and inexpensive with no radiation exposure.
2. **PSA (prostate-specific antigen):** A precautionary blood test is necessary to check your PSA levels for the possibility of prostate cancer. But don't think you have cancer just because your prostate is enlarged and you're having trouble urinating. It's very much more likely to be BPH, which is benign. With BPH, changes occur in the inner part of the prostate, whereas cancer usually develops on the outer part of the prostate. The cancer thus occurs a fair way from the urethra, so it doesn't usually cause urinary symptoms in its early stages.

3. **Regular check-up.** Men need check-ups to help detect BPH or prostate cancer early – not just with regular PSA tests, but with rectal examinations by the doctor. Those much-feared but quick, straightforward examinations involve a doctor inserting a gloved finger into the rectum and pushing gently forwards so that the prostate can be felt. If a doctor feels small, firm, isolated areas of enlarged prostate, it may be cancer. If the area of enlargement is softer, larger and evenly enlarged, it's probably BPH.

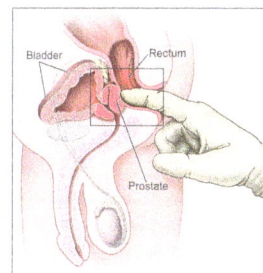

PROSTATE CHECK
National Cancer Institute

Surgical and Non-Surgical Management

1. **Trans-urethral resection of the prostate (TURP)** involves inserting an instrument through the penis via the urethra and cutting out the enlarged prostate sections near the urethra. Hospital discharge usually occurs within one or two days after surgery, sometimes with a catheter for a few days. This bypasses any initial swelling or inflammation problems that have been making the passing of urine difficult. Other less common side-effects include:

· A long-term side effect is the release of semen during ejaculation into the bladder, rather than out of the penis.
· Difficulty getting an erection.
· Heavy bleeding occurs sometimes with larger prostates.
· Loss of bladder control.
· Infection is possible after any surgical prostate procedure.
· Recurrence of BPH over time, possibly requiring another surgical procedure.

2. **Prostatic artery embolisation (PAE) is a non-surgical procedure** usually performed by a radiologist. It's typically done without an overnight hospital stay, involving

the injection of tiny spheres into prostate-feeding blood vessels to shrink the inner part of the prostate. Unlike traditional surgery like TURP, PAE preserves sexual function, is less costly, and has minimal side effects (2–5%). This is often due to some difficulty in identifying the tiny arteries feeding the prostate that facilitate the embolisation of the prostatic arteries. While long-term outcomes are still being studied, PAE shows promise, particularly for men seeking to avoid erectile dysfunction complications associated with surgery.

3. **Alpha blocker drugs** like Tamsulosin relax the smooth muscles in the prostate and bladder neck, improving urine flow and reducing blockage. Duodart, a common initial treatment, combines dutasteride and tamsulosin hydrochloride to reduce prostate size. However, these drugs and Cialis can potentially impact mood due to their interactions with neurotransmitters. Natural options like saw palmetto and nettle root may not consistently alleviate urinary symptoms associated with BPH.

CANCER OF THE PROSTATE

Prostate inflammation (prostatitis) and benign enlargement of the prostate occurs as men age and a common cause of non-cancerous high PSA (prostate-specific antigen). A PSA blood test may tell you that something bad is going on with the prostate – but that 'something' isn't necessarily cancer. Using the PSA for the diagnosis of cancer is very imprecise because both prostate cancer and benign or non-cancerous conditions can increase the PSA levels. The PSA levels alone won't tell you which cancers are aggressive and need treatment, or slow-growing and need to be managed more conservatively. Some urologists now suggest that any increase in PSA by 40% in any one year requires exclusion of prostate cancer as the cause, usually via biopsy. Blood test results greater than 4.0 nanograms per millilitre of blood need to be checked regularly.

Risk Factors	Protective Factors
Older men with a family history of prostate cancer	Fresh fruit and veg – tomato lycopene, green tea, soy phytoestrogens, pomegranate seed, curcumin, resveratrol (red grapes and red berries)
Excess weight	
High saturated-fat diet	Fish and flaxseed oil
Red meat and dairy	Vitamins D and B6
Acrylamide (bread/potato etc) cooked on high temperatures	Minerals – selenium, zinc with vitamin E
Pesticides, some PCBs (paints, plastics, etc)	Herbs – saw palmetto from ripe berries and stinging nettle
Arsenic and cadmium exposure	

Treatment of Prostate Cancer

1. Watchful waiting – even the aggressive type is often slow growing.
2. Surgery – robotic instruments are passed through keyhole incisions to allow the surgeon to remove the prostate and nearby tissues with great precision.
3. Hormone therapy.
4. A mix of the above.

Is Avoiding Surgery an Option: We sometimes opt not to disturb the protective capsule around the prostate or any prostate tissues, especially in older patients with elevated PSAs and potential cancer on MRI. While controversial, avoiding biopsy can reduce the rare risk of tumor seeding, particularly for certain biopsy procedures. Prostate cancer progression can be slow, and observation is increasingly emphasised over surgery, especially for younger patients. Impotence following BPH surgery or prostate cancer treatment is a significant concern. Many patients with mildly elevated PSAs undergo annual review with examination, PSA reading, and MRI, with an understanding that many may live with prostate cancer rather than die from it.

The *Financial Review* (2019) quotes Professor Declan Murphy, director of genito-urinary oncology at the Peter MacCallum Cancer Centre, Melbourne. He referred to the situation when men consult him for a second opinion about their treatment for prostate cancer, and it's not unusual for them to become uncomfortable. Professor Murphy explained, "They'll tell me that their surgeon says there is an 80% likelihood of recovering their erections after surgery. I tell them I am surprised and that, in their case, the likelihood may be no more than 20%.' The professor then summarises in the article: 'Sometimes they get angry, but that's the reality.'"

BENIGN PROSTATIC HYPERTROPHY AND PROSTATE CANCER

ACTION PLAN – CHECKLIST

- Check PSA yearly in males from age 50 years.
- Urinary symptoms require full medical assessment.
- Consider surgical and non-surgical options for BPH.
- Exercise regularly and consider the Mediterranean diet.
- Slow-growing prostate cancer may require careful observation only.
- Fast-growing cancer requires surgery and a mix of general medical treatments.

References:

Bosland, M. C. (2000). Chapter 2: The Role of Steroid Hormones in Prostate Carcinogenesis.

Margo, J. (2019). The truth about surgery for prostate cancer. *The Financial Review*. https://www.afr.com/ companies/healthcare-and-fitness/the-truth-about-surgery-for-prostate-cancer-20190827-p52l8d

Pais, P., Villar, A., & Rull, S. (2016). Determination of the potency of a novel saw palmetto supercritical CO_2 extract (SPSE) for 5α-reductase isoform II inhibition using a cell-free in vitro test system. *Research and Reports in Urology*, *8*, 41-49. https://doi.org/10.2147/RRU.S96576

Welk, B., McArthur, E., Ordon, M., Anderson, K. K., Hayward, J., & Dixon, S. (2017). Association of Suicidality and Depression With 5α-Reductase Inhibitors. *JAMA internal medicine*, *177*(5), 683–691. https://doi.org/10.1001/jamainternmed.2017.0089

Chapter 19

HEALING THE GUT

*"The road to health is paved with
good intestines!"*

SHERRY A. ROGERS

We consider the firewall in our computer necessary to keep the system safe from infections and viruses, but now it is time to look at the firewall in our gut, which does a much more complex job.

We are not the first to latch on to the comparison between the firewall in our computer and the need for a strong mucosal barrier in the gastrointestinal system, protecting us against toxins and unfriendly pathogens. We do have a secondary firewall in the liver to capture the bacteria that have breached the initial barrier system. We may need to debug the system at times and build a better defence. The strength of our firewall or gut barrier not only protects our immunity, but also influences our quality of life.

In 2012, the US National Institute of Health initiated the groundbreaking Human Microbiome Project, aiming to comprehensively understand the diverse array of microbes residing within us. Our gut flora alone comprises over eight hundred known species, with countless more yet to be discovered, collectively weighing about 0.2kg. Beyond bacteria, our bodies harbor fungi, viruses, protists, archaea, and microscopic animals and plants, all crucial for maintaining optimal health. While there exists a shared core microbiome among individuals, each person possesses a unique microbial profile. Microbes are distributed throughout the body, with the gut hosting the largest population. While the microbiota of the large intestine remains relatively stable, the composition of the small intestine is influenced by various factors such as diet, genetics, and even prenatal development. Loss of microbial diversity can profoundly impact growth, development, and metabolism, affecting not only the gastrointestinal tract but also the immune, circulatory, endocrine, and central nervous systems.

FUNCTIONS OF YOUR MICROBIOME

- Absorbs nutrients.
- Encodes for the enzymes that break down indigestible fibre.
- Produces vitamins.
- Produces neurotransmitters.
- Helps to keep blood glucose and body weight under control.
- Processes foreign substances (e.g. drugs and carcinogens).
- Generates energy – up to 10% of our energy is via fermentation.
- Protects the gut wall barrier – beneficial bacteria crowd out the harmful bacteria.
- Helps the immune system – 80% of the immune system resides in the gut.
- Produces short-chain fatty acids that reduce inflammation.
- Regulates communication between the gut, brain and the rest of the body.

The gut is the body's 'second brain'. The two share many of the same chemical messengers (hormones and neurotransmitters) and form part of the one integrated, responsive system. What happens in the brain affects the gut and vice versa. A good example is migraines, which don't just stop at headaches – they can also cause vomiting. Chronic stress interferes with both brain and gut function. Gut bacteria play a crucial role in producing chemicals that communicate with the brain and influence mood, movement, and immunity. For instance:

· Propionic acid boosts serotonin release, affecting memory, learning, and mood.
· Spore-forming bacteria produce 5-hydroxy tryptophan (5-HT), a precursor to serotonin, soothing and elevating mood.
· Bifidobacterium genera create mood-stabilizing GABA and B vitamins.
· Lactobacillus genera influence memory, muscle contraction, and produce GABA and histamine.
· Bacillus strains produce dopamine, impacting motivation and movement, as well as noradrenaline.

Factors like antibiotics, stress, or poor diet, can affect brain function. Research into the gut-brain relationship, particularly in autism, highlights the significance of gut microbes in behaviour and cognition, with potential therapeutic implications. See Chapter 16)

GROWING THE MICROBIOME

Your unique collection of microbes starts with the bacteria you inherit from your mother during pregnancy. After birth, your diet and surroundings further shape this microbial profile.

A mother's nutrition and gut bacteria during pregnancy greatly influence her baby's microbiome. Babies born through vaginal delivery tend to have healthier microbial communities compared to those born via caesarean-section who initially pick up bacteria from the skin and hospital. Premature or low-weight babies often have less friendly bacteria and weaker immune systems. They have less acid in their stomachs, which leaves them more prone to infection, food allergies and sensitivities

Breastfeeding, avoiding unnecessary antibiotics and maintaining a clean environment are crucial for a newborn's microbial health. If antibiotics are necessary, it can take a few weeks for the microbial balance to return, and even longer for premature babies.

A Midwife's Tips for Caesarean Delivery

1. Use probiotics during pregnancy if possible.
2. Expose the newborn to the mother's vaginal and faecal bacteria by using a sterile piece of gauze soaked in normal saline. Fold the gauze like a tampon and insert into the mother's vagina and leave it there for one hour before caesarean surgery. Then put the gauze in a sterile glass container. Immediately after the birth, swab the baby's mouth, face and body with the gauze swab.
3. Breastfeed the baby.

Breastfeeding can help restore and build gut health because the breast milk contains nutrients that stimulate and improve microbial growth. Breast milk is said to contain more than seven hundred species of bacteria. *Bifidobacterium* and *Lactobacillus* are the main probiotic microorganisms present in the gut, creating an acidic environment that is rich in short-chain fatty acids. Thus, the ability to produce vitamins and digestive enzymes while stimulating the mucous secretions to protect the gut wall is enhanced. Formula-fed babies typically have lower levels of Bifidobacterium in their gut compared to breastfed infants.

Probiotics offer benefits for both mothers and children, potentially reducing the risk of gestational diabetes and preterm births. Lactating women can use Lactobacillus fermentum CECT5716 alongside antibiotics to manage mastitis. Introducing probiotics, especially those high in Bifidobacterium, can benefit preterm infants and those on formula.

As children transition to solid foods, their gut flora diversifies, resembling that of adults within two years. Interventions during this crucial period can help mitigate the risk of allergies, coeliac disease, diabetes, and obesity later in life.

WHEN YEAST TAKES OVER

The fungus *Candida albicans* belongs to a family of yeasts that is part of the normal microbial population in humans. But it can proliferate to a point where it can become harmful and uncommonly difficult to treat. Pregnancy, nutritional deficiencies, high-sugar diets, diabetes, low immunity, medications such as antibiotics and corticosteroids have all contributed to the rise in *Candida* infections.

Once considered a disease more of the elderly, it is relatively common in pregnancy and can be seen in very young babies born to a mother with candida vaginitis caused by *Candida albicans*. While Candida albicans prefers glucose as a nutrient source, it can indeed adapt to utilise fats and proteins when glucose is scarce. It can also alter the pH level of its environment to facilitate its growth. Candida albicans is commonly found in various locations in the body, including the blood, digestive tract, and vagina.

Three out of four women suffer vulvovaginal candidiasis (thrush in the vagina and vulva) in their lifetimes, and many are infected during pregnancy due to higher pro-gesterone levels and higher glycogen content in vaginal secretions. These infections can occur without the usual symptoms of vulval soreness, itchiness or discharge, so the expectant mother may be none the wiser. The take-home message is that *candida* infections are not simple and superficial fungal infections; they should be treated immediately on diagnosis, especially among pregnant women.

Are You at Risk of Yeast Infections?

· Have you taken a repeated course of antibiotics?
· Have you ever taken the pill?

· Do you suffer from vaginitis?
· Is there a history of yeast infections in the family?
· Do you have chronic skin conditions?
· Is zinc intake adequate? Zinc deficiency can be a driver of yeast infections.
· Have you been diagnosed with diabetes mellitus, pre-diabetes or gestational diabetes?
· Has recent chemotherapy lowered the number and efficacy of your white cells?
· Do you suffer from digestive complaints like pain, bloating and wind?
· Do you suffer from muscle aches or joint pains?

Fighting the Fungus

Treating Candida albicans infections typically involves antifungal medications, such as Fluconazole, itraconazole, or Voriconazole, which can be taken orally or administered intravenously depending on the severity of the infection and the individual's overall health condition. Topical antifungal creams or ointments may also be used for localised infections, such as those affecting the skin or mucous membranes.

1. Reduce the intake of refined carbohydrates, which promote Candida albicans
2. Increase probiotic-rich foods to support a balance of gut flora.
3. Check zinc and glucose levels. Add zinc 30mg a day if levels are low.
4. Add oat bran and other dietary fibres, ginger and garlic to the diet.
5. Avoid laxatives and antacids medications where possible.
6. Wear cotton underwear.
7. Herbs with oregano oil, ginger, grapefruit extract, turmeric, and ashwagandha are effective against candida.

SMALL INTESTINAL BACTERIAL OVERGROWTH (SIBO)

Bacteria are fewer in the small intestine due to stomach acid, bile, and food movement. However, when things go wrong, trouble starts.

The Causes of SIBO:

1. Low hydrochloric acid in the stomach and long-term use of antacid medications

2. Pancreatic enzyme deficiency.

3. Multiple courses of antibiotics which disrupt the small intestine microbiome.

4. Functional problems, such as adhesions that fail to move the contents through the digestive tract in a timely manner.

5. Chronic constipation, cause the bacteria to migrate from the colon into the small intestine.

The Symptoms: These resemble many other digestive complaints such as irritable bowel syndrome, inflammatory bowel disease or even coeliac disease, with symptoms of pain, bloating, fatigue, constipation or diarrhoea.

The Diagnosis: Diagnosis may be made with a hydrogen and methane breath test, but the more accepted test for SIBO is a culture of luminal contents of the small bowel. Coeliac and Crohn's diseases need to be ruled out. A GP might initiate a trial of antibiotics (rifaximin) and see if it works – which is the easier option. Imaging tests like

X-rays, CT scans, or MRI scans may be used to assess the structure and function of the digestive tract, although they are not typically used specifically to diagnose SIBO.

The Treatment: Antibiotics are used depending on the culture of the aspirants, supplement any nutritional deficiencies and, of course, add back probiotics – *Saccharomyces boulardii*, *Bifidobacterium lactis* or *Lactobacillus acidophilus*. Try the FODMAP diet (below). High-fibre foods are not helpful at the start and can make the symptoms of SIBO worse. Try not to have snacks in the day as this, too, can make the symptoms worse.

Check out a study from John Hopkins Hospital in Baltimore (USA) that found a mix of herbs works just as well as triple antibiotics. Researchers noted antibiotics can cause harmful side effects like colitis and diarrhea and can negatively affect the gut's bacteria. Plus, antibiotics are pricey in the USA, with a month's supply of rifaximin costing about $1200 compared to $120 for the herbs in 2014. The herb mix is interesting as it includes oil of oregano, berberine extracts, wormwood, lemon balm, red thyme, olive-leaf extract and horsetail plant aiming to fight a wide range of bugs from contaminated food.

THE 'LEAKY' PERMEABLE GUT

The gut lining acts as a protective shield between our digestive system and the rest of our body. It's made up of a thin layer of cells and a mucus layer that renews every few days, allowing nutrients to pass through while keeping harmful substances out.

Zonulin, a protein, helps keep these cell barriers strong. Our gut bacteria also help by making mucus and managing zonulin levels. But if this barrier gets weak, harmful toxins can slip through, causing issues like tummy troubles, skin problems, allergies, mood swings, and inflammation.

A weak gut barrier is often linked to conditions like irritable bowel syndrome (IBS), small intestinal bacterial overgrowth (SIBO), and inflammatory bowel diseases (IBD) such as Crohn's disease and ulcerative colitis. If you're not sure what's causing your symptoms, a stool test like the Calprotectin test can give helpful clues, helping tell the difference between inflammatory bowel disease (IBD) and irritable bowel syndrome (IBS).

TESTING FOR PATHOGENS, PARASITES AND INFLAMMATION

Most colonic and small bowel diseases are due to low-grade inflammation and will test positive for calprotectin. Calprotectin can predict and identify untreated inflammatory bowel disease (IBD). Values of 500 to 600 µg/mg would indicate inflammation. Drugs like Naproxen (NSAIDs) or alcohol can cause low-grade inflammation with calprotectin levels up to 300 µg/mg.

Crohn's disease may have lower activity levels because the small bowel bacterial load is far less than in the colon, with less intense inflammation. Other gut-related issues are not as damaging as Crohn's disease, and with time and patience these can be relieved.

IRRITABLE BOWEL SYNDROME (IBS)

Irritable bowel syndrome (IBS) is the most diagnosed gastrointestinal condition, affecting about 12% of people worldwide. A range of factors are at play here because of the gut-brain connection, e.g. the interactions between psychological, behavioural, and environmental factors.

There are various causes of IBS, and much of it has to do with inflammation, genetics, immunity, psychosocial factors and, of course, the diet, which can impact upon the speed with which food moves through the gut. About 30% of IBS cases are a result of viral, bacterial and parasitic infections which can leave persisting symptoms after the initial infection has resolved.

The Symptoms: The key symptoms of IBS include bloating, abdominal pain, and changes in bowel habits, often leading to either diarrhea or constipation due to carbohydrate fermentation. Pain may ease after a bowel movement, but you might still feel like your bowels aren't completely empty. Additionally, fermentation in the colon can produce methane, which slows down digestion and can result in constipation. These changes in bowel habits can cause discomfort, fatigue, and may even contribute to feelings of depression or anxiety.

Check for Causes: The conundrum for the doctor and the patient is that on abdominal examination there may just be a slight tenderness. Further testing will be required if there is anaemia, weight loss or a high temperature. Coeliac disease should be ruled out through blood tests and stool tests to cover a range of bacteria, along with screening for bowel and ovarian cancer. A hydrogen breath test can be used to check for carbohydrate malabsorption, but simply reducing fermentable sugars in the diet may be sufficient.

Here are practical things one can do to reduce the symptoms and heal the gut:

1. **Reduce fermentable carbohydrates.** Most people manage to cut these down for a short period of time. Called a FODMAP diet, this diet is low in the short-chain carbohydrates – oligo-, di- and monosaccharides and polyols – which cause the wind and pain problems.

2. **Check for food sensitivities** which may irritate the gut. Allergy tests are useful here, but you may also need to see whether there are additives like MSG or other chemicals irritating the gut. Lactose intolerance is relatively common as well and is part the FODMAP diet below.

3. **Antibiotics such as neomycin and rifaximin** are used to treat resistant irritable bowel syndrome, stopping bacteria from producing methane if there is bacterial

overgrowth. Not everything can be sorted with medications, and certainly a low FODMAP diet is helpful in reducing the symptoms.

4. **Iberogast** very useful for the nausea, bloating, pain and reflux with no prescription required. The dose for adults is 20 drops three times a day, half the dose for children under twelve years, and even babies under three months can take three drops where there is reflux and colic. Ginger tea may also help. Add probiotics like VSL#3 (Australia), Vivomixx (USA) and Visbiome (Europe), which are useful in treating IBS in the long term.

WHAT YOU NEED TO KNOW ABOUT FERMENTABLE CARBOHYDRATES

Most foods – apart from meat, fish and eggs – have a mix of these carbohydrates. And yes, there is an app for your phone for those who wish to go on the diet, which will help with the shopping. The Monash University FODMAP diet app works by swapping foods high in fermentable carbohydrates (FODMAPs), with low FODMAP alternatives.

The diet is not a long-term solution and its usefulness should be sorted in the quickest possible time because a side effect is a reduction of diversity of the gut microbes, including the healthy *Bifidobacterium*.

In the table attached we have the basics of the FODMAP diet. The diet is primarily used to manage symptoms of gastrointestinal disorders, particularly those associated with irritable bowel syndrome (IBS) and other functional gastrointestinal disorders. Foods with high fermentable carbohydrates are reduced to see if the symptoms reduce significantly. Not all types of the fermentable foods cause gut issues. We strongly recommend you see a dietitian first to guide you through the process of eliminating and then reintroducing various foods to test their effect on your symptoms. For example, if you're only lactose-intolerant, there is no necessity to cut foods with fructose.

Sources of Fermentable Carbohydrates

FERMENTABLE CARBOHYDRATES	SOURCES TO AVOID
Monosaccharides	Fructose (fruit sugar): Honey, fresh fruit (e.g. apples, mangos, pears, watermelons and peaches), dried fruits (e.g. prunes, figs, dates and raisins) and high-fructose corn syrup.
Disaccharides	Lactose (in dairy): Milk, ice cream, custard, dairy desserts, condensed and evaporated milk, milk powder, yoghurt. Minimal amounts in soft unripened cheeses (e.g. cottage and ricotta).
Oligosaccharides	Fructans: Wheat (white bread, pasta, pastries and cookies), rye, onions, artichokes, asparagus, beetroot and leeks. Galactans: Legume beans (e.g. baked beans and kidney beans), lentils, chickpeas, cabbage, and brussels sprouts.
Polyols (sugar alcohols)	Apples, apricots, avocados, cherries, lychees, nectarines, pears, plums, prunes, mushrooms, and the food additives sorbitol (420), mannitol (421), xylitol (967), maltitol (965) and isomalt (953).

For those who are interested in following the diet without professional help there are many sources for a low FODMAP diet on the interned in pdf format. Here are some tips that might help.

Working Out the Problem: You do need to keep a diary; it is just too hard to remember the symptoms (if any) during the elimination period and the outcome of the challenges when all is done.

1. Avoid the foods high in fermentable carbohydrates three weeks. The phone app will help with the shopping.
2. If the diet worked for you, you need to reintroduce the foods back again to see which of the fermentable carbohydrates gave a problem. There is no point on being on the complete FODMAP diet if only one or two of the foods cause a problem.

The Challenges: If you feel better on the diet and symptom-free, first bring back the foods that are high in fructose for three to four days to see whether there are problems.

1. If problems occur after just one or two days, don't continue to punish yourself.
2. Go back on the low FODMAP diet until you are again symptom free.
3. Add the lactose-containing foods into the diet for three days and see the effects.
4. Go back on the low FODMAP diet for a few days as the effects can be cumulative.
5. Add the fructans – wheat and onions. Often a problem!
6. Go back to the elimination diet, even if there is no effect.
7. Bring in the legumes. Beans are known to be windy foods for many.
8. Follow the protocols above, then add the foods with polyols – apples, etc.

When all the challenges for the fermentable carbohydrates are finished, have a look over your diary and see what has given you the most grief. Bring all the foods that had no negative consequences back into the diet and see if you remain symptom free. Challenge the problem foods again later and see whether the problem persists. The diet need not be permanent!

INFLAMMATORY BOWEL DISEASE

Inflammatory bowel disease (IBD) and irritable bowel syndrome (IBS) differ significantly in symptoms and severity. IBD symptoms include colicky abdominal pain, diarrhea, weight loss, and rectal bleeding, persisting for over four weeks and requiring early, accurate diagnosis. Endoscopy and imaging show inflammation, with ongoing risks of psychological issues and cancers.

The three main types of IBD are Crohn's disease (CD), ulcerative colitis (UC), and unclassified IBD (IBD-U), mostly diagnosed in adults but also in about 20% of children. It stems from an abnormal immune response to environmental triggers, with genetic and environmental factors at play.

Food and chemical sensitivities exclusion can be helpful, as diet triggers play a role, however **the management necessarily involves gastroenterology specialists, aiming to control inflammation with drugs and surgery for severe cases.** Malnutrition is common, so intravenous nutrient injections and oral supplements are recommended. Probiotics like Escherichia coli and Saccharomyces boulardii or VSL#3 may aid in treatment. The disease is stressful for the patient and supporting carers, and psychological support is often necessary.

HELICOBACTER PYLORI

Helicobacter pylori (H. pylori) infection can cause persistent symptoms like burping, pain, bloating, bleeding, and anemia. It's a major bacterial culprit behind chronic gastritis, ulcers, and even stomach cancer. Designated as a cancer-causing agent by the WHO, H. pylori is prevalent in lower socio-economic areas, infecting about half of the world's population. It spreads easily within families through oral or fecal routes, making reinfection common even after treatment.

Symptoms of H. pylori infection: They can vary or may not show at all, but commonly include stomach pains, worsened by an empty stomach, nausea, poor appetite, and gastrointestinal issues.

Diagnosis: To diagnose the infection, doctors may conduct blood, stool, urea breath tests, or endoscopy, often requiring medication cessation during testing.

Treatment protocols: These involve a combination of antacid medicines, antibiotics, and bismuth to protect the stomach lining, but prolonged antibiotic use may disrupt gut balance, leading to other issues like Candida albicans or Clostridium difficile infections. In addition to medication, dietary changes can aid in management. Reducing high sugar and salt intake, consuming brassica vegetables, berries, fish oil, and blackcurrant seed oil, and incorporating fermented foods and probiotics post-infection resolution can help support eradication efforts.

The earlier treatment protocols eradicating this infection were devised in conjunction with Barry Marshall, who won the Nobel Peace Prize for Medicine in 2005 (with Robin Warren). They discovered the bacterium *Helicobacter pylori* and its role in inflammation and peptic ulcer disease. The story caused a bit of media frenzy at the time because Marshall drank the bacterial broth to prove his point –debunking the theory at the time that gastric ulcers were caused by stress and spicy food.

PROTOCOLS FOR HEALING THE GUT

1. **Remove** offending toxins and irritating food.
2. **Replace** with healing foods and digestive support.
3. **Repair** with bitter herbs, foods, zinc, glutamine, vitamin D.
4. **Re-inoculate** to restore healthy balance of gut microflora.

1. **Remove Toxins or Irritating Chemicals and Foods**: Gluten and infection can affect the gut barrier and trigger the release toxins. Proton pump inhibitors (PPIs) block gastric acid secretion. The many functions of hydrochloric acid play an important role in protecting the gut:

- Cleanses the food generally.
- Stops unfriendly bacterial colonisation of the gut.
- Helps the breakdown of proteins into simple amino acids.
- Helps prevents allergies and autoimmunity from undigested proteins.
- Facilitates nutrient absorption including vitamin B12.
- The acidity stimulates alkaline secretions from the pancreas to further assist protein digestion and stimulates carbohydrate and fat digestion.

As we age, we naturally lose stomach acid, and taking drugs that reduce stomach acid can cause various problems including reduced vitamin B12, calcium and magnesium absorption. It's best not to use them all the time; only take one when symptoms arise. Newer drugs like Nexium and Pariet work quickly, which might make this approach easier. Antibiotics can also disrupt the balance of good and bad gut bacteria. Painkillers like aspirin and non-steroidal anti-inflammatory drug can cause stomach ulcers and bleeding. All of these issues have an impact on the gut barrier, with a loss of the epithelial cell mass and a weak barrier wall.

2. **Replace with Healing Foods for Digestive Support**: The good news is that the gut barrier can be treated, and its integrity restored. Slippery elm powder in water last thing at night can help coat and heal the gut lining without competing with other foods. Include fermented foods, ginger tea through the day, replace red meat with fatty fish; adding at least 30g of fibre per day is a good starting place.

3: **Repair the Damage**: Betaine hydrochloride, gentian root and apple cider vinegar all increase acidity of the stomach and if taken before meals will stimulate digestive juices to help absorption. During illness, the immune cells utilise large amounts of glutamine which exceeds the amount we can produce in the body. This is why gastro-enterologists often supplement glutamine after radiation and surgery.

Your body needs zinc to make hydrochloric acid, but you need hydrochloric acid to absorb zinc! A wide range of nutrients are required to repair the gut wall and should include the minerals selenium, chromium, manganese and magnesium, along with vitamins A, C, E, D, all the B vitamins. The Mediterranean diet is ideal for providing these nutrients.

4. Re-Inoculate and Defend: If gluten (for example) has been eliminated as a necessity, it is good to add *Lactobacillus* and *Bifidobacterium*, since both protect the epithelial cells from damage caused by gluten. *Saccharomyces boulardii* or *Lactobacillus rhamnosus GG* may help prevent diarrhoea when antibiotics are prescribed. *Saccharomyces boulardii* is also useful in *candida* infections. *Lactobacillus GG* and *L. casei* might be useful if you are thinking of travelling where food hygiene may be suspicious. Adding these 'prescriptive' probiotic supplements will increase the numbers substantially, rather than depending solely on yoghurts and fermented foods.

FAECAL TRANSPLANT – WHY DO IT?

Faecal transplants have a long history, dating back to the fourth century in China and gaining traction in the USA during the 1950s. Today, they're a highly effective treatment for various gastrointestinal issues, with success rates around 90%. Faecal transplants quickly introduce a rich community of beneficial microbes from a healthy donor to the colon.

Donors must be healthy and free of disease or recent antibiotic use. The procedure involves mixing faecal matter with salt water and transferring it to the colon, usually via colonoscopy.

Studies have shown promising results for conditions like ulcerative colitis. While results for irritable bowel syndrome are positive, caution is advised as it may not work for everyone. For Clostridium difficile-associated diarrhoea, faecal transplants are more effective than antibiotics. They also show potential for treating conditions like multiple sclerosis, autism, and obesity.

Although treating Crohn's disease with faecal transplants is challenging, some small studies suggest remission is possible, but more research is needed.

HEALING THE GUT

ACTION PLAN – CHECKLIST

- Check allergy load, gluten sensitivity, *Helicobacter pylori* and infections.
- Do a stool PCR test to identify any infections.
- Check calprotectin levels to discriminate between IBS and IBD.
- Remove allergens, toxins and fast foods from your diet.
- Avoid medicines that decrease hydrochloric acid in the stomach.
- Check for nutrient deficiencies, and supplement as necessary.
- Consider nutrient injections if gut absorption is poor and deficiency severe.
- Consider if fibre is appropriate, add fish oils, probiotics.
- Use the FODMAP diet if wind and bloating persist.
- Bitter herbs, slippery elm, zinc, glutamine and vitamin D can heal the gut and help the immune system.

References:

Grover, M. (2014). Role of gut pathogens in development of irritable bowel syndrome. The *Indian Journal of* Medical *Research*, *139*(1), 11–18.

Bjarnason, I. (2017). The Use of Fecal Calprotectin in Inflammatory Bowel Disease. *Gastroenterology & Hepatology*, *13*(1), 53–56.

Brüssow, H. (2019). Probiotics and prebiotics in clinical tests: an update. *F1000Research*, *8*, Article F1000 Faculty Rev-1157. https://doi.org/10.12688/f1000research.19043.1

Chedid, V., Dhalla, S., Clarke, J. O., Roland, B. C., Dunbar, K. B., Koh, J., & Mullin, G. E. (2014). Herbal therapy is equivalent to rifaximin for the treatment of small intestinal bacterial overgrowth. *Global Adv Health Med*, *3*(3), 16–24. https://doi.org/10.7453/gahmj.2014.019.

Cleminson, J., Austin, N., & McGuire, W. (2015). Prophylactic systemic antifungal agents to prevent mortality and morbidity in very low birth weight infants. *Cochrane Database of Systematic Reviews*, https://doi.org//10.1002/14651858.CD003850.pub5.

Gearry, R. B., Irving, P. M., Barrett, J. S., Nathan, D. M., Shepherd, S. J., & Gibson, P. R. (2009). Reduction of dietary poorly absorbed short-chain carbohydrates (FODMAPs) improves abdominal symptoms in patients with inflammatory bowel disease-a pilot study. *Journal of Crohn's & colitis*, *3*(1), 8–14. https://doi.org/10.1016/j.crohns.2008.09.004

Kang, DW., Adams, J.B., Gregory, A.C. *et al.* (2017*).* Microbiota Transfer Therapy alters gut ecosystem and improves gastrointestinal and autism symptoms: an open-label study. *Microbiome* 5, 10 (2017). https://doi.org/10.1186/s40168-016-0225-7.

Monash FODMAP Diet; (2024). The official FODMAO App; https://apps.apple.com/au/app/monash-fodmap-diet/id586149216

Borody, T. J., Brandt, L. J., & Paramsothy, S. (2014). Therapeutic faecal microbiota transplantation: current status and future developments. *Current opinion in gastroenterology*, *30*(1), 97–105. https://doi.org/10.1097/MOG.0000000000000027

Chapter 20

PROBIOTICS AND THEIR FRIENDS

"The secret of change is to focus all your energy, not on fighting the old, but on building the new."

SOCRATES

Probiotics are live microbes that normally reside in the digestive tract and are essential for good health and immunity. For many millennia, different cultures have used live bacterial strains, originally cultured from humans to ferment dairy, soy or vegetables into foods as varied as cottage cheese, buttermilk, miso, tempeh, natto, kimchi, sauerkraut and pickles. The strains in these foods mostly belong to two genera, *Lactobacillus* and *Bifidobacterium*, which already occur in the gastrointestinal or vaginal tracts.

PREBIOTICS – KEEPING YOUR MICROBES HAPPY

Different types of prebiotics share a common trait - they're all indigestible but essential for our gut microbes. Some dissolve easily, while others add bulk to stool. Though fermentation might cause discomfort, persistence benefits your gut health and keeps those essential epithelial cells happy. Western diets typically have about 23 gram of fibre per day, but ideally we should have at least 30 gram per day. Friendly bacteria produce short-chain fatty acids from these prebiotics, providing energy, up-lifting mood, reducing inflammation and help ward off diseases like obesity, diabetes, and certain cancers. Check out the table below for probiotics, prebiotics, and resistant starches.

PROBIOTICS	PREBIOTICS	RESISTANT STARCH
Yoghurt (dairy)*	Legumes	Haricot beans
Cottage cheese (dairy)*	Chicory root	Red kidney beans
Buttermilk (dairy)*	Onions	Split peas
Miso and tempeh (soy bean)	Garlic	Cornflakes
Natto and soy sauce	Leafy greens	Rye bread
Kombucha (tea)	Jerusalem artichokes	Oat cakes
Kimchi, sauerkraut	Flax	Brown wholemeal bread
Kefir (grain)	Oatmeal	
Pickles (vegetable)	Leeks	
Sourdough bread (wheat)	Asparagus	

*Pasturisation destroys probiotics in dairy foods. Fermentation with bacterial cultures are then added back.

WHY YOU NEED PROBIOTICS

The advantages of using probiotics relate to their positive effect strengthening the gut barrier while crowding out the bad bacteria. The brain is also supported as the bacteria produce mood enhancing neurotransmitters and vitamins. Microbial diversity in the gut protects against bowel disease and cancer and reduces the symptoms of irritable bowel syndrome.

Yoghurt, for example, is mostly made from homogenised milk, with lactic acid bacteria *Streptococcus thermophilus, Lactobacillus bulgaricus* and other probiotic (bio-yoghurt) cultures added to the fermentation process. For yoghurts to work as probiotics, they should have live active cultures in the order of one hundred million colony-forming units per gram. When buying yoghurts, be sure to look at the 'best before' date because the quality will diminish over time. Some sweetened yoghurts are more snack food than health food and have little or no probiotic benefit.

CHOOSING A PROBIOTIC

Different probiotics are used to treat different health conditions, depending on their bacterial strain. For example, *Lactobacillus acidophilus* has been shown to inhibit the growth of harmful bacteria such as Salmonella, Listeria and Yersinia. However, a combination of *Bifidobacteria* and *Lactobacillus* strains are used for irritable bowel syndrome and high doses of the probiotic VSL#3 (which includes a multitude of strains) are used for ulcerative colitis. Here are some of the well-known strains that support many general medical health conditions.

Probiotic Strains Supporting General Health

Immune support	*Lactobacillus acidophilus, Lactobacillus rhamnosus GG**
Allergy	*Escherichia coli, Bifidobacterium bifidum, Bifidobacterium lactis*
Premature babies and toddlers	*Bifidobacteria, Lactobacillus acidophilus, Lactobacillus casei, Bifidum longum*
Antibiotic-associated diarrhoea	*Bifidobacterium strains, Lactobacillus rhamnosus GG, Lactobacillus acidophilus, Lactobacillus brevis, Saccharomyces boulardii*
Irritable bowel syndrome	*Bifidobacterium animalis, Bifidobacterium infantis, Lactobacillus planatarium, VSL#3*, Saccharomyces boulardii*
Ulcerative colitis	*Bifidobacterium longum, Escherichia coli strain Nissle, Lactobacillus acidophilus, Streptococcus thermophilus*
Infantile colic	*Lactobacillus reuteri*
Vaginal candidiasis	*Lactobacillus rhamnosus GR-1, Lactobacillus reuteri RC-14*
Urinary tract infection	*Lactobacillus rhamnosus GR-1, Lactobacillus reuteri RC-14*

Traveller's diarrhoea	*Lactobacillus GG, Saccharomyces boulardii*
Diarrhoea caused by Clostridioides difficile	*Bifidobacterium animalis, Lactobacillus acidophilus, Saccharomyces boulardii, Streptococcus thermophilus*
Helicobacter pylori	*Bifidobacterium animalis, Lactobacillus acidophilus, Lactobacillus johnsonii, Streptococcus thermophilus, Saccharomyces boulardii*
Constipation	*Lactobacillus casei strain Shirota, Lactobacillus plantarum*
Crohn's disease	*Lactobacillus casei GG, Saccharomyces boulardii, VSL#3**
Ulcerative colitis	*Escherichia coli Nissle, Bifidobacterium, VSL#3*, Saccharomyces boulardii, Escherichia coli strain Nissle*
Pouchitis	*VSL#3*, Lactobacillus acidophius*
Urogenital infection	*Lactobacillus acidophilus, Saccharomyces boulardii*
Urogenital cancer	*Lactobacillus casei strain Shirota*
Cancer	*Lactobacillus paracasei, Lactobacillus plantarum, Lactobacillus rhamnosus GG,* *Bifidobacterium adolescentes*

Stress, anxiety and depression	*Lactobacillus acidophilus, Lactobacillus casei, Bifidobacterium bifidum, Bifidobacterium longum, Bifidobacterium infantis*
Neuromuscular	*Lactobacillus paracasei*
Tooth decay	*Lactobacillus rhamnosus GG, Bifidobacterium lactis*
Obesity	*Lactobacillus paracasei*
Eczema	*Bifidobacterium breve, Bifidobacterium infantis, Lactobacillus acidophilus, Lactobacillus casei*
Stress, Depression	*Lactobacillus helveticus R0052, Bifidobacterium longum*

*VSL#3 is a combination of *Bifidobacterium breve, Bifidobacterium longum, Bifidobacterium infantis, Lactobacillus acidophilus, Lactobacillus plantarum, Lactobacillus paracasei, Lactobacillus bulgaricus* and *Streptococcus thermophilus*.

TAKING A PROBIOTIC

Probiotic supplements are regulated in Australia as 'functional foods' by Food Standards Australia and New Zealand, and by the Therapeutic Goods Administration.

Criteria for a Probiotic

- The organism must be identified (genus, species and strain).
- It must be safe – not causing disease or carrying a gene for antibiotic resistance.
- It must survive transit in the intestines and tolerate bile acid.
- It must adhere to the mucosal surface and colonise the intestine (even briefly).
- It must have documented health effects –it must kill or inhibit microorganisms or disease-causing bacteria.

Length of Treatment

While probiotic foods may be eaten long-term, there's less consensus about how long you should be on a probiotic supplement. Normally, probiotic supplements are taken for six to eight weeks, with or after meals, but always follow the instructions on the bottle.

Dose

Prevention of antibiotic-associated diarrhoea in children – minimal dose ≥5 billion colony-forming units (CFU) per day.

The minimum effective dose for an adult to maintain gut health – 10 billion colony-forming units (CFU) per day.

Minor gut problems – 20 to 30 billion CFU. The concentration depends on the bacterial strain in the probiotic and how it's delivered.

The dose depends on the strain and the medium. If probiotics are given in milk (which many are), the number of colony-forming units needed to detect the strain in stool are reduced.

Side Effects

There are few side effects – mostly gas and bloating – which decrease over time.

It is a good idea to take the time to **check the label for the strain and the number of colony forming units (CFU)** cited. Yoghurts with *Lactobacillus acidophilus, Bifidobacterium* and *Lactobacillus casei* with over 300 million CFU per 100 g are readily available. *Lactobacillus casei* strain Shirota (LcS) is available in a 65 ml container (Yakult) with 6 billion CFU, which may help constipation. Stay away from yoghurts with added sugar and no mention of the added culture on the label.

PROBIOTICS AND THEIR FRIENDS

ACTION PLAN – CHECKLIST

- Consume fruit, vegetables and grains with high fibre content.
- Add fermented foods – e.g. yoghurt, sauerkraut, miso and sourdough bread.
- Buy yoghurts with the probiotic strains labelled.
- Use probiotics with not less than 20 billion colony-forming units after antibiotic therapy.

References:

Amara, A. A., & Shibl, A. (2015). Role of Probiotics in health improvement, infection control and disease treatment and management. *Saudi pharmaceutical journal : SPJ : the official publication of the Saudi Pharmaceutical Society*, 23(2), 107–114. https://doi.org/10.1016/j.jsps.2013.07.001

Czerucka, D., & Rampal, P. (2019). Diversity of *Saccharomyces boulardii* CNCM I-745 mechanisms of action against intestinal infections. *World Journal of Gastroenterology*, 25(18), 2188–2203. https://doi.org/10.3748/wjg.v25.i18.2188

Floch, M., Walker, W., Sanders, M., Nieuwdorp, M., Kim, A., Brenner, D., & Brandt, L. (2015). Recommendations for Probiotic Use – 2015 Update: Proceedings and Consensus Opinion. *Journal of Clinical Gastroenterology*, 49(1), S69–S73.

Górska, A., Przystupski, D., Niemczura, M. J., & Kulbacka, J. (2019). Probiotic Bacteria: A Promising Tool in Cancer Prevention and Therapy. *Current Microbiology*, 76(8), 939–949. https://doi.org/10.1007/s00284- 019-01679-8

Oranusi, S., Adedeji, O. M., & Olopade, B. K. (2014). Probiotics in the Management of Diseases: A Review. *International Journal of Current Research and Academic Review*, 2(8), 138–158.

Wallace, C., & Milev, R. (2017). The effects of probiotics on depressive symptoms in humans: a systematic review. *Annals of General Psychiatry*, 16, 14. https://doi.org/10.1186/s12991-017-0138-2

Chapter 21

DIABETES

"To lengthen life, lessen thy meals."

ROBERT FRANKLIN

Diabetes is the end result of chronically high blood sugars. Millions of people have been diagnosed with diabetes but there are millions more who have the disease and are yet to be diagnosed. The consequences of a high sugar diet and a sedentary lifestyle will often deliver a cruel fate if not addressed early.

Diabetes dramatically increases the risk of other major health problems, with almost two-thirds of people with diabetes going on to die of heart disease. Those with diabetes are also far more likely than others to go blind, suffer a stroke, kidney failure or limb amputation, be diagnosed with depression and anxiety, or suffer worse outcomes from an acute viral illness.

Insulin resistance precedes type 2 diabetes. It occurs early on in the piece when muscle, fat and liver cells don't take up glucose from the blood as they should. The pancreas then makes more insulin to help overcome the rising blood glucose levels.

TYPES 1, 2 AND YOU

Type 1 diabetes is an autoimmune disease: This is a disease where the pancreas is unable to produce insulin. Without insulin, the body is unable to take the blood glucose into the cells to use as energy. There is no cure, and the person must take insulin for a lifetime. There is no known cause of type 1 diabetes but there is a genetic link in some families, and it may occur after a viral infection. This type of diabetes usually has its onset in childhood.

Type 2 diabetes is usually a progressive condition: The body loses its sensitivity to insulin or doesn't produce enough insulin to reduce the glucose in the blood to a safe level. Over time, excessive glucose in the blood causes damage to many organs. Around 3% of people with diabetes will develop a foot ulcer, from this group around 25% will require an amputation, other risks are stroke, heart attacks, kidney disease and blindness.

Gestational diabetes occurs in pregnancy. It occurs typically between twenty-four and twenty-eight-weeks' gestation, and generally disappears after the baby is born. It occurs due to hormonal changes and the increasing need for insulin as the foetus grows. Normally the condition can be managed by diet and exercise, but sometimes injections of insulin are required. There is also an increased risk of developing type 2 diabetes some 10-20 years later.

Too much insulin can prevent your body from burning fat. If you keep eating lots of sugary foods over time, your body can become less sensitive to insulin, and your blood sugar levels may stay high. This can lead to serious health issues like obesity, diabetes, heart disease, and cancer. Over time, your pancreas may produce less insulin, making it harder for your body to control blood sugar levels. When this happens, you might experience weight gain, belly fat, inflammation, fatigue, dizziness, headaches, and strong cravings for sugar.

The Symptoms of Diabetes

Symptoms of Type 1 Diabetes	Symptoms of Type 2 Diabetes
	Frequent urination
Excessive urination	Extreme thirst
Loss of appetite	Increased hunger
Constant thirst	Nerve pain or numbness
Weight loss	Slow wound healing
Nausea and vomiting	Poor vision
Tiredness	Dark skin patches
Blurred vision	Feeling tired and lethargic
Tingling lips	Itching groin, genitals
Itchy skin around genitals	Skin infections
Regular infections of thrush	Gradual weight gain
Slow wound healing	Mood swings
Drowsiness	Headaches
Altered consciousness	Feeling dizzy
	Leg cramps

METABOLIC SYNDROME

Metabolic Syndrome is the medical term for a complex health problems characterised by abnormal blood fats, abdominal obesity, and elevated blood glucose. This syndrome is the result of inflammation over many years of insulin resistance. Such an outcome needs to be avoided but is more likely if there is a family history of heart disease and diabetes. Adherence to a healthy diet and healthy weight, no smoking and checking along the way for heart disease and high blood pressure (see Chapter 22) will reduce the risk factors enormously.

MANAGING DIABETES

Treatment for Type 1 Diabetes	Treatment for Type 2 Diabetes	Treatment for Gestational Diabetes
Insulin injections. Monitor blood sugar. Maintain levels between 4.0 and 7.8 mmol/L. Mediterranean-style diet. Take probiotics. Exercise and control weight. Do not smoke. Control stress. Manage infection early. Check urine for protein every six months.	Maintain a healthy weight. Exercise daily. Eat a Mediterranean diet. Add probiotics. Avoid artificial sweeteners. Do not smoke. Treat wounds early. Check urine and kidneys every six months.	Eat a Mediterranean diet. Exercise daily. Measure blood glucose levels regularly. Take probiotics. Keep weight within the normal parameters for pregnancy.

CAN YOU REVERSE TYPE 2 DIABETES?

Yes, possibly. In the past we took for granted that once you have type 2 diabetes you have it for life. This may not be the case. In a small UK study (Steven et al., 2016) of just thirty people, those on a very low-calorie diet (600–700 calories per day) were able to lower their fasting blood glucose within days after their liver fat decreased. Those that did not have this initial rapid weight loss were barred from the continuing the study.

After about eight weeks on the diet, the participants not only produced more insulin, but their sensitivity to insulin improved. Thirteen of the group saw their blood glucose levels return to normal non-diabetic levels. The remission continued for the next six months, even after they switched from the strict diet to a normal, healthy but weight-controlled diet.

Obviously, everyone worked really hard on the program, and they lost around 14 kg along the way. But not everyone had remission. Those with the better results were younger and had a diagnosis of diabetes for less than four years compared to ten years for those who failed to gain remission.

DRUGS FOR MANAGING DIABETES

These are common methods for managing blood sugar levels in diabetes care. Insulin injections and pumps deliver insulin directly into the body to regulate blood sugar, while oral medications can help control blood sugar levels in different ways.

1. **Insulin Pumps**: These are small devices worn outside the body that deliver insulin in bursts through a small needle inserted under the skin. They provide a more continuous and adjustable way to administer insulin compared to injections.
2. **Types of Insulin**: Insulin comes in various types, including long-acting and short-acting. Long-acting insulin helps control blood sugar levels between meals and overnight, while short-acting insulin is used to manage blood sugar levels at mealtime. There are also combinations of these insulins available.
3. **Ultra-Fast Acting Insulin and Insulin Pumps**: These are typically not used in insulin pumps due to the technology's limitations. Insulin pumps primarily use rapid-acting or short-acting insulin.

4. **Sotagliflozin (Zynquista):** Sotagliflozin is a dual SGLT1 and SGLT2 inhibitor that was approved for the treatment of type 1 diabetes in certain populations. It works by blocking the absorption of glucose in the intestines and promoting glucose excretion in the urine, thereby lowering blood sugar levels.

5. **Insulin Glargine/lixisenatide (Soliqua):** This is a combination of insulin glargine (a long-acting insulin) and lixisenatide (a GLP-1 receptor agonist) that was approved for the treatment of type 2 diabetes. It provides both basal insulin coverage and postprandial glucose control in a single injection.

6. **Insulin Degludec/liraglutide (Xultophy):** Similar to Soliqua, Xultophy is a combination product containing insulin degludec (a long-acting insulin) and liraglutide (a GLP-1 receptor agonist) for the treatment of type 2 diabetes.

7. **Ertugliflozin (Steglatro):** Ertugliflozin is an SGLT2 inhibitor that was approved for the treatment of type 2 diabetes. It works by inhibiting glucose reabsorption in the kidneys, leading to increased glucose excretion in the urine and improved blood sugar control.

New Drugs on the Market for Diabetes and Weight Loss

Semaglutide (Ozempic, Rybelsus): Semaglutide works by mimicking the action of a hormone called glucagon-like peptide-1 (GLP-1). It regulates appetite and food intake by slowing down gastric emptying, promoting feelings of fullness and reducing food cravings. It is administered as a weekly injection and has been shown to lead to significant weight loss in people with obesity or overweight. It was initially designed to treat type 2 diabetes but has gained approval for weight management under the brand name Wegovy.

Mounjaro/ Zebound is the brand name for a different drug called tirzepatide. The drugs work in similar ways to reduce appetite, but there are some differences. Mounjaro activates two receptors at the same time. That's why it's called a "dual-agonist" glucagon-like peptide-1 (GLP-1) and glucose-dependent insulinotropic polypeptide (GIP). Mounjaro is administered weekly by injection.

Blood Sugar Management and Lifestyle: While insulin therapy and medications can help manage blood sugar levels, it's important to remember that diet and physical activity remain essential components of diabetes management. Balancing medication with healthy lifestyle choices is key to effective diabetes care and blood sugar control.

THE HIGHS AND LOWS OF DIABETES

There are common complications from the blood-sugar highs and lows when managing diabetes:

Somogyi Effect: When a low overnight blood sugar is followed by a high morning blood sugar level. The cause may be due to missed meals or ill timed insulin injection prompting stress hormones to raise sugar levels again by morning.

Dawn Phenomenon: Morning blood sugar levels rise due to hormones that trigger the release of glucose from the liver.

Yeast Infections: Thrive in high sugar environments, common in diabetes. Antifungals, low-sugar diets, and probiotics aid treatment.

Nerve and Blood Vessel Damage: Chronic high sugars damage nerves and vessels, leading to organ complications.

Foot Ulcerations: Reduced blood flow and sensation due to high sugars, leading to foot wounds. Proper shoes, supplements, and treatments are crucial.

Pain: Nerve damage causes sensations like burning or tingling, managed with supplements like fish oil and B vitamins. Ideally, one can add zinc, glutamine and arginine to support wound healing. Hyperbaric oxygen delivered in a pressurised environment is very helpful in diabetic feet. Exercise also increases blood flow.

Constipation: Nerve damage can affect digestion, leading to constipation. Hydration and high-fiber foods help.

Bladder Symptoms and Sexual Function: Nerve damage may cause bladder and sexual function issues, including incontinence and erectile dysfunction, especially in older men with diabetes. Erectile dysfunction (discussed in detail in Chapter 17) occurs in four out of five men over the age of fifty who have diabetes.

Infections and stress raise blood sugar, which can be difficult to control. Antifungal medicines along with low-sugar and low-carbohydrate diets with high-dose probiotic supplements are the mainstays of yeast control. Chapters 19 and 20 deal with the gut and probiotics.

HYPOGLYCAEMIA

Hypoglycemia occurs when blood sugar drops below 4.0 mmol/L, often due to not eating enough carbohydrates or increased exercise. Problems can arise diabetes medication is excessive or timed poorly. Symptoms include nervousness, weakness, brain fog, shaking, and sweating.

Managing Hypoglycaemia

1. Check your blood sugar if possible.
2. Consume fast-acting carbs like jellybeans or fruit juice (about 15g).
3. Check sugar levels again; if still low, have more carbs.
4. Adjust insulin if needed.
5. Taking 500 mg of vitamin C twice daily might help manage blood sugar spikes in type 2 diabetes.

REACTIVE HYPOGLYCAEMIA

The brain represents 2–3% of our body weight but uses 20% of the sugar from our blood. If the brain is starved of sugar even for short periods it may respond poorly, with the possibilities of lower cognition, depression, irritability, weakness, headaches and fatigue. A sugar-rich meal with simple carbohydrates such as soft drinks gives you a quick 'high' as blood sugars rise. In response, insulin levels can spike telling the cells to absorb the circulating sugar (glucose) from the blood. Glucose levels may then fall sharply, leaving you feeling tired, weak, irritable and muddle-headed.

If you notice signs of low blood sugar, like shakiness or dizziness, it's smart to consult with your doctor. They can help rule out diabetes. To keep blood sugar steady, try eating balanced meals with whole grains and protein-packed foods such as eggs or yogurt. And don't forget the good fats like avocado! Consider trying the Mediterranean diet mentioned in Chapter 30.

NOT ALL CARBS ARE CREATED EQUAL

Carbohydrates are the sugars and starches that break down into glucose as fuel for the body. They are found in fruits, grains (such as pasta, rice and bread), vegetables (e.g. potato and corn) and dairy products.

Simple carbohydrates are made up of just one or two molecules. Single-molecule carbohydrates such as glucose and fructose can break down in the body in three to five minutes, while two-molecule carbohydrates such as sucrose in table sugar and lactose in milk take about twelve to fifteen minutes.

Complex carbohydrates have the advantage of being large molecules containing three or more glucose molecules, as well as fibre. Examples are beans, legumes, oats and corn. They break down gradually over three to four hours. They maintain a steady flow of energy to the cells, avoiding the sugar or insulin spikes and hypoglycaemia.

NATURAL WAYS TO IMPROVE BLOOD GLUCOSE CONTROL

Diet: Focus on whole foods, nuts and seeds, virgin-pressed olive oil and fish.

Exercise is the very best way to control blood sugar levels and keep fit.

Maintain a healthy weight.

Stress management should be addressed where this is an issue.

Support the immune system; infection can drive up blood glucose levels.

Focus on specific nutrients that may help you smooth out your blood-sugar highs and lows.

Nutrient	Action	Source
Fish oils	Reduce inflammation, for prevention of heart disease and associated risk of diabetes.	Best source: fresh fish, especially mullet, salmon, tailor, mackerel.
Probiotics	*Lactobacillus acidophilus and Bifidobacterium bifidum* reduce diabetic markers.	Fermented dairy or high-potency probiotics.
Cinnamon	Cinnamon helps lower blood sugar levels.	Half a teaspoon is the usual dose.
Vitamin C	Vitamin C improves immunity, glucose tolerance and guards against infections.	Sources: green vegetables, berries and citrus. Amount: 1 g/day.
Chromium	Helps insulin work better, improves blood-sugar control and weight loss.	Sources: broccoli and red wine. Amount: 250 mcg chromium /day.

Zinc	Improves immunity and can reduce risk of diabetes complications.	Source: meat and oysters. Amount: 20 mg/day.
Carnitine	Carnitine assists fat metabolism and improves insulin sensitivity.	Sources: steak, chicken, dairy. Amount: 2 g/day
Coenzyme Q_{10}	An antioxidant, important for energy metabolism. Beneficial in insulin sensitivity.	Source: meats, sardines, peanuts. Amount: 150 mg/day.

DIABETES

ACTION PLAN – CHECKLIST

- Check blood glucose levels regularly if your diagnosed is diabetes.
- Check levels of zinc, vitamin D and B12.
- Focus on whole foods with a Mediterranean diet.
- Exercise to control blood sugar levels daily.
- Manage stress.
- Don't smoke.
- Treat yeast infection early.

References:

Forouhi, N. G., Misra, A., Mohan, V., Taylor, R., & Yancy, W. (2018). Dietary and nutritional approaches for prevention and management of type 2 diabetes. *The BMJ, 361*, Article k2234.

Steven, S., Hollingsworth, K. G., Al-Mrabeh, A., Avery, L., Aribisala, B., Caslake, M., & Taylor, R. (2016). Very Low-Calorie Diet and 6 Months of Weight Stability in Type 2 Diabetes: Pathophysiological Changes in Responders and Nonresponders. *Diabetes Care, 39*, 808–815. https://doi.org/10.2337/dc18-er06.

Chapter 22

HEART DISEASE

"Nothing is impossible to a willing heart."

JOHN HEYWOOD

Despite the remarkable advancements in modern medicine, cardiovascular disease still holds the unfortunate title of being the world's leading cause of death. Heart disease and stroke, arising from issues within our cardiovascular system, pose significant challenges to our health. Many of these fatalities can be prevented through simple lifestyle changes like staying active, eating well, and steering clear of smoking.

Yet, navigating the realm of heart health isn't easy. Now, while the solutions might seem as simple, the journey of managing heart issues is a rollercoaster, with drug companies and food giants throwing in their two cents. We're here to remind you that heart health isn't just about cholesterol and blood pressure – there's much more to the story!

HOW HEART DISEASE CUTS OFF YOUR LIFE BLOOD

Heart disease, primarily coronary artery disease, develops when plaque builds up in blood vessels, restricting blood and oxygen flow to the heart. This can lead to angina or, if severe, a heart attack. If a blockage occurs in blood vessels to the brain, a stroke can result. While our focus is on heart disease, the advice provided here can also reduce the risk of stroke.

F.A.S.T is Key for Stroke

F – **Face:** Ask the person to smile. Does one side of the face droop?
A – **Arms:** Ask the person to raise both arms. Does one arm drift downward?
S – **Speech:** Ask the person to repeat a phrase. Is the speech slurred or strange?
T – **Time:** If you see any of these signs, call 000 right away.

RISK FACTORS FOR HEART DISEASE

1. Family history – genetics.
2. High blood pressure.
3. High cholesterol.
4. Diabetes and prediabetes.
5. Excess weight.
6. Poor diet – trans fats and high carbohydrate.
7. Age fifty-five and over.
8. High homocysteine levels.
9. Systemic lupus erythematosus (lupus).

10. Respiratory viral or bacterial infection.

11. Low levels of vitamin K2?

Still worried? Seek a simple, non-invasive, computerised tomography (CT) scan which takes about 30 minutes. This is called a **Coronary Artery Calcium Score**. It is a great predictive test for heart complications. It checks the current calcium build-up as an indicator of plaque in your coronary arteries. The cost is moderate at about $200.

Coronary Artery Calcium Score	Calcification Grade = Risk of Coronary Event
0	Nil
0-10	Minimum
11-100	Mild
101-400	Moderate
>400	High Risk

The coronary calcium score is a valuable tool for assessing heart attack risk. A score of 0 indicates less than 1% risk of cardiovascular events over the next ten years, while a score over 400 suggests a 20% risk. A score over 100 may prompt further evaluation, especially in older individuals. Even a score of 90 in a thirty-year-old warrants attention.

The score helps identify coronary artery disease, guiding further tests like ECG stress tests or angiograms to pinpoint the site and the extent of nay blockages. For high-risk cases, angiograms can locate blockages, aiding decisions on treatments like stents or surgeries to improve blood flow. Great modern medicine!

The angiogram is a very useful test if there are high risk factors. The angiogram can locate the blockage and is helpful if you have chest pain and restricted blood flow to the heart. However, other tests and historical evidence come into play when a cardiologist offers a recommendation on a stent, or indeed on the need for more complex procedures to surgically enhance coronary artery blood flow.

THINGS YOU CAN AND CANNOT CHANGE

Age, sex, and genetics play a significant role in heart disease risk. While you can't change your age or family history, understanding their impact can help you mitigate other risk factors. If you're over fifty-five, your risk of heart disease rises. Genetic factors affecting around 30% of heart disease cases may include malfunctioning genes leading to cholesterol build-up in arteries, visible sometimes as yellowish deposits on the eyelids. While women have lower heart disease risk due to oestrogen during reproductive years, it becomes a major threat later on for both genders.

Avoiding smoking is crucial as it doubles heart disease risk, especially with high blood pressure or cholesterol. Quitting also reduces risks of cancer and other diseases.

Regular exercise lowers heart disease risk by boosting 'good' cholesterol. Managing stress is also vital as chronic stress significantly increases heart disease and stroke risks.

Consider adding Vitamin K2 to your routine. Vitamin K2 controls how calcium is used and stored in the body. One function is to stop the hardening of the walls of the arteries and blood vessels with calcium. Vitamin K2, is primarily produced by bacteria; good sources are nattō, a fermented soybean dish, along with liver, eggs, and dairy products like hard cheeses.

Check homocysteine levels: High levels of homocysteine, an amino acid, pose risks for stroke and heart disease by hardening blood vessel walls and increasing blood pressure and inflammation. Genetics and certain medical conditions contribute to elevated levels, but factors like drugs, smoking, and nutritional deficiencies can also play a role. The metabolic pathway for homocysteine involves B vitamins like folic acid, vitamins B6 and B12. Deficiencies in these vitamins can lead to increased homocysteine levels. Supplementing with B vitamins and betaine can help lower homocysteine levels, reducing the risk of cardiovascular issues.

Managing High Homocysteine

Supplement mg/day	Diet
B6: 2-50mg/day B12: 0.02-1mg/day Folic Acid: 0.5-5mg/day	Wholegrains Green leafy vegetables Oranges Beans
Betaine (from beet) 750mg twice/day	

DIET TO PREVENT HEART DISEASE?

1. **Preventing heart disease starts with avoiding junk foods** loaded with added sugars, especially fructose, which can raise blood pressure, obesity and diabetes risks. Trans fats found in baked goods and some margarines are not for you as they raise both bad cholesterol and triglycerides. Opt for whole foods like colorful vegetables, garlic, ginger, turmeric, beetroot, and mushrooms, as well as unrefined grains, avocado, nuts, and seeds to support heart health.
2. **Incorporate foods rich in vitamin K2,** like nattō and certain cheeses (Gouda, Edam, Jarlsberg), eggs and liver.

3. **Maintain a healthy weight**, focusing on waist measurement, get adequate vitamin D from sunlight.
4. **Consider supplementing** with CoQ10, especially if taking statin drugs, to mitigate potential side effects.
5. **Include fish** for omega-3 fats, limit red meat consumption, and watch salt intake, avoiding processed foods high in sodium. Here we will see the percentage omega 3 fat content in Australian seafood: *Source:* Sahar et al. (2008). *Asia Pacific Journal of Clinical Nutrition*, 17(3), 385–390

Fish	Omega-3 mg/100g
Southern Bluefin Tuna	230
Coral Trout	270
Barramundi	276
Northern Whiting	302
John Dory	315
Deep Sea Cod (Ribaldo)	340
Snapper (Bight Redfish)	357
Prawn (shrimp)	373
Australian Salmon	476
Ocean Trout	921
Atlantic Salmon	2252
Swordfish	2571

Address other health issues that can increase heart disease risk: People with **diabetes** are up to four times more likely to experience heart attacks and strokes. Systemic **lupus erythematosus (lupus)** is a is chronic inflammatory condition accelerates plaque buildup in arteries, tripling the risk of cardiac events. **Chest infections, viruses,**

and **streptococcus pneumoniae** can trigger heart attacks and strokes, especially in individuals with existing heart disease or diabetes.

While **cholesterol** levels remain controversial, individuals with existing heart conditions may need to lower cholesterol. Genetic screening tests, supported by Medicare, can help diagnose genetic predispositions to high cholesterol, though costs can be around $1200. However, it is worth having a look at the cholesterol controversy to see, in perspective, the current issues in this area of medicine.

THE CHOLESTEROL CONTROVERSY

Times have changed and we now know that not all fats are villains, and not all sugars are good. Plus, low-cholesterol diets might not be the life-savers we thought they were. Cholesterol is actually vital for our health, playing a role in making the essential hormones, oestrogen, testosterone, and more. Plus, it helps digest fats and absorb important vitamins A, D, E and K.

Lipoproteins: High density (HDL) is the better than low density (LDL) while cruising through your arteries keeping them clear. LDL can team up with fat and calcium, leading to plaque buildup. Then there's the triglycerides, born from excess carbs (especially fructose) and causing problems as they get stored as fat. So, here's the plan: lower LDL, boost HDL, and keep those triglycerides in check.

You Want More	You Want Less	You Want Less	Why Numbers Count
High-Density Lipoproteins (HDL)	Low-density Lipoproteins (LDL)	Triglycerides	Cholesterol Measures
High-density lipoproteins carry cholesterol from your tissues to your liver, reducing fatty build-up in your arteries.	Low-density lipoproteins carry cholesterol from your liver to your tissues, contributing to build-up in your arteries.	If you consume more calories than you need, the excess is stored in triglycerides in fat cells until the body needs it.	Total cholesterol measures high-density (HDL) and low-density (LDL) lipids in your blood. By dividing your total cholesterol by the HDL will give the risk (ratio). A ratio below 3.5:1 is good.

CHOLESTEROL DRUGS & 'STATINS' – WHY THE FUSS?

Statin drugs have been a hot topic in the medical world, stirring up quite the controversy. The US National Cholesterol Education Program had a big say in who should be popping these pills for heart health. But it turns out, those that made these recommendations had a vested interest in the drug game.

In the UK, doctors weren't having it anymore. They were fed up with so-called 'experts' pushing statins left and right. Then, in 2020, BMJ Evidence Based Medicine took a deep dive into the cholesterol saga. What they found? A messy system of drug regulation with no clear oversight.

Statins are known for their side effects: think diabetes, muscle pain, memory fog, and more. Despite reports of people feeling off, these issues often flew under the radar because pharmaceutical companies were promoting their own research. Do statins even add years to your life? Not really. Kristensen (2015) and colleagues calculated the average length of time they postponed death was by a median of 3–4 days.

Another study by Ravnskov (2016) and colleagues found that seniors with high cholesterol might actually outlive their low-cholesterol counterparts. So, here we now are, Australian guidelines recommend that you take statins only if you are at higher risk of a cardiac event or have already had an event. Seems fair.

THE DIET DILEMMA

Remember the saga of cholesterol and eggs! The poor egg was kicked to the curb for years, all because of their cholesterol content. We swapped butter for margarine, chased low-fat everything, without any health improvement.

Then, in 2015, the US Dietary Guidelines gave eggs a redemption arc. Suddenly, we learned that a dozen eggs a week won't send our cholesterol levels soaring. It was like the comeback story of the century for the poor old egg famer!

All that said, atherosclerosis is a chronic inflammatory condition causing deposits of cholesterol (and fibrous tissues) inside the arteries, narrowing the lumen. Cholesterol oxidation products (COPs) are partially responsible for triggering atherosclerosis and other conditions through inflammation. Oxidation products occur through heating/ cooking, dehydration, and irradiation but even more so when foods are subsequently reheated. Any fatty food cooked on a high heat is a source of future inflammation. So, while our bogeyman for heart disease is now sugar/fructose because it builds up fat stores and stiffens the blood vessels, we are not free to consume deep fried foods or 'trans' fats without paying some price in the future.

And don't even get us started on carbohydrates! A study published in JAMA Internal Medicine in 2014 found a direct correlation between higher sugar consumption and an increased risk of dying from heart disease. Fast forward to 2017, and Harvard's 2019 revelation about sugar-sweetened beverages further shook up the nutrition, medical, and food industries. Suddenly, low-fat, high-sugar products were thrown off the grocery shelves. The study revealed that the more sugar-sweetened beverages people consumed, the greater their risk of premature death from cardiovascular disease, and to a lesser extent from cancer.

THE TRUTH OF THE MATTER

We might take you back just a few years to 2016, when the news broke with damning evidence of monetary exchange between the sugar industry and some of the major universities, including MIT, Harvard and Yale. Money was paid to cast doubt on the role of sugar and point the finger at fat. Cristin Kearns, unearthed secrets from dusty old boxes at Colorado State University. The Sugar Association was playing defense, dead set on keeping sugar in our diets. The sugar industry's playbook reads like a page-turner from the tobacco days. They knew their sweet stuff was causing trouble, yet they peddled it anyway.

But the tides are turning. Slowly but surely, people are waking up to the sugar shenanigans. There's finally some recognition that maybe, just maybe, the sugar industry shouldn't have a stranglehold on dental research and health policies. It's like a revolution! But we still have some health problems to sort through.

HIGH BLOOD AND THE NEW 'NORMAL'

High Blood Pressure can signal trouble. If your heart is pushing your blood around your body with too much force, it can make your arteries less flexible or more prone to rupture. Believe it or not, some research now suggests high blood pressure may be linked to lack of diversity of gut bacteria and inflammation. Which is all very likely, but there are many causes of high blood pressure, including age, obesity, high salt/low potassium diet and chronic medical conditions.

When it comes to reading blood pressure monitor, the top number (systolic) measures the blood flow as your heart squeezes, while the bottom one (diastolic) tracks the pressure when the heart muscle relaxes. Doctors used to debate which number mattered most, but it seems the insurance industry had it pegged right with their focus on the top number.

Guidelines evolve like everything else; the Royal Australian College of General Practitioners has its finger on the pulse, recommending medication only if your blood pressure hits 140/90 mm Hg and you've got a moderate risk of heart issues.

LOWERING BLOOD PRESSURE – JUST ADD A DASH

Potassium, an electrolyte, partners with sodium to regulate fluid balance and blood volume. It's crucial for nerve impulses, blood pressure regulation, and muscle function including the heart. Potassium can help counter cardiovascular issues like high blood pressure and stroke, balancing out sodium's effects. Where sodium in the diet can raise blood pressure, potassium can bring it down and can help your kidney function along the way.

Now, how much should you aim for? Well, that depends on factors like your lifestyle, where you live, and how much salt you add. Firstly, try the Mediterranean diet with whole foods, high in minerals and fibre with no *added* salt. To that you can add a dash of about 3 grams of potassium a day.

NITRIC OXIDE

In 1998, three brilliant US scientists won the Nobel Prize for uncovering the wonders of nitric oxide. It's not your typical drug, vitamin or mineral – it's a gas. The gas sends messages to your nervous system, opens up blood vessels, and even helps fight infections. Nitric oxide is made in the lining of your arteries, keeping blood pressure in check and preventing clots. It is not stored, but simply diffuses to receptors in nearby cells and has a half-life of about one millisecond, so we need to make it constantly.

Here is where it gets interesting: nitrites and nitrates. They have some chemical differences. Your mouth bacteria work on nitrate-rich foods like beetroot and kale, turning them into nitrite. Then, when it hits the stomach's acidic environment nitrite reacts and generates nitric oxide gas.

Certain things such as antibiotics kill oral bacteria, and in doing so they inhibit the nitric oxide production. So too, if the stomach acid is depressed and not acidic, you can't generate nitric oxide. So, how do we keep our nitric oxide levels up?

- · Avoid mouthwashes .
- · Eat nitrite/nitrate-rich veggies like beetroot and spinach.
- · Consume bitter foods like lemons, kale and radishes to increase stomach acidity.
- · Consider adding L-citrulline supplements (found in foods like watermelon). The body converts it into another amino acid called L-arginine - which just happens to be the building block for nitric oxide production.

LOW BLOOD PRESSURE

Of course, blood pressure does not go in just one direction. Low blood pressure occurs when the systolic blood pressure is <90 mm Hg and the diastolic <60 mm

Hg. The symptoms are dizziness, tiredness and poor concentration. If it falls too far confusion can set in, along with clammy skin and rapid or shallow breathing.

Causes of Low and High Blood Pressure

What Will Push It Up?	What Will Help Lower It?	Drugs to Lower Blood Pressure
Coronary Calcium Score over 100 Obesity and stress Animal protein, fats. Salt and coffee Liquorice herb Heavy metals Thyroid disease Antidepressants Pain medications Herbs – licorice, arnica Low magnesium Calcium supplementation	Coronary calcium score less than 100 Exercise – aerobic Fish oils Magnesium Garlic Potassium Vitamins D and C Mediterranean diet Relaxation therapy	Diuretics – fluid tablets increase urinary output. ACE (angiotensin-converting enzyme) inhibitors – dilates blood vessels. Calcium-channel blockers – relax blood vessels. Beta blockers – reduce the stress hormone signals (adrenaline) and reduces the heart rate and the force of the blood being pumped around the body.

Some causes of low blood pressure, such as dehydration, are easily fixed. But low blood pressure can also signal chronic underlying health problems and maybe an over-enthusiastic treatment of raised blood pressure. Sometimes high doses of blood pressure medication can inadvertently push blood pressure too low, leading to light-headedness or nausea, especially when transitioning from sitting to standing. Chronic conditions like Chronic Fatigue Syndrome might also contribute to low blood pressure woes. All of these conditions will see you make an appointment to see your doctor ASAP.

HEART DISEASE

ACTION PLAN – CHECKLIST

· Check the health of your coronary arteries with a calcium CT score.
· Check your risk factors, including homocysteine levels.
· Add foods with magnesium and potassium, and cut down on sugar and salt.
· Add vitamin K2, CoQ10, vitamin D, and B vitamins.
· Use a Mediterranean diet and add fermented foods.
· Exercise and maintain healthy body weight.
· Manage stress.

References:
Soltan, S., & Gibson, R. (2008). Levels of Omega 3 fatty acids in Australian seafood. *Asia Pacific Journal of Clinical Nutrition*, *17*(3), 385–390.

Geleijnse, J. M., Vermeer, C., Grobbee, D. E., Schurgers, L. J., Knapen, M. H., van der Meer, I. M., Hofman, A., & Witteman, J. C. (2004). Dietary intake of menaquinone is associated with a reduced risk of coronary heart disease: the Rotterdam Study. *The Journal of nutrition*, *134*(11), 3100–3105. https://doi.org/10.1093/jn/134.11.3100

Taylor F, Huffman MD, Macedo AF, Moore THM, Burke M, Davey Smith G, Ward K, Ebrahim S, Gay HC. Statins for the primary prevention of cardiovascular disease. Cochrane Database of Systematic Reviews 2013, Issue 1. Art. No.: CD004816. DOI: 10.1002/14651858.CD004816.pub5. Accessed 18 May 2024.

Seth, A., Mossavar-Rahmani, Y., Kamensky, V., Silver, B., Lakshminarayan, K., Prentice, R., Van Horn, L., & Wassertheil-Smoller, S. (2014). Potassium intake and risk of stroke in women with hypertension and nonhypertension in the Women's Health Initiative. *Stroke, 45*(10), 2874–2880. https://doi.org/10.1161/STROKEAHA.114.006046

Yang, Q., Zhang, Z., Gregg, E. W., Flanders, W. D., Merritt, R., & Hu, F. B. (2014). Added sugar intake and cardiovascular diseases mortality among US adults. *JAMA internal medicine, 174*(4), 516–524. https://doi.org/10.1001/jamainternmed.2013.13563

Kristensen, M. L., Christensen, P. M., & Hallas J. (2015). The effect of statins on average survival in randomised trials, an analysis of end point postponement. *BMJ Open, 5*, Article e007118. https://doi.org/10.1136/ bmjopen-2014-007118

Kearns, C. E., Schmidt, L. A., & Glantz, S. A. (2016). Sugar Industry and Coronary Heart Disease Research: A Historical Analysis of Internal Industry Documents. *JAMA Internal Medicine, 176*(11), 1680–1685. https://doi.org/10.1001/jamainternmed.2016.5394

Ravnskov, U., et al. (2016). Lack of an association or an inverse association between low-density-lipoprotein cholesterol and mortality in the elderly: a systematic review. *BMJ open, 6*(6), e010401. https://doi.org/10.1136/bmjopen-2015-010401

Unruh, L., Rice, T., Rosenau, P. V., & Barnes, A. J. (2016). The 2013 cholesterol guideline controversy: Would better evidence prevent pharmaceuticalization?. *Health policy (Amsterdam, Netherlands), 120*(7), 797–808. https://doi.org/10.1016/j.healthpol.2016.05.009

Dehghan, M., Mente, A., Zhang, X., Swaminathan, S., Li, W., Mohan, V., Iqbal, R., Kumar, R., Wentzel-Viljoen, E., Rosengren, A., Amma, L. I., Avezum, A., Chifamba, J., Diaz, R., Khatib, R., Lear, S., Lopez-Jaramillo, P., Liu, X., Gupta, R., Mohammadifard, N., ... Prospective Urban Rural Epidemiology (PURE) study investigators (2017). Associations of fats and carbohydrate intake with cardiovascular disease and mortality in

18 countries from five continents (PURE): a prospective cohort study. *Lancet (London, England), 390*(10107), 2050–2062. https://doi.org/10.1016/S0140-6736(17)32252-3

Wise J. Sugar industry paid for dietary research in 1960s, analysis shows *BMJ* 2016; 354 :i4936 doi:10.1136/bmj.i4936

Saiz, L. C., Gorricho, J., Garjón, J., Celaya, M. C., Erviti, J., & Leache, L. (2018). Blood pressure targets for the treatment of people with hypertension and cardiovascular disease. *The Cochrane Database of Systematic Reviews, 7*(7), Article CD010315. https://doi.org/10.1002/14651858.CD010315.pub3

Malhotra. A. (2019) Do statins really work? Who benefits? Who has the power to cover up the side effects? *European Scientist.* https://www.europeanscientist.com/en/features/do-statins-really-work-who-benefits-who-has-the-power-to-cover-up-the-side-effects/

Diamond, D. M., Alabdulgader, A. A., de Lorgeril, M., Harcombe, Z., Kendrick, M., Malhotra, A., O'Neill, B., Ravnskov, U., Sultan, S., & Volek, J. S. (2021). Dietary Recommendations for Familial Hypercholesterolaemia: an Evidence-Free Zone. *BMJ evidence-based medicine, 26*(6), 295–301. https://doi.org/10.1136/bmjebm-2020-111412

Unger, T., Borghi, C., Charchar, F., Khan, N. A., Poulter, N. R., Prabhakaran, D., Ramirez, A., Schlaich, M., Stergiou, G. S., Tomaszewski, M., Wainford, R. D., Williams, B., & Schutte, A. E. (2020). 2020 International Society of Hypertension Global Hypertension Practice Guidelines. *Hypertension (Dallas, Tex. : 1979), 75*(6), 1334–1357. https://doi.org/10.1161/HYPERTENSIONAHA.120.15026

Chapter 23

DEMENTIA AND
COGNITIVE DECLINE

*"It takes courage to stay young
when you are growing old."*

RHONDA WHITE

The fascinating world of the brain is like no other. It's like the ultimate power station, with billions of nerve cells buzzing around and organising themselves into intricate networks. Think of it as the control center, processing heaps of information to keep the show on the road – telling us how we feel and nudging us toward certain behaviours. But there is a twist - while the brain is this complex machine, our understanding of central nervous system disorders hasn't quite caught up to speed. We are still unraveling the mysteries of this incredible organ.

The relationship between genes, environment, and the aging process can throw a few curveballs, leading to social, psychological and economic consequences for the elderly. Dementia has become the second-leading cause of death in Australia and has taken the top spot among Australian women in 2021 edging out heart disease. In fact, dementia is among the top causes of disability and dependency among older adults worldwide.

DEMENTIA AND ALZHEIMER'S DISEASE: WHAT'S THE DIFFERENCE?

Memories help us make sense of the present and help make mindful choices for the future by prioritising information. We learn from experience, we have identity and social connections. so when we struggle to lay down new memories and fail to recall recent events we could perhaps be on the unenviable slippery slope to dementia.

Dementia is a broad term for the decline in cognitive function affecting memory, thinking and social abilities. Alzheimer's disease on the other hand, is a specific type of dementia characterised by progressive memory loss and cognitive decline.

Dementia is not a normal part of ageing, nor is it a psychiatric disorder. It's a syndrome of cognitive decline that affects memory and reasoning, with changes of personality and behaviour, and erosion of the capacity to function and communicate. People with dementia can lose their drive for life, withdraw socially, show little empathy for others or insight into their own behaviour. They act compulsively, obsessively or in socially unacceptable ways. It is often a personal, spiritual, and physically distressing journey for the sufferer and family.

Alzheimer's disease accounts for up to 70% of all cases of dementia. It is the most common of these illnesses, followed by vascular dementia and Lewy body dementia. Lewy bodies are protein deposits that develop in the nerve cells in the part of the brain that controls thinking, memory and movement control. Alzheimer's disease starts slowly and gets worse with time, with a life expectancy of three to nine years from time of diagnosis.

There can be a **rare genetic mutation** called **dominantly inherited Alzheimer's disease (DIAD)** that causes memory loss and dementia in people typically in their 30s to 50s. The disease affects less than 1% of the total population.

If you have dementia, you are likely to have more illness and hospital admissions. *The Lancet* (2017) concluded that 65% of the factors contributing to dementia are preventable with factors such as age, genetics and brain shrinkage out of our control.

Preventable Risk Factors for Dementia

- Less education
- Hypertension
- Heart disease
- Diabetes
- Obesity
- Depression
- Excessive alcohol
- Excessive dietary linoleic acid (seed oils/canola oil)
- Hearing impairment
- Smoking
- Physical inactivity
- Low social contact
- Traumatic brain injury
- Air pollution

PROBLEM PROTEINS IN THE AGEING BRAIN

Brain nerve cells can live over a century, with new neurons forming in adult brains to support learning and memory. While these newborn neurons often don't survive, the outdated idea that brain cells don't renew after birth has been debunked. Neurogenesis, the development of new adult neurons, is influenced by age and hormone levels. However, these new cells are vulnerable to age-related diseases and treatments like cancer therapy and irradiation.

Infection and inflammation are risk factors but so too are diabetes, heart disease and depression. Vascular dementia, for instance, occurs due to compromised blood supply to the brain caused by stroke and high blood pressure. Additionally, certain proteins contribute to dementia.

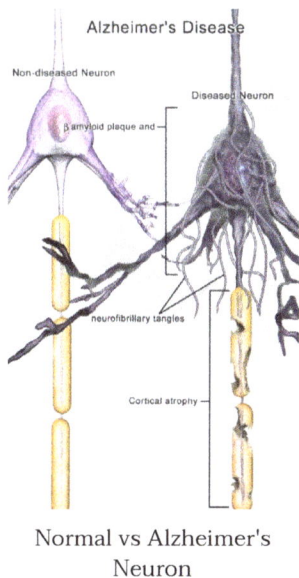

Normal vs Alzheimer's
Neuron
*Image by Bruce Blaus, courtesy
of Wikimedia Commons*

Beta amyloid: Beta amyloid forms amyloid plaques, which are clumps of protein that clog the areas between brain cells, causing communication problems and cell death. Normally in a healthy brain, the plaques are removed as waste, but in Alzheimer's disease the immune cells in the brain (microglia and monocytes) become less efficient at removing waste. A scanning technique known as positron emission tomography (PET) can produce images showing where beta-amyloid and tau have accumulated in the brain.

Tau: Tau has a function in transport and signalling within the brain. Tau normally helps stabilise brain nerve cell structure, but when too much tau accumulates, it detaches from these structures and collapses into insoluble, twisted fibres inside the cells disrupting the functions of the neurons.

High Homocysteine: Homocysteine is a risk factor for dementia in older people. It stirs up inflammation creating more plaque and tangles. Homocysteine metabolism is reliant on the vitamins B6, B12 and folic acid, so supplementation is necessary, see Chapter 22.

For the genetically susceptible we would recommend herbs and mushrooms that might help stave off brain inflammation. The herb that stands out is curcumin, as it crosses the blood brain barrier, binds to the plaques and has been shown to help clear them. Sprinkle in some black pepper for an extra boost.

Malfunctioning Neurotransmitters

1. **Acetylcholine (Ach):** Aging can significantly reduce Ach production, dropping by up to 90% in Alzheimer's patients. Vital nutrients like choline, found in eggs, soy lecithin, liver and meat, are crucial for its production. Ach deficiency is linked to fatigue, memory loss and mood disorders. The drug Aricept helps prevent its breakdown, sometimes helping to treat mild to moderate dementia symptoms.
2. **Glutamate:** This neurotransmitter aids memory and learning but can harm or kill brain cells if in excess, known as glutamate excitotoxicity. It is associated with Alzheimer's, stroke, and Parkinson's. Monosodium glutamate (MSG) exacerbates the problem, earning it the title of "the taste that kills."
3. **Brain-derived neurotrophic factor (BDNF):** This is a nerve-growth-factor protein found at the nerve terminals in the brain and spinal cord. This protein promotes the health, survival and growth of your nerves, signals transmission and aids memory and learning. It also regulates glucose and energy metabolism, and is useful in prevention and management of diabetes. The problem is that BDNF decreases as you age. Lower levels indicate a higher risk of dementia, Parkinson's disease, multiple sclerosis and Huntington's disease.

The good news is that dark chocolate (flavonoids), light exercise and niacin (vitamin B3) all stimulate BDNF. Unsurprisingly, when rats are treated with an MSG additive, they have less BDNF. More good news is that the mushroom lion's mane (*Hericium erinaceus*) can also help produce the nerve-growth-factor hormone.

Inflammation and Nerve Damage: Excessive free radicals can trigger inflammation and disease, including neurological degeneration. Antioxidants, both endogenous and from the diet, may keep inflammation in check. Chronic diseases like diabetes and cigarette smoke are known culprits. Lesser known is the damage caused by refined vegetable oils that can remain in the body for up to seven years. Canola and other seed oils have been linked to Alzheimer's disease because of their negative effects on cell membranes and chronic toxicity. Infections like Epstein Barr virus and severe influenza, alongside poor sleep and high stress, compound negative effects.

Procedures Precipitating Cognitive Decline: Left heart catheterisation, often associated with heart disease, poses risks to mental function. While necessary for diagnosing heart issues, the procedure, sometimes with surgery and stent insertion, may harm cognitive capacity, especially in the elderly. It's a catch-22 situation since untreated heart disease increases the likelihood of dementia. In fact, it's common for people who have heart problems to lose some of their mental sharpness even before they undergo heart procedures. Surgery and anaesthetics, especially if prolonged may deal a heavy hit to cognitive capacity in the elderly.

Drug Therapies and Dementia: Some geriatricians have observed remarkable improvements in dementia patients by discontinuing all medications after initial assessment. Statins, known for side effects like memory loss, hinder both cholesterol production crucial for myelin, the protective sheath around nerve fibers, and coenzyme Q10, leading to inflammation and reduced cerebral energy.

Older drugs like Aricept, which preserve acetylcholine breakdown, offer temporary relief but carry side effects. Acetylcholine is vital for thinking and memory, it is also used for depression and conditions like muscle spasms and overactive bladder, yet its use in the elderly can lead to memory loss and confusion exacerbating cognitive decline. Antidepressants, linked to dementia risk further complicate the picture.

Despite billions spent, the failure rate for new Alzheimer's drugs stands at a staggering 99.6%. Over 300 compounds are in various stages of development, with newer drugs such as the following targeting harmful brain protein plaques:

1. **Aducanumab (Aduhelm):** The drug targets amyloid beta plaques in the brain, which are characteristic of Alzheimer's disease. Its approval has been controversial due to limited evidence of its effectiveness.
2. **Lecanemab (BAN2401):** An antibody therapy designed to target and clear amyloid beta plaques in the brain.
3. **Donanemab:** Another antibody therapy targeting amyloid beta plaques.
4. **ALZ-801:** This is a modified form of an existing Alzheimer's medication designed to enhance its effectiveness in targeting amyloid beta plaques. It is currently in clinical trials.
5. **Tau-based Therapies:** Some drugs in development aim to prevent the formation or spread of tau tangles in the brain.

DIAGNOSIS, EARLY SYMPTOMS, AND BEYOND

As we age, our thinking skills may slow down a bit, typically by about 1–2% each year after the age of forty-five to fifty-five. However, in dementia, this decline can accelerate to 6% -10% each year or even faster in some cases. Memory loss is often serves as an early warning sign for those progressing towards dementia. Other symptoms like confusion, poor decision-making, and changes in personality or behavior can also appear over time.

Typically, symptoms of dementia become noticeable about three years before an official diagnosis. By this time, the process of brain degeneration may have been underway for two or three decades. It isn't always easy to identify because other conditions like head injuries, medication side effects, infections, and depression can cause similar symptoms. Currently dementia is typically diagnosed after it's onset, primarily through the exclusion of other disorders and by addressing declining memory capacity with the following:

1. **Medical Referral:** Consultation with a geriatrician involves gathering detailed medical and family history, as well as input from close relatives regarding concerns.

2. **Assessment:** Evaluating cognitive abilities, social functioning, and behavior.

3. **Physical Examination:** Checking overall health, including gait, strength, hearing, eye movements, cardiovascular health, and psychological well-being.

4. **Neurological Testing:** Utilizing imaging techniques like CT, MRI, and PET scans to identify brain abnormalities.

5. **Blood Tests:** Screening for inflammatory markers and nutrient deficiencies like vitamin B12, homocysteine, magnesium, zinc, and vitamin D.

6. **Neurological Focus:** Addressing issues related to sleep, medication and pain.

7. **Hair Mineral Analysis:** Particularly useful in high-exposure areas for environmental toxins, testing for arsenic, lead, mercury, and cadmium levels, as well as identifying mineral deficiencies.

Symptoms of Dementia

Early Dementia Symptoms	Dementia Progression	Advanced Stage Dementia
Gradual memory loss Problems with time Unsettled with non-performance Gets lost easily	Confused Repeat questions Inadequate hygiene Poor decision-making Loss of intellect	Depression Aggression Smell and speech disturbance Inability to carry out purposeful movements Hallucinations
Alzheimer's	**Alzheimer's Progression**	**Advanced Alzheimer's**
Destruction of neurons in areas of memory	Destruction of areas to do with speech, language, reasoning and social behaviour	Loss of ability to live and function

A DOZEN THINGS TO CONSIDER

Early assessment, including biomarker exploration, is crucial for diagnosing dementia. Current drug therapies focus on neurotransmitters like acetylcholine. Managing conditions such as high blood pressure and heart disease is vital, with additional strategies ranging from anti-inflammatory drugs to hormone therapy. Lifestyle changes also play a key role in reducing risk:

1. **Stay Connected:** Social engagement is vital. Join clubs, play games, and maintain regular social interactions to keep your brain stimulated.
2. **Protect Against Head Injuries:** Avoid activities with high risks of head injuries, such as boxing or certain contact sports.
3. **Moderate Alcohol Consumption:** Excessive alcohol intake can harm nerve cells and impair cognitive function. Limit alcohol consumption to avoid cognitive decline.
4. **Minimize Toxin Exposure:** Reduce exposure to brain-toxic substances like herbicides, lead, mercury, and arsenic, while ensuring adequate vitamin D from sunlight or supplements.
5. **Train Your Brain:** Engage in cognitive exercises to strengthen neural networks and improve memory, attention, and reasoning skills.
6. **Manage Stress:** High cortisol levels from stress can impair memory and brain function. Find stress-relief techniques to protect against cognitive decline.
7. **Regular Exercise:** Physical activity improves blood flow to the brain, promotes the growth of brain cells, and reduces the risk of cognitive decline.
8. **Prioritise Sleep:** Quality sleep is essential for clearing neurotoxic waste products from the brain, crucial for preventing dementia.
9. **Healthy Diet:** Maintain a balanced diet rich in antioxidants, healthy fats, and B vitamins to support brain health and reduce inflammation.
10. **Consider Mushrooms:** Lion's mane and reishi mushrooms have shown neuroprotective effects, benefiting cognition and mental health.
11. **Antioxidant-Rich Foods:** Incorporate foods like turmeric, garlic, green leafy vegetables, berries, dark chocolate, fish, and virgin pressed olive oil to combat inflammation and support brain health.

12.	**Probiotics:** Promote gut health with probiotics, which play a role in neuro-logical development and memory.

As we age and become more-frail, shopping and cooking are not easy. Chewing and digestion may not be ideal. A slow depletion of essential nutrients can increase the risk of dementia. We need to train the brain for the good things so you can cruise, rather than stagger, into your later years.

Apart from dark chocolate, add fish for optimal brain function, eggs to give you plenty of choline, and natural Greek-style yoghurts to keep your tummy happy. Get into the habit of shopping for berries and ripe fruit, leafy green vegetables, onions, and high-fibre cereals so you won't always need a list.

The following are some of the key nutrients and foods that may help cognition and memory as we age. Don't be discouraged by the list below. Most of the nutrients you already know about, but some might remind you why they are important.

Neurotransmitters and Hormones

Acetylcholine	Derived in part from the nutrient choline; it effects memory, learning, alertness, and concentration as well as movement, coordination and muscle tone.	Source: Fish, eggs, liver, soy-beans, peanuts and other nuts. Dose: 420 mg two to three times/day.
Melatonin	Taken long-term (2–3 years) can improve cognition.	Dose: 6 - 10 mg/day an hour before bed for sleep.

Herbs and Mushrooms

Ginkgo biloba	*Gingko biloba* may help memory, improve circulation and blood flow to the brain.	Amount: 240 mg/day (*Ginkgo biloba* extracts).
Lion's mane (*Hericium erinaceus*)	Also known as Yamabushi-take, it supports nerve growth and helps repair nerve cells.	Dose: 750 mg/day tablets containing 96% of Yamabushitake.
Brahmi (*Bacopa monnieri*)	Inhibits the breakdown of acetylcholine acting in a similar to drugs such as Aricept.	Dose: 300 mg/day.
Reishi mushroom *Ganoderma lucidum*	Shown to reduce age-related oxidation and plaque formation.	Dose: 1800 mg/day
Curcumin from turmeric	Anti-inflammatory effects. It may protect against plaque deposit.	Dose: 400 mg/day.
Sage	Sage/ salvia - antioxidant, anti-inflammatory properties and protects against the breakdown of acetylcholine (animal studies).	Dose: 60 drops of *Salvia officinalis* daily (1:1 alcohol 45%).

Other Nutrients

Lipoic acid	Antioxidant, helps to boost levels of acetylcholine and reduce inflammation.	Source: Spinach, organic meats, broccoli, and tomatoes. Dose: 600 mg/day.
Grape seed polyphenols	Polyphenols are considered better than vitamin E and vitamin C in protecting against ageing.	Source: Grape seeds. Dose: 1 g/day.
N-acetyl-cysteine (NAC)	A modified form of the amino acid L-cysteine, helps to reduce inflammation, improve immunity, and protect the brain. It is a precursor to glutathione, often depleted in Alzheimer's disease.	Source: Meat, fish, chicken and eggs, beans, lentils, garlic, onions, and broccoli. Dose: 600 mg/day along with other antioxidants.
Probiotics	Lactobacillus and Bifidobacterium genera have been used most in the studies supporting cognition and memory.	Source: Fermented dairy supplements for greater than 4 weeks.

DEMENTIA AND COGNITIVE DECLINE

ACTION PLAN – CHECKLIST

- Check for early symptoms of dementia in your middle years.
- Focus on neurological issues, sleep, drugs and pain.
- Manage or avoid stressful situations.
- Test for inflammatory markers and nutritional deficiencies.
- Manage coexisting conditions.
- If concerned, get cognitive assessment with a neurologist or geriatrician.
- Coordinate care among physicians and other caregivers.
- Stay connected to family and friends.
- Devise a strategy for future advanced management care.
- Test for toxic metals with a hair mineral analysis.
- Use Mediterranean diet with low alcohol.
- Use probiotics, herbs, acetylcholine, N-acetyl-cysteine.
- Get plenty of exercise and sleep and good hydration.
- Maintaining a sense of self identity and relationships with others.

References:

2023 Alzheimer's disease facts and figures. (2023). *Alzheimer's & dementia : the journal of the Alzheimer's Association*, *19*(4), 1598–1695. https://doi.org/10.1002/alz.13016

Birks, J., & Evans, G. J. (2009). Ginkgo biloba for cognitive impairment and dementia. *Cochrane Database of Systematic Reviews*, *1*, Article CD003120.

Blaylock, R. L. (1996). *The Taste That Kills*. Health Press.

Cardinali, D. P., Furio, A. M., & Brusco, L. I. (2010). Clinical aspects of melatonin intervention in Alzheimer's disease progression. *Current Neuropharmacology*. *8*(3), 218–227.

Chaudhari, K. S., Tiwari, N. R., Tiwari, R. R., & Sharma, R. S. (2017). Neurocognitive Effect of Nootropic Drug *Brahmi* (*Bacopa monnieri*) in Alzheimer's Disease. *Annals of Neurosciences*, *24*(2), 111–122. https://doi.org/10.1159/000475900

Goosens, K. A., & Sapolsky, R. M. (2007). Stress and Glucocorticoid Contributions to Normal and Pathological Aging. In D. R. Riddle (Ed.), *Brain Aging: Models, Methods, and Mechanisms* (Chapter 13).

Hara, Y., McKeehan, N., Dacks, P. A., & Fillit, H. M. (2017). Evaluation of the neuroprotective potential of N-acetylcysteine for prevention and treatment of cognitive ageing and dementia. *The Journal of Prevention of Alzheimer's Disease*. http://dx.doi.org/10.14283/jpad.2017.22

Chapter 24

CANCER

"Cancer affects all of us, whether you're a daughter, mother, sister, friend, co-worker, doctor, or patient."

JENNIFER ANISTON

When President Richard Nixon signed the US National Cancer Act into law in 1971, it was like a call to arms against cancer. The media buzzed with excitement, heralding a declaration of war on this formidable foe. With the birth of the National Cancer Institute came a flood of funding, injecting billions of dollars into research initiatives and sparking hope for a brighter future.

Fast forward nearly fifty years, and the battle rages on. Personalised cancer vaccines from the '70s were pioneered blazing a trail into the unknown, laying the groundwork for the incredible advancements we see today.

There is no denying—cancer is tough. The treatments we throw at it—surgery, radio-therapy, chemotherapy—they can be brutal. They strip away life's pleasures, leaving a trail or pain, nausea and weakness. Yet, amidst the struggle, there is hope. New break-throughs bring us closer to a world where cancer is not a life sentence but a challenge that can be overcome.

ARTIFICIAL INTELLIGENCE AND CANCER TREATMENT

Artificial intelligence (AI) is poised to revolutionise the field of medicine, particu-larly in the realm of cancer treatment. With its ability to analyse vast quantities of data swiftly and accurately, AI holds the promise of ushering in an era of precision medicine, tailored to the individual characteristics of each patient.

In the realm of oncology, where every cancer presents with challenges and com-plexities, AI stands to play a pivotal role in identifying the most effective treatment strategies. AI algorithms can pinpoint optimal therapies, maximising the chances of successful outcomes while minimising potential side effects. The synergy between health professionals and technology in the modern era offer significant improvements in precision medicine, risk assessment and diagnostic efficiency— and hope.

HOW CELLS TURN CANCEROUS

Every cell in your body has its own set of instructions encoded within its genes. These instructions, made up of about 1,700 building blocks called nucleotides, guide the cell's activities, with around fifty of these blocks replicating every second. Some-times mistakes happen during this replication process, whether by chance or due to outside factors like viruses, chemicals, or radiation.

Some types of cancer, e.g. breast cancer, have a stronger link to family history, such as the BRCA gene mutation. If someone carries this mutation, they may have a higher risk of developing breast, prostate, or other cancers.

While about 10% of cancers are thought to be caused by inherited gene mutations, the vast majority—around 90%—are believed to be triggered by factors in our environment and lifestyle. Childhood cancers, on the other hand, often stem from gene mutations and typically affect tissues like blood, lymph, brain, bone, and liver.

When a gene mutates, it can disrupt the cell's normal growth and reproduction, leading to uncontrolled division and the formation of cancerous tumors. Factors like diet and lifestyle choices can influence how these mutations progress. This means there's a chance to intervene before a tumor forms, potentially changing the course of the disease for the better.

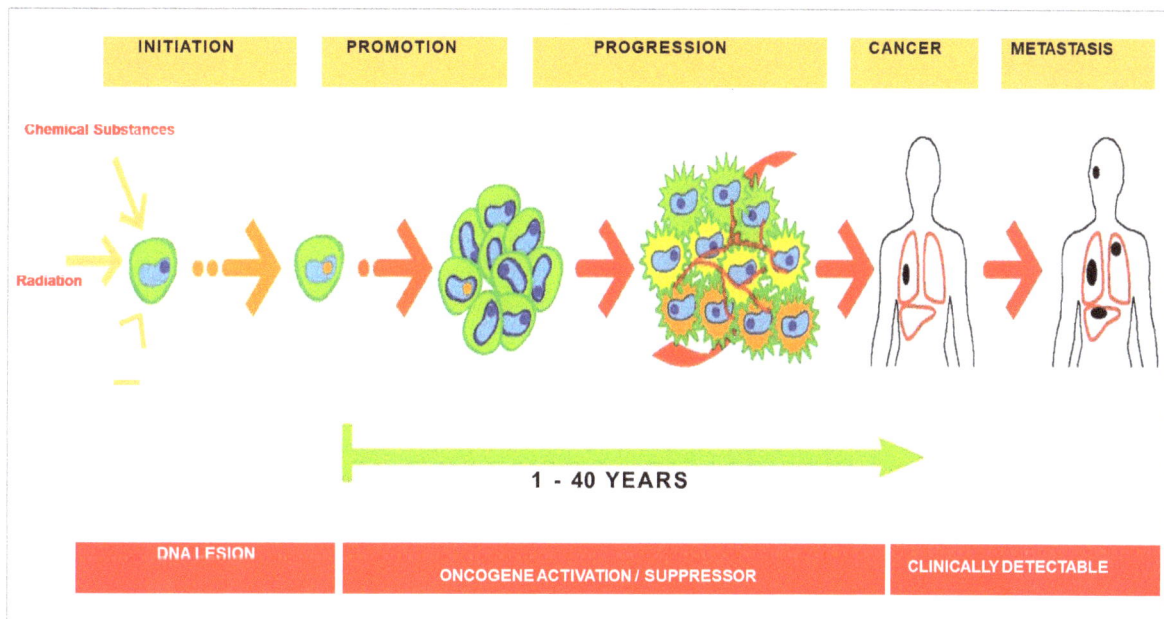

Béliveau, R., & Gingras, D. (2007). Role of nutrition in preventing cancer. Canadian Family Physician, 53(11), 1905-1911

HOW CANCER DIFFERS FROM NORMAL CELLS

- They replicate endlessly.
- They avoid normal programmed cell death.
- They grow blood vessels to supply nutrients.
- They invade other organs and form tumours elsewhere in the body.
- They change genetically to adapt to the environment when the need arises.
- They promote tumours through inflammation.
- They reprogram their energy supply to meet demand, e.g. supply glucose at twenty times the rate required by normal cells.

CANCER DOESN'T WORK ALONE

Most cancers are diagnosed after the age of sixty-five, since the biological processes behind ageing can drive the development of cancer. The cumulative impact of oxidative stress, inflammation and ageing chromosomes can grow over time, leading to many chronic diseases such as heart disease, diabetes and cancer.

Oxidative stress: When your body uses oxygen to break down glucose for energy, it produces atoms called free radicals. These free radicals can be a bit unruly, as they have an uneven number of electrons. To stabilise themselves, they seek out other molecules, potentially causing damage along the way by altering their structure.

Antioxidants found in vitamins, minerals, and proteins neutralise the free radicals, repair any damage they've caused, and boost the immune system with their anti-inflammatory properties. However, if free radicals overwhelm the body's antioxidant defences, they can wreak havoc, damaging cell membranes potentially leading to mutations in DNA—a precursor to cancer. So, while aging may increase the risk of cancer and other diseases, a healthy diet rich in antioxidants can help mitigate some of these risks by combating oxidative stress and supporting overall health.

CANCER TRIGGERS

The World Health Organisation divides cancer-causing agents into:

1. **Physical carcinogens,** such as ultraviolet and ionising radiation.
2. **Biological carcinogens,** such as viral, bacterial or parasitic infections.
3. **Chemical carcinogens,** such as tobacco smoke, pesticides and asbestos.
4. **Endocrine disrupters,** man-made chemicals that interfere with our body hormones.

Note: Cancer is more likely to develop if you're already at risk – e.g. if you're physically inactive or obese, if you drink or smoke, or if you have a major chronic disease. Lifestyle factors, as always, are all-important.

1. **Physical carcinogens – UV rays and radiation:** Too much sun exposure can damage your DNA, and it can trigger gene mutations that eventually lead to cancer. The earth itself emits low 'background' levels of this form of energy. Radiation comes from the field of medicine - radiotherapy, X-rays and computed tomography (CT) scans. It is worth remembering that ultrasounds and MRIs involve no exposure to radiation, so if the clinical situation allows these should be preferred. While radiotherapy is a common cancer treatment, there is a lifetime dose limit for each treated area. Children who undergo CT scans are at a higher risk

of developing cancer, particularly in younger age groups, due to their increased sensitivity to radiation and longer lifespan for potential cancer development.

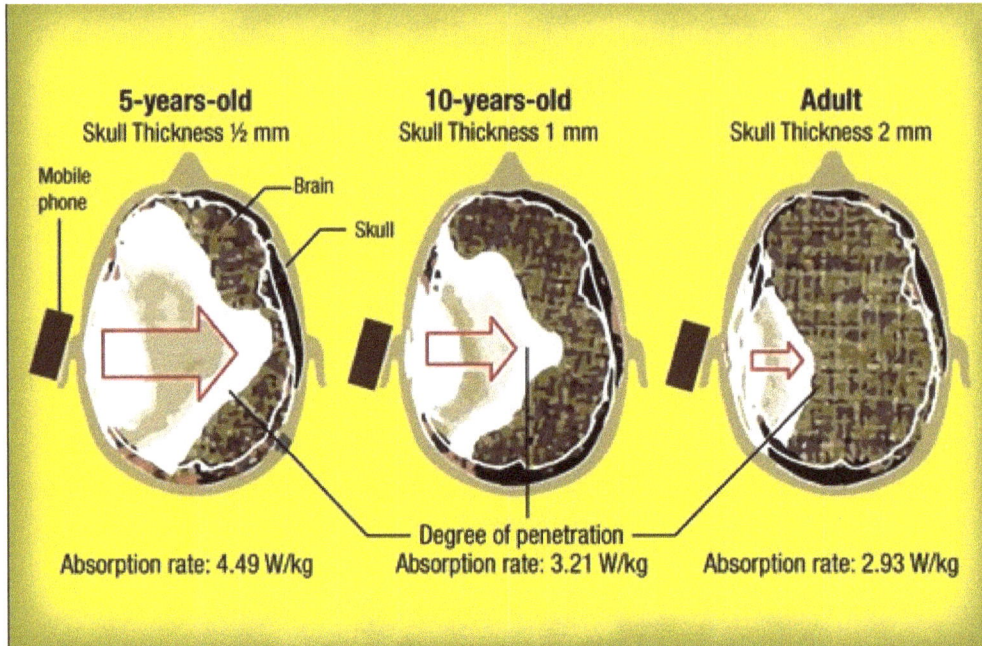

5-years-old	10-years-old	Adult
Skull Thickness ½ mm	Skull Thickness 1 mm	Skull Thickness 2 mm
Absorption rate: 4.49 W/kg	Absorption rate: 3.21 W/kg	Absorption rate: 2.93 W/kg

Used with permission from SafeSpace

Advice from the American Academy of Paediatrics: 'Smartphone use by children should be limited, and children should text more than talk when they do need a smartphone. If they do call, children are advised to keep the device an inch or more away from their heads.' **iPads belong on tables, not laps.** If they do sit on a child's/adult's lap, they should be on airplane mode. They are a two-way microwave radiating device, so they send and receive images all the time. Young children should not have smartphones.

2. **Biological Carcinogens:** Infections can trigger gene mutations leading to cancer. Long-term inflammation can promote cancer growth by suppressing the immune system. Human papillomavirus (HPV) is linked to cervical cancer, while hepatitis A and B are associated with liver cancer. Epstein-Barr virus is linked to pharyngeal cancer, and Helicobacter pylori bacteria are linked to stomach cancer. Fungal infections have also been implicated in cancer development.

3. Chemical Carcinogens: Tobacco smoke is the leading cause of chemical carcinogen-related deaths, killing millions annually. Other sources include pesticides, asbestos, contaminated foods, and personal care products. Pesticides, especially herbicides, constitute a significant portion of chemical carcinogens. Arsenical insecticides and dioxins are recognised as human carcinogens, while others are suspected.

4. **Endocrine Disrupters and Persistent Organic Pollutants (POPs):** Endocrine disrupters, like phthalates and bisphenol-A (BPA), interfere with hormone function and may contribute to breast, prostate, and thyroid cancers. POPs, such as organochlorine pesticides, dioxins, and PCBs, accumulate in body fat and pose health risks to humans and wildlife. Heavy metals like cadmium, lead, mercury, and arsenic, are toxic, fat-soluble, and bioaccumulate.

Note: Many lawsuits have dogged the makers of glyphosate herbicides (Roundup) since concerns were raised by the International Agency for Research on Cancer in 2015, which classified glyphosate as a '**probably carcinogenic to humans.**' In 2018 the US court awarded eighty million dollars to a groundskeeper who used the product and developed non-Hodgkin lymphoma. A similar award occurred in 2019 and the total payout by pharmaceutical company Bayer in settlement of the cancer claims over inadequate labelling have been in excess of 20 billion Australian dollars! A take-away message from all is that "the dose makes the poison".

Endocrine Disrupters

Polychlorinated biphenyl (PCB)	Found in paints, plastics, rubber, dyes, motor oil in hydraulic systems, tapes and floor finishes.
Polybrominated diphenyl ethers (PBDE)	Found in flame retardants, electronics, furniture and textiles.
Dioxins	From burning of wood, incineration, smelting, paper bleaching, and some herbicides and pesticides.
Organochlorine pesticides	A class of pesticides that includes DDT, dieldrin and chlordane.
Bisphenol A (BPA)	An endocrine-disrupting chemical found in plastics and resins, water bottles and other containers (including epoxy resins lining cans).
Phthalates	From plastics, furnishings, floorings, toys, cleaning agents, cosmetics, hairspray, and perfume. They leech into fatty foods if microwaved.
Parabens (hydroxybenzoates)	Anti-fungal preservatives. In cosmetics, shampoos, sunscreen and some foods and beverages.

Other Problem Toxins

Tobacco smoke	Tobacco smoke contains more than seventy are known carcinogens.
Pesticides and insecticides	Care should be taken when using: glyphosate (RoundUp), malathion and diazinon. The organophosphate insecticides *tetrachlorvinphos* and *parathion* are classed as 'possibly carcinogenic'. *Mancozeb*, (used on fruit and vegetable crops), is a potential carcinogen and neurotoxin.
Perpolyfluoralkyl	Perflurooctanoic acid (PFOA) and perfluorooctane sulfonate (PFOS), occurs in everything from firefighting foam to non-stick frying pans because of its heat-resistant properties. Used in some water supplies, textiles and leather, paper coating (including food packaging), metal plating and etching, photographic materials, aviation hydraulic fluid, cosmetics and sunscreen, medical devices and as ingredients in firefighting foams. Both cause tumours in animals.
Lead	A 'probable carcinogen', found mostly in old house paints, batteries and contaminated soil.

AUSTRALIAN EXPOSURE TO AGRICULTURAL CHEMICALS

The 25th Total Australian Diet Study, published in 2019, analysed 206 agricultural chemicals across 88 food types. Agricultural chemicals were found in 42 food types, but most dietary exposures were below acceptable daily intake levels, indicating low public health risk. Bok choy had the highest number of detected chemicals (16), followed by apples and capsicum (11 each), and several other fruits and vegetables (ranging from 6 to 10). Metal contaminant levels met international standards, with seafood containing higher mercury and arsenic levels.

The 26th Total Diet Study focussed on persistent organic pollutants (POPs) including dioxins, with fatty fish containing the highest levels. The 27th study, published in 2021, evaluated per- and poly-fluoroalkyl (PFAS) compounds found in various foods. PFOS was detected in five food types, but at low levels and without public health concerns for the general Australian population.

Note on Rice and Arsenic: Rice has also been shown to have arsenic. Levels of metal contaminants were also comparable, or lower, than those found internationally. Arsenic levels in rice can be reduced by parboiling. The arsenic content is in their outer layers, by discarding the cooking water used during parboiling, the overall arsenic levels in the finished rice can be reduced.

Avoid Harmful Chemicals: Never microwave fatty foods in plastic containers meant for single use. Check the labels of products such as shampoos, deodorants and cosmetics for details of their ingredients and manufacturing processes and **choose organic produce** to minimise pesticide residues.

Minimise Your Pesticides Intake

Wash fruit and vegetables as soon as you get home. The longer the pesticides are on products, the harder it is to remove them. Buy locally so the food has short storage time. Brush soil off the skin and remove stalks from fruit and vegetables before you wash them. Washing will get rid of most pesticide residues. Peeling will get rid of more, but any nutrients in the skin of the fruit or vegetable will also be lost. Wash before peeling.

Method 1 : Soak the fruit and vegetables in a mix of one-part vinegar to two parts water for twenty minutes, then rinse thoroughly in running water.

Method 2: Soak the fruit and vegetables in 5–10% vinegar for one hour before rinsing.

Method 3: Soak the fruit and vegetables in two cups of water to one teaspoon of bi-carbonate of soda for fifteen minutes, then rinse in running tap water.

OBESITY AND CANCER

Estimates of the percentage of cancers attributable to being overweight and obese range from 4.5% in Europe to 20% in the USA. Excess weight and obesity now vie with smoking as the number one cause of cancer. Obesity is linked to around thirteen types of cancers, from endometrial, breast, ovarian, prostate, liver, gallbladder, kidney, colorectal and renal cancers, to leukemia and malignant melanoma.

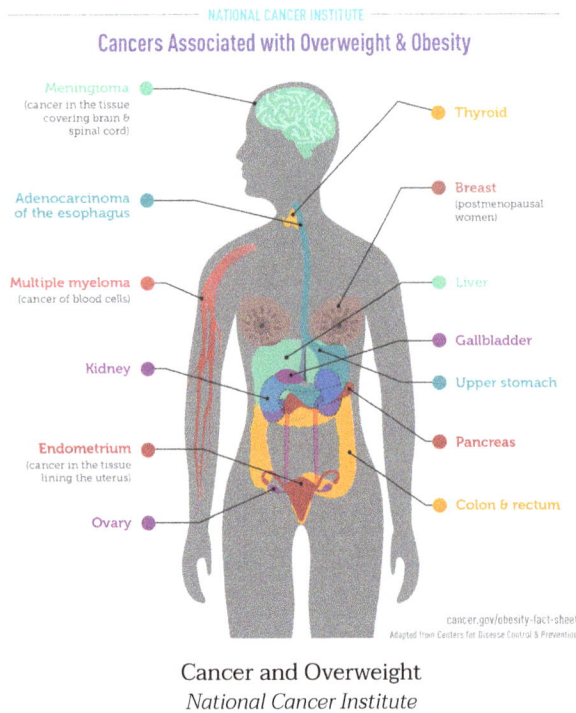

Cancers Associated with Overweight & Obesity
NATIONAL CANCER INSTITUTE

Meningioma (cancer in the tissue covering brain & spinal cord)

Adenocarcinoma of the esophagus

Multiple myeloma (cancer of blood cells)

Kidney

Endometrium (cancer in the tissue lining the uterus)

Ovary

Thyroid

Breast (postmenopausal women)

Liver

Gallbladder

Upper stomach

Pancreas

Colon & rectum

cancer.gov/obesity-fact-sheet
Adapted from Centers for Disease Control & Prevention

Cancer and Overweight
National Cancer Institute

Between 30% and 50% of cancer deaths could be prevented by modifying or avoiding key risk factors:

· Avoid tobacco products.
· Reduce alcohol consumption.
· Eat more fruit, vegetables, and fish.
· Maintain a healthy body weight.
· Exercise regularly.
· Maintain weight.
· Get adequate sleep.
· Reduce exposure to radiation.
· Reduce use of pesticides.

Diets and Cancer: Overall, plant-based diets and watching your calorie intake can help protect against cancer, as shown in studies from the UK. For strict vegans, it's important to be aware of potential nutrient deficiencies in vitamin B12, zinc, iron, and omega-3 fatty acids which are found mainly in animal products.

To fight inflammation: Adding some tasty anti-inflammatory foods to your daily meals, like curcumin, green tea, quercetin, and resveratrol. Resveratrol has been found to have some pretty good cancer-fighting properties. Fruits, veggies, whole grains, legumes, fish, and low-fat dairy can also help reduce the risk of cancer by lowering oxidative stress and inflammation.

When you're shopping for groceries, go for fresh local produce whenever you can and organic if possible. Fresh local foods tend to hold onto their nutrients for a short period. Frozen is better than canned. And remember to keep alcohol consumption in check—it's linked to several types of cancer. Try sticking to just one standard drink per day and give yourself a few alcohol-free days each week for a healthier lifestyle and cancer prevention.

Here is a table we put together highlighting the risks and advantages of foods and nutrients in the diet:

Site of Cancer	Increased Risk	Decreased Risk	Probable Increased Risk	Probable Decreased Risk
Colorectal	Alcohol Processed meat Red meat Excess weight High sugar High cooking temperatures	Low weight Folate, garlic Fruit Vegetables Wholegrains Curcumin MK4 (K2) Resveratrol Probiotics	Trans fats Low calcium	Vegetables Fibre Vitamins D, B2, B3 and B5 Magnesium Coffee Olive oil
Breast	Excess weight High sugar Alcohol > 2 units/ day Low iodine	Heathy weight < Alcohol Breastfeeding Fruit Vegetables Soy foods Vitamin D Resveratrol Probiotics	Alcohol Red meat Fried meat Low iodine Low folic acid High iron	Vitamins A and D Fibre Coffee Olive oil

Lung	Alcohol, Meat - processed	Fruit Vegetables Resveratrol	Beta carotene	Vitamin D
Stomach	Salt, pickled, foods Excess weight Low iodine Alcohol	Fruit Vegetables Vitamin C Fibre Ginger Probiotics	High-starch diets	Vitamin E Selenium
Prostate	Red meat High-fat diet Corn oil Excess weight Alcohol Milk Refined carbs Low protein High-temp cooking	Fruit Vegetables – onions, garlic and chives Fish oils Curcumin Pomegranate Green tea Coffee Resveratrol Cannabis Zinc Probiotics	Low iodine	Vitamins K and D Soy foods Fish Nuts Seeds Tomatoes Selenium Milk thistle Resveratrol

Naso-pharynx	Excess weight Alcohol Salted fish Fructose Sugars	Raw fruit Dark-green vegetables - Cruciferous vegetables High-fibre	Alcohol Hot drinks Red meat - & processed	Beta carotene, Vitamins C & E Folic acid
Pancreas	Red meat Alcohol Excess weight High-fat diet French fries (potato chips)	Fruit Vegetables Beta carotene Fibre Nuts Vitamins C & D Low cal diet Resveratrol	Sugar	
Bladder	Alcohol Meat Fat – butter Fried food Coffee Fructose Added sugar	Fruit, citrus Vegetables Tomato Vitamins C, D, E and A Green tea Yoghurt Resveratrol		

Liver	Alcohol Aflatoxin Red meat Sugar	Fruit Vegetables MK4, K2) Cereals White meat Fish & eggs Milk Yoghurt Probiotics	Fructose White bread	Coffee
Thyroid		Curcumin		
Kidney	Excess weight Meat Milk Fat	Fruit Vegetables Fibre <Magnesium Alcohol Vitamin E Nuts Fish		
Uterus, cervix, ovaries & endometrial cancer	>Weight Alcohol Meat Dairy	Green tea Resveratrol Probiotics	Saturated fat Acrylamide - >temp cooking	Vegetables and fibre Soy foods Coffee

YOUR ALLIES AGAINST CANCER

1. Fruit and Vegetables – Why Some Are Better Than Others: Resveratrol is a plant chemical found in high concentrations in purple grapes, but to a lesser extent in red wine. The richest source of resveratrol is Polygonum cuspidatum (Japanese knotweed) but it is also in ripe fruit and vegetables. Resveratrol is best known for its benefits against heart disease, but it also has anti-tumour activity and the ability to inhibit different stages of cancer development, i.e. the initiation, promotion and progression of cancer, so it's quite a powerful anticancer agent.

Resveratrol is produced by plants in the late ripening stage; it imparts a sharp, bitter flavour to help protect the plant against attack. It has a high antioxidant capacity and antimicrobial functions that protect the plant in response to various stresses such as injury, UV radiation and fungal attack. Pesticides and fungicides erode the incentive for the plant to make these protective chemicals.

Potter *et al* (2002) found that resveratrol can be processed by an enzyme (CYP1B1) found in many tumours, It produces an antileukaemic/anticancer agent called piceatannol. This resveratrol experience prompted further research to find more foods with similar anticancer agents. Here are some food sources:

- Red/purple grapes.
- Soybeans and peas.
- Berry skins and seeds – blackberry, blueberry, blackcurrant, mulberry, cranberry, pomegranate and passion fruit seeds
- Green tea

2. **Antioxidants Are Better Together:** Antioxidants, found in fruits, veggies, whole grains, nuts, and seeds, form a team against cancer. They safeguard cell membranes and work best when combined. A good mix includes glutathione, alpha lipoic acid, carotenoids, vitamins D and A, B vitamins, vitamin C, vitamin E, CoQ10, iodine, zinc, and selenium—especially crucial for specific cancers like thyroid, breast, prostate, and stomach cancers.

3. **Iodine and Cancer:** Around 29% of the world's population including Western Pacific, South East Asia and Africa live in areas of iodine deficiency. The thyroid gland contains over 70% of the body's iodine and the rest is found in tissues throughout the body. Thyroid, breast, prostate and stomach cancers have been linked to low iodine levels. Selenium works synergistically with iodine because many thyroid enzymes are selenium dependent. By keeping your iodine and selenium levels in balance you can guard against thyroid cancer and potentially other cancers.

Iodine deficiency is associated with fibrocystic breast disease. It affects women of child-bearing age. Rates of breast cancer and prostate cancer are much higher in Australia (17.3% and 15% respectively) than in iodine-rich Japan (9.2% and 10% respectively). However, overdose of iodine can occur relatively easily, so generally iodine supplementation should be under medical supervision. There are some inconsistencies in iodine recommendations worldwide.

Iodine Recommendations

Australia	USA	Europe
150 µg per day to the upper limit of 1100 µg per day.	Similar to Australia. 150ug/day	No more than 600 µg per day

Looking now at foods that are high in this key trace element, we see that dried seaweed is huge, but cooked seaweed and the broth is at least five-fold lower than dried seaweed. There are some foods (cabbage, broccoli, and Brussels sprouts) that interfere with the uptake of iodine, but typically it's not a concern for people with a well-balanced diet and adequate iodine intake.

Food	Iodine Content	Food	Iodine Content
Seaweed (dried)	4300 mg/kg	Cheddar cheese	23 ug/100g
Sushi	92 ug/100g	Eggs	22 ug/100g
Tinned salmon	60 ug/100g	Milk	13 ug/100g
Oysters (6)	160 ug/100g	Bread	3 ug/100g
Iodised salt- 76 µg/ ¼ teaspoon			

4. Vitamin D and Cancer: Some seventeen forms of cancer are associated with vitamin D deficiency, including four of the most common: prostate, breast, colon and ovary. It binds to receptors in cancer cells, enters their nuclei, and regulates the actions of genes inside. It can help prevent new cells from becoming cancerous, influence signalling between cells, recognise dysfunctional cells, block proliferation, limit the blood supply and initiate cell death. Some interesting research on vitamin D and cancer suggest far-reaching consequence should we have low levels. Blood levels below 30 nmol/L are considered insufficient. Many doctors would prefer a goal approaching 80-100 nmol/L.

· Breast cancer appears to be more aggressive, with 94% more likely to metastasise if vitamin D is deficient.
· Postmenopausal women with higher intakes of vitamin D also are less likely to develop cancer than those with lesser intakes. An increase in blood vitamin D levels by 5 nmol/l was associated with a 6% decrease in breast cancer risk.
· People with the highest intake of vitamin D are 11% less likely to develop adenomas (such as polyps), which predispose to cancers of the colon and rectum.

- Rates of prostate, breast, colon and rectum cancers and non-Hodgkin lymphoma are reduced with chronic (but not acute) exposure to UV radiation (which the skin uses to produce vitamin D).
- Blood (serum) levels of vitamin D below 30 ng/mL are associated with increased risk of colon cancer.
- Prostate cancer and multiple sclerosis have been shown to benefit from sunlight exposure, independent of the action of vitamin D.
- A toxicity threshold for vitamin D of 10,000 to 40,000 IU/day and serum 25(OH)D levels of 200-240 ng/mL, which is not possible from the sun or from food but can occur with excessive supplementation.
- Adults should have 800 International Units (IU) of vitamin D per day, and children 400 IU per day.
- High Dose to Address Vitamin D Deficiency -50,000 IU for one month only to replete stores.
- Maintenance Dose -1000 IU–2000 IU. Check in 3 months.

Food Sources	Vitamin D in IU
Egg (large)	43.5
Salmon 100 g	526
Mackerel 100 g	1006
Cod liver oil (1 teaspoon)	450
Tuna (100 g)	69

5. Vitamin C and Cancer Care: The body can only store vitamin C for about three weeks, so it's crucial to maintain regular dietary intake. Symptoms of vitamin C deficiency range from fatigue to poor wound healing.

For cancer patients, high-dose intravenous (IV) vitamin C is the most effective form for achieving anti-tumour activity. When used alongside chemotherapy, it can enhance treatment outcomes by reducing side effects and increasing drug sensitivity. IV vitamin C is typically administered before or after chemotherapy sessions due to its short half-life in the body. Studies have shown significant improvements in fatigue, insomnia, constipation, and pain with IV vitamin C treatment.

However, it's important to note that IV vitamin C may not be suitable for everyone, including those with certain medical conditions or during pregnancy. For those unable to receive IV treatment, oral liposomal vitamin C provides an alternative with improved absorption. Dietary sources of vitamin C include citrus fruits, kiwi, berries, peppers, tomatoes, and leafy greens.

6. Probiotics and Cancer: Probiotics provide another line of defence against cancer – not a cure or a fixer. A healthy colony of gut microbes will guard against pathogens that trigger gene mutations, as well as reducing inflammation and cancer promotion. Strains of *Bifidobacterium* or *Lactobacillus* in fermented milk products are well known for their beneficial effects on health. For even minor health conditions you need at least 20–30 billion colony-forming units. See Chapter 20 (Probiotics and Friends).

CANCER ACTION PLAN

CHECKLIST

- Avoid ultraviolet and ionising radiation from phones and electronics.
- Check B vitamins plus levels of C, D, iodine, iron, zinc, folate.
- Beware of any genetic predispositions for cancer.
- Keep weight within ideal healthy range.
- Use Mediterranean diet principles.
- Avoid carcinogens such as tobacco smoke, pesticides, and asbestos.
- Avoid man-made chemicals that interfere with your body's hormones.
- Reduce alcohol and red meat.
- Avoid high-temperature cooking of oils and sugars.
- Add berries, garlic, turmeric, green tea, maitake mushrooms.
- Consume and pre- and probiotics daily
- Buy organic and local produce..

References:

Béliveau, R., & Gingras, D. (2007). Role of nutrition in preventing cancer. *Canadian Family Physician, 53*(11), 1905-1911.

Aceves, C., Anguiano, B., & Delgado, G. (2013). The extrathyronine actions of iodine as antioxidant, apoptotic, and differentiation factor in various tissues. *Thyroid, 23*(8), 938–946. https://doi.org/10.1089/ hy.2012.0579

Bhaskaran, K., Douglas, I., Forbes, H., dos-Santos-Silva, I., Leon, D. A., & Smeeth, L. (2014). Body-mass index and risk of 22 specific cancers: a population-based cohort study of

5·24 million UK adults. *Lancet (London, England), 384*(9945), 755–765. https://doi.org/10.1016/S0140-6736(14)60892-8

Garland, C. F., Garland, F. C., Gorham, E. D., Lipkin, M., Newmark, H., Mohr, S. B., & Holick, M. F. (2006). The role of vitamin D in cancer prevention. *American journal of public health, 96*(2), 252–261. https://doi.org/10.2105/AJPH.2004.045260

Klimant, E., Wright, H., Rubin, D., Seely, D., & Markman, M. (2018). Intravenous vitamin C in the supportive care of cancer patients: a review and rational approach. *Current Oncology, 25*(2), 139–148. https://doi.org/10.3747/co.25.3790

Mathews J D, Forsythe A V, Brady Z, Butler M W, Goergen S K, Byrnes G B et al. Cancer risk in 680 000 people exposed to computed tomography scans in childhood or adolescence: data linkage study of 11 million Australians BMJ 2013; 346 :f2360 doi:10.1136/bmj.f2360

Potter, G. A., Patterson, L. H., Wanogho, E., Perry, P. J., Butler, P. C., Ijaz, T., Ruparelia, K. C., Lamb, J. H., Farmer, P. B., Stanley, L. A., & Burke, M. D. (2002). The cancer preventative agent resveratrol is converted to the anticancer agent piceatannol by the cytochrome P450 enzyme CYP1B1. *British journal of cancer, 86*(5), 774–778. https://doi.org/10.1038/sj.bjc.6600197

Soldati, L., Di Renzo, L., Jirillo, E., Ascierto, P. A., Marincola, F. M., & De Lorenzo, A. (2018). The influence of diet on anti-cancer immune responsiveness. *Journal of translational medicine, 16*(1), 75. https://doi.org/10.1186/s12967-018-1448-0

Song, D., Deng, Y., Liu, K., Zhou, L., Li, N., Zheng, Y., Hao, Q., Yang, S., Wu, Y., Zhai, Z., Li, H., & Dai, Z. (2019). Vitamin D intake, blood vitamin D levels, and the risk of breast cancer: a dose-response meta-analysis of observational studies. *Aging, 11*(24), 12708–12732. https://doi.org/10.18632/aging.102597

Chapter 25

CHRONIC FATIGUE SYNDROME AND FIBROMYALGIA

"To improve is to change: to be perfect is to change often."

SIR WINSTON CHURCHILL

"Chronic fatigue is when the tanks are empty" is a phrase commonly attributed to Dr. Sarah Myhill, a British physician known for her work in the field of chronic fatigue syndrome (CFS) and related conditions. Also known as myalgic encephalomyelitis (ME), it is described as a debilitating, chronic, profound and complex disorder with fatigue lasting more than 6 months.

When you're dealing with this condition, your brain's stress signals go haywire, it disrupts the body's chemistry and the never-ending tiredness that sticks around for over six months can be isolating.

SOME ATTRIBUTED CAUSES

Severe viral infection and inflammation has been attributed to CFS. In March 2024 the US Centres for Disease Control reported that COVID-19 patients were over 4 times more likely to have chronic fatigue than those without the infection. Stressful events, pre-onset of fatigue are common, as are links to underlying genetic causes. It is no surprise then that genetics, infection, physical trauma and difficulties with metabolism and cellular energy are interrelated in CFS. Some might add problems with environmental pollutants to the list. Nor is it a surprise that CFS/ME has been identified with stress, hormonal and immune disorders with poor detoxification pathways contributing.

The complexity of the syndrome relates to the variability of the illness and the unseen collateral damage to many areas in the body. Studies have tried to come up with objective markers through blood tests and even brain imaging. However, although imaging studies have shown inflammation in different brain regions and greater inflammation correlating with fatigue and cognitive defects, there are still no conclusive tests for CFS.

THE SYMPTOMS

If you have the syndrome, you're overwhelmed by fatigue and a host of symptoms that are not improved by bed rest and can get worse after physical activity or mental exertion. The disability is increased because of muscle pains, headaches, poor stamina, sleeping problems and sensitivity to noise, light and pain. You will find the word 'malaise' commonly used in CFS. Malaise refers to a general feeling of discomfort, illness, or unease, often accompanied by symptoms such as fatigue, weakness or lethargy. The term encompasses a range of physical and emotional sensations, including fatigue.

Apart from no definitive tests and no drugs, there is often no way to prove your case of chronic fatigue. Symptoms dictate how one copes with work and home life.

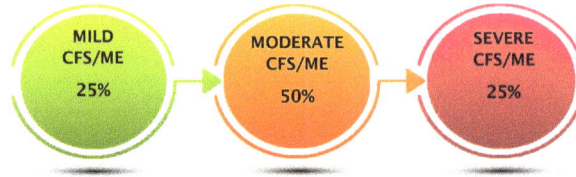

CFS affects many people differently. Some people manage a job and home life, while some 25% are severely affected.

DIAGNOSIS

Diagnosis is a process of elimination, doctors first must rule out the many other conditions with similar symptoms before diagnosing CFS/ME. One must have had severe fatigue for six or more consecutive months and the fatigue interferes with daily activities and can't be due to ongoing exertion nor other medical conditions associated with fatigue.

You must also have four (or more) of these eight symptoms:

1. Post-exertional malaise lasting more than twenty-four hours after physical or mental exercise.
2. Unrefreshing sleep.
3. Significant impairment of short-term memory or concentration "brain fog".
4. Feeling dizzy or faint when sitting up or standing (due to a drop in blood pressure).
5. Muscle aches and pain.
6. Pain in the joints without swelling or redness.
7. Headaches of a new type, pattern or severity.

8. Tender lymph nodes in the neck.

Less common conditions include: Sensitivity to light or sound, dizziness or light-headedness, digestive issues such as irritable bowel syndrome (IBS), temperature dysregulation (feeling too hot or too cold), and emotional symptoms like depression or anxiety.

We recommend the following tests and have references to our chapters in this book which might help with explanations:

Conditions to Exclude & Chapter Reference	Ask Your Doctor About These Tests
Anaemia Chapter 35	Full blood count to check for anaemia, ferritin (iron stored in the body), vitamin B12 and folate.
Thyroid -over or underactive Chapter 13	Check of thyroid-stimulating hormone (TSH), thyroid hormones T3 and for Hashimoto's disease.
Addison's disease Chapter 31	Fasting morning cortisol to test adrenal response.
Chronic diseases (excluded in these tests). Chapter 28	Electrolyte and liver function tests to check over twenty biochemical parameters.
Diabetes mellitus Chapter 21	Fasting glucose to test blood sugar levels. HbA1c to assess diabetes

Assessment of allergies Chapter 2	Tissue transglutaminase (TTG) test for gluten antibodies. RadioAllergoSorbent. (RAST) blood tests and skin prick tests to check for food allergies.
Malabsorption of nutrients Chapter 35	Measure of magnesium and zinc plus other nutrient levels to test for deficiencies
Chronic inflammation Chapter 1	Erythrocyte sedimentation rate (ESR) and C-reactive protein (CRP) tests for inflammation.
Autoimmune disease Chapter 3	Antinuclear antibodies (ANA) test to check autoimmune response. Carcinoembryonic antigen (CEA) to test for cancer antibodies. C-reactive protein (CRP) as above, re: inflammation.
Liver and renal problems Chapter 28	Normal biochemistry (electrolyte and liver function, including renal and nutrient tests _ usually some 20 items in this test.
Heart disease Chapter 28	Cardiac enzymes, ECG. Coronary Calcium Score.
Infections (e.g. glandular fever, HIV) Chapter 1	Blood tests specific to suspected virus, often 6-7 tests included.
Sleep apnoea Chapter 27	Breathing tests; trial of continuous positive airway pressure (CPAP) machine.

Habitual drug abuse Chapter 15	Liver function tests. Levels of protein and ferritin to test for deficiencies. Drug testing for drug abuse.

ISSUES IN RECOVERY FROM CFS

As you travel the next few pages of explanation, you may find it helpful to have in mind the four steps to consider in recovery from CFS/ME:

1. **The Krebs Energy Cycle:** When this energy cycle is disrupted, the key debilitating symptoms are exhaustion, brain fog and musculoskeletal aches and pains. Nutritional supports can be helpful in stimulating this energy cycle.
2. **Infection and the subsequent impairment of the immune system:** Viruses and other infections are common causes of CFS/ME, and subsequent allergy/chemical problems opportunistically emerge because of a depleted immune system.
3. **Adrenal fatigue:** Not as a primary cause but seen as a result of a compromised immune system due to stress with debilitating illness, Chapter 31.
4. **An associated central sensitivity syndrome (CSS):** The nervous system becomes hypersensitive. To calm things down use nutrients and specific exercises that target the vagus nerve in an effort to balance the (autonomic) nervous system. See Chapter 27, When All Else Fails.

1. **The Krebs Energy Cycle:** There's a growing scientific consensus that there are changes occurring in the mitochondria – those parts of the cells that produce energy. It's seen as a cellular energy problem where an infection or another insult compromises the cells' capacity to generate energy, resulting in a hyper aroused immune response that makes the problem worse.

When normal chemical reactions produce energy from food via a cyclical process (the Krebs Cycle) they produce 36 units of the energy molecule – adenosine triphosphate (ATP) per cycle. The process requires vitamins, minerals and many other nutrients. If the cycle is hampered in some way (e.g Epstein Barr or Covid virus), the body reverts to a far less efficient pathway, supplying just 2 ATP energy units per cycle, rather than the usual 36 units. Lactic acid then accumulates in the tissues, making one feel like we've got a bad case of the flu, complete with brain fog, aches and pains and flu-like symptoms. In CFS, there's no "second wind" to help us bounce back. It's like our bodies are stuck in low gear, making everyday tasks feel like climbing a mountain.

2. **Infection and Inflammation:** Low-grade inflammation, infection, chemical and other stressors can damage the mitochondrial energy production. Glandular fever (Epstein-Barr virus/EBV), herpes virus and recently COVID, cytomegalovirus, toxoplasmosis and Lyme disease may be a trigger. In Australia, Ross River virus, Barmah Forest virus, Q and Dengue fever are common examples of viruses associated with chronic fatigue syndrome. Blood tests sometimes (but not always) show evidence of an immune system under stress, exhibiting antinuclear antibodies, rheumatoid factor, thyroid or other antibodies. If the immune system is compromised, other complaints such as allergies and chemical sensitivities can come to the fore. You may have been exposed to mould, dust mites, gluten or chemicals in the past without a problem, but now they literally make you sick.

3. **Adrenal Fatigue and the Stress Response:** As we have seen previously, chronic stress affects energy production in the mitochondria. When unrelenting and long-term stress occurs, cortisol rises initially to meet the crisis, but eventually the adrenal 'crashes', lowering cortisol levels. Researchers suggest that this persistent and long-term cortisol elevation can be a 'switch' to low cortisol output. This process, of course, is not only seen in CFS – any prolonged physical or emotional stress can result in this type of adrenal "exhaustion".

4. Central Sensitivity Syndrome (CSS): The characterisation of central sensitivity syndrome includes a heightened sense of pain, fatigue, less restorative sleep, memory and mood disorders, as well as sensory sensitivity. These effects can explain some of the most distressing symptoms of chronic fatigue syndrome – i.e. unusual pain, impaired working memory, slow processing speed, poor attention span and difficulty retrieving words. In CFS/ME everyday experiences can make the symptoms worse, including headaches, irritable bowel syndrome (IBS), bladder pain, and more. It's like a tangled web where the nervous, digestive, and cardiac systems all play a part. To calm things down, think psychologically and nutritionally, but also physiologically to reduce the overall hypersensitive state. We need to stimulate the para-sympathetic nervous system (PSNS) via the vagus nerve to help the body self-correct. Simple exercises can help to manage the high adrenaline output. See the section on vagal stimulation in Chapter 27 (When All Else Fails).

MANAGEMENT OF CFS/ME

Symptom Management: Addressing specific symptoms of pain, sleep disturbances, and cognitive difficulties through mindfulness, medications, lifestyle modifications, and complementary therapies is usually necessary. Aspirin and ibuprofen can help, high-dose hydrocortisone (20-30mg) has shown some improvement in CFS/ME symptoms, but the high degree of adrenal suppression makes it not ideal if prescribed long term.

Activity Management: Balancing activity and rest is necessary to avoid overexertion and post-exertional malaise - a hallmark symptom of CFS. Don't push too hard. Know when to rest and when to build strength. Breaking strenuous activities into smaller tasks with rest is ideal. Maintain a diary for symptoms and activity since the outcome of overexertion may not be seen immediately but after a few says.

Graded Exercise Therapy (GET): Gradual increasing physical activity levels serves to improve physical function and tolerance.

Cognitive Behavioral Therapy (CBT): Helps individuals cope with the psychological impact of CFS, manage stress and develop adaptive coping strategies. See Chapter 12, Mindfulness.

Medications: Managing pain, sleep disturbances, and mood disorders can be difficult because medication effectiveness can vary, and caution is needed due to potential side effects. Cabanas et al (2021) found that ME/CFS patients reported improvement in impaired thought, concentration and cognitive overload as well as other immune disturbances symptoms e.g sore throat, enlarged or tender lymph nodes, and susceptibility to colds/influenza after treatment with low dose naltrexone.

Nutritional Support: Where allergy or sensitivity exist, dietary guidance and nutritional supplementation can help address potential deficiencies and support overall health and energy levels.

Support Groups and Counseling: Emotional support, validation, and education through support groups and counseling sessions can help people feel less isolated and better equipped to manage their condition.

Complementary Therapies: Exploring alternative treatments such as acupuncture, massage therapy, and mindfulness-based interventions to alleviate symptoms and improve well-being. Additionally, it is important to check inflammatory and viral markers via blood tests. Check for nutritional deficiencies and allergies and supplement where necessary. An exercise physiologist can assist in keeping muscles toned during tough times.

Orthostatic intolerance: Symptoms are worse when standing, and better when lying down. Increase water intake to at least two litres per day and increase salt and potassium. Low blood pressure may need a medical assessment.

Light and sound sensitivity may be an issue and sunglasses and sleep masks may be helpful. Wear ear plugs when necessary.

Pain: Over-the-counter pain relievers work for many but avoidance if possible is ideal. Non-steroidal anti-inflammatory medications and PEA (palmitoylethanolamide) reduce inflammation. Low dose naltrexone has shown promise in long COVID and CFS/ME. Cannabis is in the early stages of research for CFS/ME and this many also be helpful with chronic pain. The problem with cannabis are the side effects, including cognitive impairment, respiratory issues (if smoked), dependency, and exacerbation of mental health conditions. These risks should be carefully weighed against any potential benefits in CFS. Where over-the-counter pain relievers don't work, and pain is severe, narcotic medicines (tramadol, codeine or morphine) are prescribed. See Chapter 9 on Chronic Pain.

Sleep: If unrefreshing, try slow-release melatonin (5-10 mg an hour before bedtime). (See Chapter 32).

Stay connected to family and friends as pain and fatigue can be isolating.

Detoxification: Certain supplements may support detoxification processes, including glutathione, alpha-lipoic acid, selenium, and vitamins C and E and of course plenty of fluids.

NUTRIENTS SPECIFIC FOR CFS/ME

Here we are looking to improve energy pathways, enhance gut absorption and recommend the nutrients needed to combat infections and stress which can distort and compromise energy output. When addressing Chronic Fatigue Syndrome (CFS) through nutrition the goal is often not just to fix deficiency, but to boost mitochondrial output when biochemical pathways aren't functioning efficiently. Researchers have identified key nutrients to support the energy cycle and a mix of these supplements can usually be found in the pharmacy or health food stores.

General Supplementation: Deficiencies in vitamins C and D, zinc, magnesium, B complex vitamins, folic acid, l-carnitine, glutathione, essential fatty acids and CoQ_{10} have been identified by various researchers. Multivitamin/mineral supplements have been shown to be safe and improve the quality of life in CFS/ME.

D-Ribose: When D-ribose is low, energy output is low. It increases energy and reduces the key symptoms of cramping, pain and stiffness.

Both CoQ_{10} and nicotinamide adenine dinucleotide (NADH) increase energy production in the mitochondria; a deficiency in CoQ_{10} occurs in about 30% of those with CFS/ME.

Glutathione is a critical antioxidant, but not absorbed well orally. Supplementation is best done via its precursor N-acetylcysteine (NAC).

Intramuscular vitamin B12 weekly worked better than oral dose in chronic fatigue patients in a Swedish study. Injections of methyl cobalamin, plus oral folic acid tablets (1–5 mg), were given, with good effect for chronic fatigue.

Higher dose folic acid (15-20 mg/day) worked well with those who have a genetic (MTHFR) variant.

GABA: Those affected may have low levels of GABA (inhibitory neurotransmitter) and high levels of glutamine (excitatory neurotransmitter), both of which affect mood.

GABA has a calming effect on the nervous system: it relieves stress and helps with poor mental focus and pain.

Herbs: To improve your cognition, try the herb *brahmi* (also known as *Bacopa monnieri*), along with *Ginkgo biloba* and the amino acid tyrosine (e.g. available in brain and mood formulas).

L-carnitine is an amino acid that assist the transport of fats (fatty acids) into the mitochondria to generate energy in muscles and in the brain. Benefits have been shown in chronic fatigue trials when supplemented, but this too takes time – maybe up to six months.

Selenium improves mitochondrial function as well as protecting neurons against oxidative stress.

Citrulline: An amino acid used to increase blood flow and reduce fatigue and brain fog. Usually found in powder form. A scoop (3 grams) is the daily dose.

Zinc and Omega 3 fatty acids: Trials of high doses of evening primrose oil plus fish oil (DHA and EPA) have brought about improvements in both mental and physical fatigue, but the duration of the trial in this case was three months only. **Patience is another necessary factor, and there is no pill for that!**

Intravenous injections: Often a more efficient way to kick-start a struggling energy and immune system is to bypass normal digestion and the passage through the liver. This particularly applies if there is evidence of an unreliable gut or liver dysfunction. Injections can help improve both energy and immune function. We suggest including a range of B vitamins, 5,000 mg of vitamin C and good doses of magnesium, calcium and zinc. These may be given weekly to every second week, and one should see a positive difference in four to six weeks in CFS/ME. This 'cocktail' is useful in other conditions, particularly where exhaustion and immune deficit coexist.

Faecal transplant: Sixty CFS/ME individuals were given faecal transplants and followed up 15–20 years later. 50% presented significant symptom improvement. In other studies, there have been some relapses in the condition as time goes by.

Try These Nutrients for Brain Fog and Muscle Aches

D-ribose – 10–15 grams three times per day for energy, pain and stiffness.

CoQ_{10} with a daily dose of 150–200 mg per day for better energy. Best taken in the morning.

Sodium bicarbonate can be taken at night can help reduce acidity and inflammation. Start with a quarter of a teaspoon and build up to half a teaspoon in a glass of water at night for 3 weeks and see if it makes a difference. Don't use it long-term.

CHRONIC FATIGUE SYNDROME/ MYALGIC ENCEPHALOMYELITIS

ACTION PLAN – CHECKLIST

- Early diagnosis, tests, and exclusion of other causes of fatigue.
- Check out the triggers and determine the major symptoms.
- Determine the dominant causes of fatigue symptoms and personalise care.
- Supplement to improve energy metabolism.
- Treat the symptoms with and without drugs.
- Educate patients, family and friends about CFS/ME.
- Team management with psychological, exercise and dietary guidance.
- Monitor progress.
- Maintain social and work contacts.
- Give yourself an energy score out of ten regularly so you can check it against treatment initiatives.

FIBROMYALGIA (FM)

Too Sore to Move, Too Tired to Think – Fibromyalgia or Chronic Fatigue?

Fibromyalgia is a condition known for causing persistent pain in the joints and muscles, along with several tender spots on the body that are extra sensitive. It often comes with other central nervous system issues like trouble sleeping, fatigue, irritable bowel, headaches, memory lapses, concentration problems (often called "fibro-fog"), and sometimes numbness or tingling in the hands and feet.

Symptoms of Fibromyalgia

· Widespread pain lasting three months.
· Extreme tiredness (fatigue).
· Unrefreshing sleep.
· Digestive problems – abdominal pain, bloating and constipation.
· Tingling or numbness in hands and feet.
· Thinking and memory problems.
· Symptoms vary from day to day and from person to person.

Ninety per cent of those who suffer are women. Most develop the condition between age thirty and sixty, but it can appear at any age. Fibromyalgia shares many of the same features and symptoms as chronic fatigue syndrome. They are a collection of symptoms that are difficult to manage, rather than a disease. Both have central sensitisation of the central nervous system (CSS). They both occur more often in people with a history of viral infection, inflammatory arthritis, depression or stress and both have a genetic influences.

Again, you get problems with the energy cycle and often you get depleted thyroid, adrenal and sex hormones. The lactic acid that would normally be turned into glucose if the body's energy cycle was working smoothly seems to inflame the muscles instead. FMS has some autoimmune features thus rheumatic disease, mental health and neurological conditions (e.g. multiple sclerosis) should be ruled out.

DIAGNOSING FIBROMYALGIA

Fibromyalgia differs from chronic fatigue syndrome in that pain, rather than fatigue, often presents as the prominent symptom. Tests have highlighted problems with microcirculation in painful muscles, poor energy and reduced muscle relaxation rates. As with CFS, there's a lot to be ruled out before you reach a diagnosis of fibromyalgia. Consider asking your doctor for the following tests to exclude other conditions:

· Full blood count and erythrocyte sedimentation rate (ESR) and CRP tests of inflammation.
· Antinuclear antibody test for rheumatoid arthritis and lupus.
· Thyroid function test.
· Coeliac gene test (HLADQ2,8), and allergy tests.
· Check hormone status.
· Check nutrients, e.g. vitamin D, magnesium, iron, iodine, vitamin B12 and zinc.

There are many diagnostic tools on the internet that may be easily downloaded. The American College of Rheumatology a specific diagnostic criteria for FMS. A pain index relies on the patient gently pressing nineteen chosen points (several focused around the neck) and marking the number of body parts experiencing pain over the last week. The diagnostic criteria for fibromyalgia must meet the following criteria:

1. Widespread Pain Index (WPI) score ≥ 7 and a Symptom Severity (SS) score ≥ 5 OR the WPI score is 4–6 and the SS score is ≥ 9.
2. Generalized pain, defined as pain in at least 4 of 5 regions, must be present.

3. Symptoms have been generally present for at least 3 months.
4. Jaw, chest, and abdominal pain are not included in generalized pain definition.

PAIN in last week*				SYMPTOMS in last week*	
Region	Centre	Right	Left	Symptom	Score [0-3]
Neck	☐			Fatigue	☐0 ☐1 ☐2 ☐3
Jaw		☐	☐	Wakening unrefreshed	☐0 ☐1 ☐2 ☐3
Shoulder girdle		☐	☐	Cognitive symptoms	☐0 ☐1 ☐2 ☐3
Upper arm		☐	☐	Other symptoms+	Headache ☐1 Abdominal pain ☐1 Depression ☐1
Lower arm		☐	☐		
Chest	☐			Tick appropriate box and count 0 = no problem 1 = slight or mild problems, generally mild or intermittent 2 = moderate, considerable problems, often present and/or at a moderate level 3 = severe, pervasive, continuous, life disturbing problems	
Upper back	☐				
Lower back	☐				
Hip		☐	☐	TOTAL SYMPTOM SEVERITY SCORE [SSS = 0-12] ☐	
Abdomen	☐				
Upper leg		☐	☐	Fibromyalgianess score = WPI ☐ + SSS ☐ = ___	
Lower leg		☐	☐		
WIDESPREAD PAIN INDEX SCORE [WPI = 0-19] ☐				Fibromyalgia diagnosis = WPI ≥7 ☐ PLUS SSS ≥5 ☐ OR WPI ≥3 ☐ PLUS SSS ≥9 ☐ Criteria filled = YES / NO * Symptoms present at similar level for 3 months + No other explanatory diagnosis	

New modified ACR diagnostic criteria for fibromyalgia
https://www.racgp.org.au/afp/2013/october/fibromyalgia

WHAT'S NEXT

1. Look for a Cause of the Inflammation

- Check for inflammation markers via blood tests.
- Rule out statin drug myopathy with sensitivity to anti-cholesterol drugs.
- Check blood for medical conditions that affect mood, such as thyroid disorders, vitamin deficiencies (e.g., vitamin D, vitamin B12), hormonal imbalances, or inflammatory markers. Additional tests may be performed based on individual symptoms and medical history.
- Check for allergies via RAST (blood) and skin scratch tests. Check for food and/ or chemical allergens and sensitivities that may aggravate the condition (see Chapter 2 Allergies).
- Get rid of junk food, alcohol, gluten, legumes, and other foods that may exacerbate chronic inflammation.
- Lose weight - obesity can cause increased sensitivity to pain because of inflammation.
- Detoxification with clean air, clean water, organic food where possible, and non-toxic body and household products.

2. Manage Pain

- Exercise and psychological support are keys to improvement.
- Stress management, mindfulness, meditation, music and biofeedback all help.
- Try some natural therapies before jumping into heavy-duty pain killers. Magnesium for muscle spasm and fish-oil supplements together with other strategies such as acupuncture, massage, hydrotherapy and relaxation techniques, and a graduated return to activity and formal exercising.

- Optimal levels of serotonin, dopamine and GABA decrease pain levels. S-adenosyl-L- methionine (SAMe) has antidepressant, anti-inflammatory and analgesic properties. The oral dose is 400 mg/day twice a day for six weeks.
- Trigger point therapy is very useful. Painful 'knots" are injected with local anaesthetic or cortisone, a mix of both or perhaps botox injections.
- The conservative management for pain commonly include anti-inflammatory medications (Celebrex), Lyrica/ (pregabalin) for neuropathic pain, anti-depressants which help with sleep and pain and then the SSRI's like Prozac.
- Cannabis has been used in some small trials. It has anti-inflammatory and analgesic effects so it useful in chronic pain. Side effects and dosing is an individual thing, and you need the support of a doctor experienced in prescribing cannabis.
- Palmitoylethanolamide (PEA) is an analgesic and seems to have an indirect effect on pain and inflammation. The usual dose for chronic pain is 400–500 mg by capsule or powder three times a day. See Chapter 9.
- Pregnenolone is a steroid hormone precursor made from cholesterol. It has anti-inflammatory, and antidepressant effects and has positive effects on pain and cognition. It is best taken in the morning because it may have a negative effect on sleep.

3. **Sleep Well:** The herb Withania (ashwagandha) is ideal to support the immune system, stress symptoms and sleep. Consider melatonin 3-6 mg at night, as poor sleep heightens the sensation of pain. Stilnox script may be necessary. See Chapter 32.

4. **Exercise Often:** Swimming and low-weight-bearing exercises are good, as are stretching, walking and strength training – don't overdo it! Since central sensitivity syndrome (CSS) is a feature of both CFS and fibromyalgia, there is a need to reduce sensitisation through vagal stimulation. See the section on vagal stimulation in Chapter 27, When All Else Fails.

5. **Diet is Important:** Avoid low blood sugars. A Mediterranean diet will guard against hypoglycaemia. Identify the triggers for irritable bowel and digestive symptoms

– gluten, FODMAP and lactose (see Chapter 2). Add probiotics and supplement with magnesium and vitamin D, CoQ10 and the B vitamins.

There's a lot you can do to help identify the triggers and address your symptoms. Start by reviewing the strategies, include a formula with the nutrients we suggested for chronic fatigue syndrome and you can adjust them to give more emphasis to your symptoms.

FIBROMYALGIA

ACTION PLAN – CHECKLIST

- Exclude other conditions, e.g. rheumatoid arthritis and lupus.
- Check for food and chemical sensitivities as causes of inflammation.
- Check inflammatory markers to quantify the degree of inflammation.
- Consider pregnenolone to reduce inflammation.
- Try PEA, magnesium, acupuncture, massage and trigger point injections for pain management.
- Prescription medications are necessary when pain is severe.
- Try sodium bicarbonate at night to help balance acidity and reduce inflammation.

References:

Centers for Disease Control and Prevention. (2019). *Myalgic Encephalomyelitis/Chronic fatigue Syndrome: IOM 2015 Diagnostic Criteria.* https://www.cdc.gov/me-cfs/health-care-providers/diagnosis/iom-2015-diagnostic- criteria.html

Cabanas, H., Muraki, K., Eaton-Fitch, N., Staines, D. R., & Marshall-Gradisnik, S. (2021). Potential Therapeutic Benefit of Low Dose Naltrexone in Myalgic Encephalo-myelitis/Chronic Fatigue Syndrome: Role of Transient Receptor Potential Melastatin 3 Ion Channels in Pathophysiology and Treatment. *Frontiers in immunology*, *12*, 687806. https://doi.org/10.3389/fimmu.2021.687806

Bjørklund, G., Dadar, M., Pen, J. J., Chirumbolo, S., & Aaseth, J. (2019). Chronic fatigue syndrome (CFS): Suggestions for a nutritional treatment in the therapeutic approach. *Biomedicine & Pharmacotherapy*, *109*, 1000–1007. https://doi.org/10.1016/j.biopha.2018.10.076

Castro-Marrero, J., Sáez-Francàs, N., Santillo, D., & Alegre, J. (2017). Treatment and management of chronic fatigue syndrome/myalgic encephalomyelitis: all roads lead to Rome. *British Journal of Pharmacology*, *174*(5), 345–369.

Picard, M., & McEwen, B. S. (2018). Psychological Stress and Mitochondria: A Conceptual Framework. *Psychosomatic medicine*, *80*(2), 126–140. https://doi.org/10.1097/PSY.0000000000000544

Harte, S. E., Harris, R. E, & Clauw, D. J. (2018). The neurobiology of central sensitization. *Journal of Applied Behavioural Research*, *23*, Article e12137.

Mahoney, D. E., Hiebert, J. B., Thimmesch, A., Pierce, J. T., Vacek, J. L., Clancy, R. L., Sauer, A. J., & Pierce, J. D. (2018). Understanding D-Ribose and Mitochondrial Function. *Advances in bioscience and clinical medicine*, *6*(1), 1–5. https://doi.org/10.7575/aiac.abcmed.v.6n.1p.1

Tennant, F. (2019). Hormone Treatments in Chronic and Intractable Pain: An Emerging Practice. *Practical Pain Management*, *5*(3). https://www.practicalpainmanagement.com/treatments/hormone-therapy/ hormone-treatments-chronic-intractable-pain.

Chapter 26

THE HYPERSENSITIVE
PERSON

*"The ship in harbour is safe, but
that is not what ships are built for."*

JOHN A. SHEDD

The hypersensitive person (HSP) is a delightful individual who just happens to have a low tolerance for the not-so-pleasant parts of life, whether they be physical or psychological stressors. They are like emotional barometers, keenly attuned to the vibes around them, and their heightened awareness means they can spot both opportunities and threats faster than most.

Brain scans of these highly sensitive people show greater activity in the regions involved in awareness and sensory integration. This hypersensitivity is believed to have genetic roots, a sort of evolutionary perk for survival. However, It comes with its own set of pros and cons. On the upside, HSPs are incredibly perceptive, but on the downside, this heightened state can be taxing on both mind and body.

Over the years, health professionals have come up with a slew of names for this unique group, such as 'strong reactor,' 'universal reactor,' and more recently, 'highly sensitive person.' Regardless of the label, the common thread is clear: HSPs experience the world in a profoundly intense way. Sensitivity isn't a weakness. For a highly sensitive person, a drizzle can sometimes feel like a full-blown monsoon, but that's just part of their unique charm.

THE STRONG OR UNIVERSAL REACTOR

Most strong reactors tend to be women. They are sensitive, perfectionist, pleasant, intelligent, and giving, often with some artistic streak. A hallmark is their intuition, their sixth sense, giving them a greater awareness of subtlety. They 'just know' things without necessarily understanding how. But their sensitivity can work against them in their response to health treatments. Strong reactors may need much lower doses of drugs than the average person and often react poorly when given drugs or general anaesthetics.

The term 'universal reactor' was another name coined by environmental medical colleagues for patients who suffered major symptoms at low levels of exposure to foods, food chemicals, environmental chemicals and drugs. Universal reactors, or strong reactors, or hypersensitive persons (HSPs, see below) – whichever descriptor suits their situation – make up some 15–20% of the population. They may feel lethargic and unwell in a particular climate and more likely than their peers to suffer autoimmune diseases and multiple chemical sensitivities.

THE HYPERSENSITIVE PERSON (HSP)

The psychologist Professor Elaine Aron came up with this term in a book of the same name that went on to sell millions of copies. Aron found that highly sensitive people have traits that make them visionaries, artists, or inventors, as well as conscientious, cautious, wise and intelligent people, and more often they are women.

She and her colleagues have looked at brain scans of HSPs. She found stronger activation in regions involving awareness and responsiveness, which could be predicted from the personalities of those tested. Their traits allow them to process at a deeper level, have better concentration, have better vigilance, can spot errors and have the innate ability to be in tune with their own body and with the emotions of others.

The Good	The Not-So-Good
Pleasant personality. Physiologically alive, ticklish. Sensitive to light and sound. Sensitive to other people's moods. Engages brain systems involved in sensory information processing and integration, action planning, and overall awareness.	Low pain threshold. More vulnerable to emotional stress. Sensitive to immune triggers – allergies/sensitivities, chronic fatigue and infections. Prone to blushing, shaking and tensing of muscles. Often hypoglycaemic, needing to 'graze' during the day. Can't say "no" without feeling guilty. Inappropriately labelled with psychological disorders or neurosis. Unnecessarily strong drugs and treatments can exacerbate their health problems.

Aron concedes the difficulties of being over-aroused, with feelings of being out of control and failing to perform at one's best. The risk is exhaustion, and there is a need for quiet times to control over-stimulation. HSPs are often not well understood and could be considered unfairly as neurotic by those who don't know them well. Without a quiet time to recover, they can show physical symptoms of arousal, such as blushing, trembling, sweating, a pounding heart, shaking hands and tense muscles. With lower stress thresholds and higher sensitivity, HSPs must work harder to manage their stress, but it's achievable.

UNDERSTANDING THE TOTAL LOAD CONCEPT

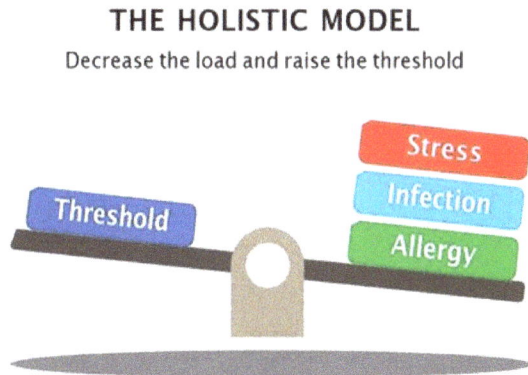

THE HOLISTIC MODEL

Decrease the load and raise the threshold

Threshold

Stress
Infection
Allergy

The scientific model of medicine acknowledges multiple causes for illness, but conventional treatments often don't suit hypersensitive individuals. Doctors prefer a straightforward cause-and-effect approach, which doesn't address why germs or immune failures occur. For example, antihistamines are prescribed for allergies without investigating the specific allergen or the reason for the reaction.

The holistic model takes a thorough approach, examining why the immune system failed and what increased the body's stress. For instance, a hypersensitive person might tolerate some wheat when healthy, but stress or lack of sleep can lower their threshold, making even one slice of bread cause symptoms. Immunologists understand the concept of a patient's 'total load,' though it's not widely recognised.

This approach isn't a quick fix but aims to address the root causes of health issues.

HYPERSENSITIVE PERSON

ACTION PLAN – CHECKLIST

· Check for food and chemical sensitivities or allergies.
· Decrease the toxic burden with a clean diet.
· Use gentle treatments like acupuncture, massage and mindfulness.
· Have time out and a good personal space.
· Say 'No' without feeling guilty.
· Decrease your 'load' and increase your 'threshold'.
· Avoid generic drugs that perhaps have additives which are often more sensitising.

References:

Acevedo, B. P., Aron, E. N., Aron, A., Sangster, M. D., Collins. N., & Brown, L. L. (2014). The highly sensitive brain: an fMRI study of sensory processing sensitivity and response to others' emotions. *Brain and Behavior*, 4(4), 580–594.

Chapter 27

WHEN ALL ELSE FAILS,
WHAT ARE YOUR OPTIONS

"Use what talent you possess; the woods would be very silent if no birds sang there except those that sang best."

HENRY VAN DYKE 1852–1933

Doctors agree that when usual treatments for CFS and fibromyalgia fail, further investigation is needed. Is the issue the diagnosis, the treatment, or both? Here are six alternative options to explore.

1. Is it a mould infection or a mould allergy?

2. Have you ever thought about Lyme disease?

3. Could it be mast cell activation syndrome (MCAS)?

4. Are you being over medicated?

5. Is the sympathetic nervous system (SNS) activating stress and inflammation, and would vagus nerve stimulation help?

6. Is sleep apnoea causing fatigue?

1. IS IT A MOULD INFECTION OR MOULD ALLERGY?

Most people will not experience any health problems from coming into contact with mould. However, those with lowered immunity, asthma, allergies, or other breathing conditions may be more sensitive to mould. Studies on mold exposure show a wide range of symptoms, including fatigue, cognitive impairment, muscle pain, headaches, and mood changes, all linked to the duration of exposure.

Continuous moisture creates an ideal environment for mold. Beyond financial costs and lack of home insurance, residents often report poor health due to mold. People inhale toxins from mold and bacteria found in dust, carpets, wallpaper, heating, ventilation, and air conditioning systems.

The links between damp indoor spaces and respiratory or neurological problems is well documented. Mold can cause allergies, infections, and produce mycotoxins, which can lead to diseases like fibromyalgia and Alzheimer's. Skin prick tests and specific IgE blood tests can diagnose common mold allergens, but limited mycotoxin testing is available in Australia.

Four Common Moulds Warrant Testing

Aspergillus is the most common mold in the environment and often linked to indoor air problems. It spreads through inhalation and grows on starchy foods like grains, bread, and nuts. Aflatoxin from Aspergillus mainly targets the liver, causing symptoms such as diarrhea, jaundice, low-grade fever and loss of appetite. It can also cause cancer.

Alternaria is found both indoors and in soil, and can spoil crops. It grows on paper, wood, cardboard, ceiling tiles, and shoes.

Penicillium soil fungi can enter homes through dust or food from moist environments or water-damaged buildings. Some species are used in cheese production and anti-biotics, but others produce harmful mycotoxins causing symptoms including cough, fatigue, joint pain, headaches and rash.

Cladosporium is an indoor and outdoor mold. While less toxic than others, it can cause sensitivity problems, especially in asthmatics.

GETTING RID OF MOULD

If the house has been flooded, it is best to call professionals to do the remediation. Mould needs to be uprooted at the core and harmful fungal spores, fragments and my-cotoxins can be extremely difficult to destroy. Mould experts can tell if there is mould or debris in the air with equipment that measures particulate numbers and sizes. Infra-red cameras can check behind walls if necessary. If specialist assistance is not possible or practical, here are a few tips to consider before embarking on the job yourself:

- Wear mask and gloves before entering the mouldy area.
- Put anything from contaminated area in a plastic bag – toys, clothes, furnish-ings, etc.
- Don't brush the area to avoid releasing the mould spores. Vacuum the area first using a HEPA filter vacuum.

- There are 2 methods of cleaning: Clean surfaces with a mixture of 4 litres of hot water, 1 tablespoon bicarb of soda and half a cup of vinegar. Scrub the surfaces and leave for an hour, then wipe clean.
- Or, mix one teaspoon of clove oil per litre of water and put it in a spray bottle, lightly mist the mouldy surface. Leave overnight, then vacuum the area and and wipe with a wet cloth. Repeat the process.
- It may take between twenty-four and forty-eight hours for the mould spores to dry and drop off.
- Vacuum the area again while using a mask and gloves.
- Make sure the place is completely dry.
- Clove oil effectively kills mold spores and prevents their regrowth. Also unlike some chemical cleaners, clove oil leaves a pleasant, spicy scent.

Medical Treatment

- Check for mould and other allergies through skin prick tests and blood tests – avoid exposure.
- Avoid other allergic triggers (dust mites and other environmental allergens) that further compromise immune responses.
- Avoid further exposure to water-damaged areas.
- Beware that some treatments, such as antibiotics and steroids, can predispose people to fungal infections, so be careful of overtreatment.
- The treatment is more complex when mycotoxins are identified. Sequestering agents are used for binding toxins as they circulate between the gut and liver before expulsion via the faeces. The purpose is to reduce the body burden of toxins. This requires professional help since there are several sequestering agents such as cholestyramine (CSM), charcoal or sodium bentonite that may be suitable.
- Intravenous injections of antioxidants bypass the gut, so this may be best the way of supplementation when using sequestrants.

· Support the immune system with zinc and vitamins A, E and C. NAC and gluta-thione alone or in combination have been shown to mitigate the oxidative effects of mould.
· N-acetyl-cysteine (NAC) is a powerful antioxidant. It also is a precursor to gluta-thione which detoxifies toxic chemicals.
· Do a diary to identify improvement over time – or not.

Beware of Mould Exposure and Treat Aggressively

Outdoors	Indoors
Improve any drainage so water drains from the home.	Use a dehumidifier and empty water reservoirs regularly.
Check for seepage and leaky pipes.	If there is poor drainage or risk of flooding, get rid of carpets.
Ensure there are no loose water in containers around the home.	Repair any water leaks; check and repair for damp spots.
Avoid trees that prevent sunlight from entering the home.	Ensure good airflow, keep curtains or windows open to sunlight.
Remove rubbish and leaves.	Check air conditioners and filters for mould.
Check the roof gutters for leaves and debris that harbour mould.	Check for ventilation the washing machine and clothes dryer.
Wear a mask when mowing or gardening.	Use exhaust fans in the bathroom/shower and laundry.
	Pot plants are best outside.
	Avoid or limit fish tanks.
	Use moisture-absorbing crystals in damp areas.

2. HAVE YOU EVER THOUGHT OF LYME DISEASE

Lyme disease has a controversial reputation in Australia – a reputation shared with other countries. Infectious disease medical specialists in Australia (with very few exceptions) will not entertain the diagnosis, declaring quite courageously that while people can come into Australia with Lyme disease, no one has ever contracted the illness in this country. Australia has many species of ticks, the most notable being the paralysis tick (*Ixodes holocyclus*) and the bush tick (*Haemaphysalis longicornis*). However, there has been no definitive evidence that these ticks carry *Borrelia burgdorferi*. Despite disagreement around the science, there is considerable evidence supporting a significant number of Australians who suffer from this often serious tick-borne illness.

Lyme disease is caused by bacteria transmitted through tick bites, and symptoms can appear quickly after infection. Unlike Chronic Fatigue Syndrome, which develops slowly, Lyme disease symptoms may include fatigue, headaches, muscle/joint pain, sore throat, and gastrointestinal issues, and can emerge weeks, months, or even years later. Not everyone develops a rash, but a history of tick exposure and rapid symptom onset should raise suspicion. The early onset and the history of tick bite should make one consider Lyme disease. In a French study by Perthame at al, (2023) the manifestations from over three thousand reported cases of Lyme disease identified 62% with skin complaints, 26% had neurological complications, about 7% had joint issues, and almost 2% had eye problems and just over 1% cardiac conditions.

Testing for Lyme disease can be tricky due to potential false negatives, and clinical diagnosis based on symptoms and history is often necessary.

Treatment typically involves oral antibiotics like doxycycline, amoxicillin, or cefuroxime for 3-8 weeks, sometimes followed by intravenous antibiotics if symptoms persist or progress. Nutritional management can complement antibiotic treatment.

Chapter 25 on Chronic Fatigue provides additional guidance on this aspect.

3. COULD IT BE MAST CELL ACTIVATION SYNDROME (MCAS)

Have you ever run your fingernail up your arm and found that you have left a red mark in its place? It's known as 'dermographia' and occurs in about 76% of people with mast cell activation syndrome (MCAS). You feel tired, perhaps bruise easily, or get a rash and maybe have resistant gut pain.

Mast cells are white cells that are part of your immune system, with a primary function to defend the body against toxins and infectious agents. Mast cells are found in most tissues including the brain, but are more prominent in cells of the skin, mouth, nose, conjunctiva, lungs and digestive tract – all the organs that connect to the outside environment and play a role in allergy and immunity.

Mast cells have granules containing several hundred different chemicals including histamine that signal to the immune system when a toxin or infectious agent enters the body. The mast cells then release chemicals to neutralise the danger. When the immune system is hyper-aroused, the mast cells may become overactive. And, rather than releasing the appropriate amounts of biochemical substances in a measured and self-limiting fashion, they become completely disorganised, resulting in a wide range of symptoms. While MCAS has recently been recognised as an important driver of chronic inflammation and/or allergy, there are often problems recognising the condition because of the various presentations – fatigue, itchy skin, swelling due to fluid, flushing, nausea, hoarseness, vomiting, diarrhoea, abdominal cramping, dizzy, racing heartbeat, wheezing, runny nose, and headache.

Major Mast Cell Chemicals	Effects
Histamine Function – Muscle cell contraction, vasodilation, mucus secretion, alterations in blood pressure, and heart rate, gastric secretion, pain and neurotransmission.	Flushing, itching, diarrhoea, hypotension (low blood pressure).
Leukotriene Function – Asthma, allergic reactions, inflammation.	Shortness of breath.
Prostaglandins Function – Hormone-like activity with many functions.	Flushing, bone pain, brain fog, cramping.
Tryptase Function – Involved in allergic reactions.	Fatigue, weight loss, enlarged lymph nodes.
Heparin Function – Blood thinning (anticoagulant).	Osteoporosis, problems with clotting and bleeding.
Tumour necrosis factor-a Function – Involved in inflammation.	Fatigue, headaches, body aches.

Normally histamine is broken down by enzymes (amine oxidases) but if the enzyme activity is low or impaired, then histamine breakdown is poor. Drugs and alcohol don't help matters as they can lead to excessive histamine release from the mast cells, mimicking an allergic reaction. Foods with high levels of histamine exacerbate the condition, and when you put all these factors together you can have problems with diarrhoea, stomach cramps, headache, runny nose and eyes, asthma, low blood pressure, fast heart rate, flushing and skin irritation. But beware, these reactions to foods are not just confined to MCAS.

Meeting diagnostic criteria: To do this, episodes of the symptoms must affect two or more organ systems. **An important criterion is a clear improvement of the symptoms when using antihistamines.** There are sophisticated tests measuring tryptase and histamine from the mast cells, but you need the input of an allergist or doctor familiar with the condition.

Symptoms of MCAS

Neurological	Respiratory – Ear, Nose, Throat	Gastrointestinal	Skeletal
Headache	Itchy nose	Diarrhoea	Bone pain
Brain fog	Nasal congestion	Nausea	Muscle pain
Poor cognition	Itchy throat	Abdominal pain	Osteopenia
Anxiety	Wheezing	Reflux	Osteoporosis
Depression	Shortness of breath		
Skin	**Cardiovascular**	**Gynaecological**	**Urinary**
Flushing	Light-headedness		
Hives	Fainting		
Skin rashes	Rapid heart rate	Urinary cramps	Bladder irritability
Itch - no rash	Chest pain	Bleeding	Urinary frequently
Itch with rash	Low/high blood pressure		

High histamine foods: High concentrations of histamines are often seen with spoiled fish – scombroid food poisoning occurs when naturally high levels of histidine in fish are converted to histamine during decomposition. The following is a list of foods with histamine and histamine-releasing properties – the lower the better in MCAS.

Fish	Meat	Cheese	Vegetables
Tuna, mackerel, mahi dine, anchovy, herring, bluefish, amberjack, and marlin, shellfish, mussels, lobster, crab and prawns.	Cured meats, ham and bacon, aged meat, salami, liverwurst, most sausages, offal and liver.	Matured cheese, hard cheese, mould cheese, gouda, kefir and sour cream.	Sauerkraut, spinach, tomatoes/concentrates, eggplant, avocados, olives, beans and soy products/tofu, and pickled vegetables.
Fruit	**Nuts and Seeds**	**Herbs**	**Dressings**
Strawberries, raspberries, lemons and oranges, bananas, pineapple, kiwi fruit, pears, paw paws and guavas.	Walnuts, cashews, peanuts, pumpkin seeds and sunflower seeds.	Nettle tea and herbal mix products, cinnamon, cloves, curry, nutmeg, thyme and anise.	Fish sauces, yeast extracts, balsamic/wine vinegar, tomato sauces, flavour enhancers (MSG), bullions and broth, soy sauce and spicy foods, carob, cocoa, brown/ dark chocolate, theobromine (energy drinks).

Other Mast Cell Triggers

Source: Mastocytosis Society (https://tmsforacure.org/symptoms/symptoms-and-triggers-of-mast-cell-activation/).

Sun or sunlight, heat, cold or sudden temperature changes	**Stress** (emotional or physical pain, or environmental changes, weather, pollution, pollen, pet dander etc)
Exercise	Fatigue
Foods or beverages, alcohol and additives	**Drugs** (opioids, NSAIDs, antibiotics and some local anaesthetics) and contrast dyes
Natural odours, chemical odours, perfumes and scents	**Venoms** (jelly fish, snakes, bees, wasps, spiders, fire ants, mosquitos and fleas, etc.)
Infections (viral, bacterial or fungal)	**Mechanical irritation**, friction, and vibration

Managing MCAS Symptoms Involves Several Approaches

1. **Medications**: Trial different antihistamines and consider drugs like Montelukast/Singulair for asthmatics. Carry an adrenaline autoinjector for anaphylaxis. Ranitidine, Famotidine, and oral sodium cromoglycate may help with gastrointestinal symptoms. Topical steroids, sodium cromoglicate, and Malizumab/Xolair can address skin, eye, and severe allergy reactions, respectively.
2. **Avoiding Problematic Drugs**: Some medications worsen symptoms by either releasing histamine or inhibiting its breakdown. These include anti-inflammatories, narcotics, certain antibiotics, cimetidine, diuretics, and some antidepressants.
3. **Supplements**: Quercetin, rutin, vitamin B6, copper, vitamin C, zinc, and manganese may help manage symptoms by inhibiting histamine production or supporting its breakdown.

4. **Therapies**: Cognitive behavior therapy, pain management with PEA, and immunotherapy can be beneficial. Vagal nerve exercises and mindfulness-based techniques can address nervous system hyper-arousal.

5. **Dietary Modifications**: Adopting a low-histamine diet, guided by a dietitian, can help manage symptoms. Fermented, aged, or processed foods tend to have higher histamine levels and should be avoided.

6. **Medication Management**: Be cautious of over-medication and its potential side effects, especially given that many drugs contain fillers that may be harmful to hypersensitive individuals. Chapter 37 (Medicate Carefully) discusses the risks of polypharmacy, particularly in vulnerable populations.

By exploring these above strategies and teaming up with a knowledgeable healthcare provider, we hope you can navigate your symptoms on your quest for better health.

4. ARE YOU BEING OVER-MEDICATED?

It's true that individuals who are unwell are often prescribed multiple medications to alleviate their symptoms, and they may accept them eagerly in hopes of finding relief. Unfortunately, side effects are indeed common with many medications.

It's also accurate that up to 80% of drugs contain fillers, which are inactive ingredients used to bulk up the medication or aid in its delivery. While these fillers are generally considered safe for most people, they can potentially trigger adverse reactions in hypersensitive individuals. In Chapter 37 (Medicate Carefully) we discuss how 'polypharmacy' is problematic.

5. WOULD VAGUS NERVE STIMULATION (VNS) HELP?

The vagus nerve is a key part of the parasympathetic nervous system (PNS), primarily transmitting messages from the gut to the brain and influencing immunity, mood, digestion, and heart rate.

The sympathetic nervous system (SNS), fueled by adrenaline and cortisone, often leads to overdrive and overreactions, resulting in increased pulse rate, blood pressure, and muscle tension and potentially leading to inflammation and various discomforts.

The parasympathetic nervous system (PNS) slows pulse rate and blood pressure, relaxes muscle tension, and supports gastrointestinal function. By supporting the PNS via the vagus nerve, you can help calm the SNS, influence stress response, and reduce inflammation and pain.

The vagus nerve communicates with organs involved in various functions like taste, heart function, digestion, and hormone regulation. Lifestyle factors, stress, fatigue, and certain health conditions can affect its function, highlighting the importance of supporting vagal tone for overall well-being.

Non-invasive Vagal Nerve Stimulation (VNS) Techniques

1. **Exercise:** Fitness is key. Moderate aerobic activity or even tai chi or yoga are excellent.
2. **Stress reduction:** Mindfulness and meditation. (Chapter 12).
3. **Breathing:** Deep, slow diaphragmatic breathing, reducing from typically ten to fourteen breaths per minute to five to seven breaths per minute. You can achieve this by counting the inhalation to five, holding briefly, then exhaling to a count of ten.

4. **Acupuncture:** Acupuncture points that are located on the ear concha and lower half of the back of the ear produce clinical benefits via vagus nerve stimulation (VNS).

5. **Music:** Listen to Mozart's music. Singing, humming, chanting, and gargling can activate these muscles and stimulate the vagus nerve.

6. **Valsalva manoeuvre:** A physiotherapist or exercise physiologist can assist with this exercise. The idea is to generate increased pressure within the chest cavity and trigger a slowing of heart rate that may stop an abnormal rhythm.

7. **Diving reflex:** Water immersion of the face and neck for five minutes at 14°C. Splashing cold water or using ice cubes in a zip-lock bag applied to the right lateral neck and the cheek areas increases heart-rate variability and vagal stimulation.

8. **Devices:** Non-invasive devices can be worn as an ear bud with an attachment about the size of an iPhone (costing about AUS $1300). A surgically implanted device in the neck is used for people with treatment-resistant epilepsy and depression. It is programmed by the physician, and the battery is changed every six years. These devices are currently being assessed for chronic inflammation, depressive illness, heart disease, Crohn's disease, stroke, tinnitus, diabetes, migraine and irritable bowel syndrome.

IS SLEEP APNOEA CONTRIBUTING TO FATIGUE?

Forty per cent of adults snore occasionally. Seventy-five per cent of regular snorers have sleep apnoea. It occurs commonly in men over thirty-nine years, particularly those with large necks (collar size over 44 cm) and a large tongue.

Being overweight or having excessive alcohol may dump some individuals in the high-risk category. It is often missed in a person living and sleeping alone without the benefit of someone reporting on snoring and abnormal breathing. It is worth checking out if you have fatigue or nod off during the day. See Chapter 32, Sleep Well.

WHEN ALL ELSE FAILS

ACTION PLAN – CHECKLIST

- Check for allergies to mould and identify sensitivities to foods and chemicals.
- Check for Lyme disease as a cause of chronic fatigue, joint aches and neurological symptoms. An interested doctor is needed for diagnosis and testing.
- Check out MCAS when itchy skin/flushing, fatigue and brain fog persist.
- Improve vagal tone with exercises and actions to balance adrenaline overdrive.
- Check for sleep apnoea as a major cause of fatigue or exhaustion.

References:

New South Wales Government, Environmental Health. (2022) Mould (Fact Sheet). https://www.health.nsw.gov.au/environment/factsheets/Pages/mould.aspx

Perthame, E., Chartier, L., George, J. C., Varloud, M., Ferquel, E., & Choumet, V. (2024). Case presentation and management of Lyme disease patients: a 9-year retrospective analysis in France. *Frontiers in medicine, 10,* 1296486. https://doi.org/10.3389/fmed.2023.1296486

Akin, C., Valent, P., & Metcalfe, D. D. (2010). Mast cell activation syndrome: Proposed diagnostic criteria. *The Journal of allergy and clinical immunology*, *126*(6), 1099–104.e4. https://doi.org/10.1016/j.jaci.2010.08.035

Johnson, R. L., & Wilson, C. G. (2018). A review of vagus nerve stimulation as a therapeutic intervention. *Journal of inflammation research*, *11*, 203–213. https://doi.org/10.2147/JIR.S163248

New South Wales Government, Health. (2014) Lyme disease – testing advice for NSW clinicians. https://www.health.nsw.gov.au/Infectious/factsheets/Documents/lyme-disease-testing-advice.pdf

Peacock, B. N., Gherezghiher, T. B., Hilario, J. D., & Kellermann, G. H. (2015). New insights into Lyme disease. *Redox Biology*, *5*, 66–70. https://doi.org/10.1016/j.redox.2015.03.002

Steinemann, A. (2018). Prevalence and effects of multiple chemical sensitivities in Australia. *Preventive Medicine Reports*, *10*, 191–194. https://doi.org/10.1016/j.pmeDr2018.03.007

Chapter 28

LOVE YOUR LIVER

"Dear wine, we had a deal, you were to make me funnier, sexier, smarter and a better dancer. I saw the video, we need to talk".

ANONYMOUS

In traditional Chinese medicine, the liver has held the esteemed title of the 'general of the army' for over two thousand years, playing a crucial role in safeguarding health. Despite its significance, this hard-working organ is about the size of your two fists and sits snugly on the right side of your upper abdomen. It wears many hats, processing your meals, storing and releasing energy in the form of glucose, producing essential chemicals, detoxifying your body, and bolstering your immune system.

Opting for a turmeric latte over your usual gin and tonic might earn you some brownie points with your liver, but testing its function may identify some lifestyle changes that may need to be addressed.

RED FLAGS IN LIVER FUNCTION TESTS

1. **Bilirubin**: Elevated in jaundice or Gilbert's Syndrome.
2. **Serum Alkaline Phosphatase (SAP)**: Increases with bile obstruction.
3. **Transaminases (SGPT, SGOT)**: Rise in acute liver conditions or fatty liver disease.
4. **GGT (Gamma-Glutamyl Transferase)**: Selectively raised with alcohol or drug abuse.

Features in suboptimal liver function:

1. **Jaundice**: Due to impaired bile pigment processing.
2. **Swollen Ankles**: Related to fluid overload, often from poor albumin production.
3. **Appetite Changes**: Loss of appetite or unexplained weight loss.
4. **Diarrhea**: May indicate significant liver damage.
5. **Strange Bruises**: Resulting from impaired vitamin K conversion.
6. **Dark Urine**: Indicates bile abnormally reaching the urinary tract.
7. **Intense Exhaustion**: Due to waste buildup in the liver.
8. **Right Shoulder Pain**: Resulting from liver swelling irritating surrounding muscles.
9. **Abdominal Pain**: Associated with liver pressure on the abdomen or ribs.

FUNCTIONS OF THE LIVER

Nutrient Metabolism: One of the main functions of the liver is to make and store glycogen as a fuel source for the body. When required, it breaks down the glycogen to glucose for energy. But, like all multi-taskers, when you are under pressure one or two jobs may fall by the wayside.

A frequent scenario involves women of child-bearing age, when the liver takes on additional tasks each month. During the latter half of the menstrual cycle as hormone levels surge in preparation for menstruation, the liver's role is to metabolise and eliminate these hormones. While occupied with this process, the liver's ability to break down glycogen into glucose may be hindered. This can result in low blood sugar levels, leading to symptoms such as irritability, anxiety, fatigue, difficulty concentrating, and cravings for sweets.

Nutrient Storage: The liver stores vitamins (particularly vitamins B1, B2, A, D, E and K), minerals (especially iron and copper), amino acids that form proteins, glycogen for glucose and cholesterol, and fatty acids required for many cell functions. So, the liver often needs a rest from the likes and dislikes of alcohol and sugary or fatty foods.

Digestion: Bile acids are produced in the liver, then concentrated and stored in the gall bladder to be released when the body needs to digest fat. If your liver doesn't work properly, your digestive system will struggle with fats. You miss out on the fat-soluble vitamins A, D, E and K, which can only be absorbed by the body if they're dissolved in fat first.

Immune Support: Almost a quarter of the cells in the liver are Kupffer cells, which specifically assist the immune system. Kupffer cells engulf dead or damaged cells, break down old red blood cells and help recycle the iron from haemoglobin.

Detoxification: The liver is the body's great detoxifier. To do its job properly, the liver must convert some of its fat-soluble toxic substances into a water-soluble form that can thus be excreted by the kidney. It depends on proteins, water, vitamins, and minerals to achieve this. If it doesn't, toxic substances fail to get neutralised and can end up harming the cells. Protect it with berries, garlic, beetroot, water, green tea, fibre, probiotics and coffee.

TOXINS TO AVOID

Drugs: Paracetamol otherwise known as Panadol or Tylenol is toxic when taken a dose higher than 200mg/kg over a 24-hour period. More than 8 tablets per day is toxic. These drugs deplete the production of the potent antioxidant glutathione (GSH) and the antidote N-acetylcysteine to replenish the GSH stores and protect against liver poisoning.

Alcohol: Your body typically processes about 170 to 240 grams of alcohol daily. For a 70 kg individual, this translates to roughly 7 grams per hour, or one drink per hour. Consuming around 200 grams of ethanol per day puts you in the 'alcoholic' category. Alcohol is eliminated through breath and liver metabolism. The body prioritises the metabolism of alcohol calories over proteins, fats, and carbs. Alcohol absorption is faster on an empty stomach, but food and antacids can slow it down by inhibiting liver enzymes.

Women tend to eliminate alcohol slightly faster than men due to higher liver volume per lean body mass. However, women may reach higher blood alcohol levels than men with the same alcohol intake due to lower body water content. Additionally, women have fewer alcohol-metabolising enzymes, especially when premenstrual, as the liver focuses on breaking down excess hormones.

Pesticides and Heavy Metals: Pesticides are metabolised in the liver and may have a carcinogenic effect. The liver also metabolises heavy metals and excretes them in the bile. The exposure of lead, cadmium and mercury have been shown to increase liver enzyme markers and liver injury.

NON-ALCOHOLIC FATTY LIVER DISEASE (NAFLD)

Non-alcoholic fatty liver disease develops when people who don't necessarily drink much alcohol, but store too much fat in the liver. The fat gets laid down abnormally in the liver cells because the body can't cope with the excess calories. Insulin resistance, high blood pressure, high abdominal (visceral) fat and high blood triglycerides go hand in hand with NAFLD.

It's a relatively new diagnosis but an increasingly common one, especially among middle-aged, obese women. It is now the most common cause of liver disease in the world. The main cause of death in those with NAFLD is coronary heart disease. Around 80% of people with chronic heart failure have liver disease. The diagnosis is made with blood tests for liver function, an abdominal ultrasound, a CT scan and/or MRI scan. 20–30% of cases with NAFLD progress to liver scarring which blocks/impairs blood flow compromising the detoxification processes and causing a more severe condition – non-alcoholic steatohepatitis (NASH).

Fructose, A Major Cause Of NAFL: Table sugar is 50% fructose and 50% glucose. The problem with fructose is that it enables you to accumulate fat in the liver, as well as blocking its conversion to energy. An interesting study by Schwarz (2015) showed that in just nine days, a high-fructose intake resulted in an increase of liver fat in healthy men who otherwise had a normal diet. Avoid these high fructose foods:

- Corn syrup, honey, maple syrup, agave and molasses.
- Apples, mangos, pears, watermelon and peaches.
- Dried fruit – figs, dates and raisins.
- Cakes and biscuits.

NON-ALCOHOLIC STEATOHEPATITIS (NASH)

The early symptoms of NAFLD may not be noticeable but as the disease progresses to NASH you may experience abdominal swelling, nausea, vomiting and/or diarrhoea, and jaundice with yellowing of the skin and the whites of the eyes. Urine may turn a darker colour, and you may become confused. If left untreated, the consequences can be cirrhosis, liver failure or liver cancer, as another chemical or a viral infection can further damage an already vulnerable liver.

Managing NASH

- Avoid any medications that harm the liver. Paracetamol, Dilantin and anti-cholesterol drugs.
- Avoid all alcohol.
- Reduce total cholesterol level.
- Aim for a healthy body mass index (BMI) or reduce weight by 10% of your body weight.
- Control blood sugars and avoid high-fructose and sweetened foods.
- Exercise regularly.
- Consume plenty of water.
- Increase high-fibre foods.
- Drink green tea.
- Use the Mediterranean diet, including beetroot, garlic and probiotics.
- Use yoga and deep-breathing exercises to massage the liver.

SUPPORTING THE LIVER

Physical support: Massage the liver and abdominal organs via yoga, tai chi, Pilates and deep breathing. If all this seems too hard, try 10 deep breaths 3 times a day.

Bioenergetic support: Try acupuncture. Activate the Liver 3 point, located on the top of the feet about 3 cm behind where the big toe and the second toe meet (? tender point there). If not acupuncture, give the area a good massage for just three minutes daily. The liver meridian pathways extend around the Liver 3 points, up the front of the legs and abdomen to the liver area.

Support the Liver Biochemically

Vitamins and Minerals	Useful Herbs and Foods
Avoid deficiencies in vitamins A, D, E and K and B. **Zinc:** Helps metabolise alcohol and protein. **Selenium:** Important in detoxification. **L-carnitine:** Helps transport fatty acids. **Alpha lipoic acid:** Protects against liver damage. **Probiotics and prebiotics:** Helps reduce the overgrowth of harmful bacteria in the gut that can produce ammonia as a byproduct of their metabolism the ammonia load.	**Milk thistle:** Helps reduce inflammation and fibrosis. **Artichokes:** Contain chlorogenic acid that inhibits proliferation of liver cancer cells. **Berberine:** Helps regulate glucose and fat metabolism. **Turmeric:** Helps detoxification and is an anti-oxidant. **Dandelion:** Protects against liver damage. **Gogi berry:** Anti-cancer effects.

LOVE YOUR LIVER

ACTION PLAN – CHECKLIST

- Check liver function via blood tests regularly.
- Avoid alcohol and drugs.
- Treat other conditions: hyperlipidaemia, insulin resistance and diabetes.
- Avoid high-fructose foods.
- Modify lifestyle with diet and exercise.
- Aim for an ideal body weight or reduce body weight by at least 3% to 5%.
- Use antioxidants and specific nutrients/herbs to support the liver.

References:

Friedman, S. L., Neuschwander-Tetri, B. A., Rinella, & M., & Sanyal, A. J. (2018). Mechanisms of NAFLD development and therapeutic strategies. *Nature Medicine*, *24*(7), 908–922. https://doi.org/10.1038/s41591-018-0104-9

Schwarz, J. M., Noworolski, S. M., Wen, M. J., Dyachenko, A., Prior, J. L., Weinberg, M. E., Herraiz, L. A., Tai, V. W., Bergeron, N., Bersot, T. P., Rao, M. N., Schambelan, M., & Mulligan, K. (2015). Effect of a High-Fructose Weight-Maintaining Diet on Lipogenesis and Liver Fat. *The Journal of clinical endocrinology and metabolism*, *100*(6), 2434–2442. https://doi.org/10.1210/jc.2014-3678

Chapter 29

OBESITY IS MOSTLY ABOUT SUGAR

"Over the long term, people who consume even a single diet soft drink daily are more likely to suffer from diabetes, hypertension, stroke and cardiovascular disease".

SUSAN SWITHERS

In Australia, around 31% of adults are carrying extra weight around their waistlines, while about 25% of kids are anything but "snack-sized." In the USA, a hefty 42.4% of adults are grappling with weight issues while in the UK, 28% of adults fall into the obese category, with another 36% teetering on the edge. Canada sees approximately 27% of adults dealing with weight concerns, while across Europe, obesity rates range from 10% to 30% in different countries, offering a variety of statistics. However, in

Japan, where portion sizes are modest and diets include fresh fish and green tea, only a tiny 4% struggle with obesity, showing the power of healthy eating habits.

So, we've got a problem in the west with too much food and not much activity. Poor food choices are implicated in so many diseases. When our fat cells get too big, they don't just store extra energy from food, they also affect with our hormones, appetite, and other body functions. This can lead to inflammation and scarring, making us more vulnerable to all sorts of health issues. According to Diabetes Australia, a healthy waist size is under 80 cm for women and under 94 cm for men, at least, these are the goals. But half of us aren't hitting that mark. Over the past 25 years, the average waist size has shot up by over 10 cm for men and 7 cm for women. Despite decades of trying to cut back on fat, we're still getting bigger and sicker. Sugar is finally getting the blame it deserves for driving obesity worldwide. It's taken a while for the truth to come out, which hasn't exactly helped people trust those making health recommendations. But it's not the whole story.

SUGAR vs FAT

Almost half a century ago, one brave physiologist, Professor John Yudkin, founder and head of the Department of Nutrition at Queen Elizabeth College in the University of London, published the classic book *Pure, White and Deadly*. His research identified correlations between sugar consumption and obesity, tooth decay, heart disease, gout and diabetes. His work put him into immediate and bitter conflict with key figures in the medical establishment of the time – most notably, US physiologist Dr Ancel Keys.

Keys believed consumption of saturated fats was behind the rising rates of heart disease. While he published widely, promoting the Mediterranean diet and espousing the health benefits of unsaturated fats such as olive oil, nuts and seeds, there was no mention of the overconsumption of sugars. The American Heart Association had embraced Keys' thinking, denouncing foods high in saturated fats such as butter, lard, eggs and beef for their contribution to heart disease. At one point, the Association's president predicted that atherosclerosis (hardening of the arteries) could be conquered by the year 2000 if low-fat diets were adopted.

Keys was bitter in his attacks on Yudkin. The food industry supported Keys and joined his efforts to discredit Yudkin. American journalist Gary Taubes has written at length on the medico-political history of this misguided focus on fats, and his book *The Case Against Sugar* is well worth a read. It wasn't until around 2014 that major medical journals began questioning the fat-focused ideology, with the American Medical Association publishing a paper suggesting that added sugar significantly increased heart disease death rates. All of which, leaves us now with an obesity epidemic.

FACTORS IN WEIGHT MANAGEMENT

To maintain your weight, the energy you consume should match what you burn through activity. Your diet affects energy intake, while your activity levels mostly determine how much energy you burn. However, the weight management story gets a tad more complicated.

To lose weight and keep it off, you'll need to commit to lasting changes in your diet and activity levels. Once you reach your goal weight, your smaller body will need fewer calories, so adjust your meals accordingly. Cutting out snacks between meals can lower insulin levels, promoting fat burning.

Body shape, hormones, genetics, and gut microbes influence weight. While genetics affect body shape, you can work on achieving a leaner frame. We find that the deep visceral fat which gives the 'pot belly' appearance; it is more dangerous than the upper subcutaneous fat as it releases more of the inflammatory molecules. This fat type is a serious risk factor for diseases such as diabetes, heart disease and stroke.

High-carbohydrate diets accumulate this type of fat, but genetics, stress and hormones complicate the process.

Insulin: This hormone is intimately involved in sugar metabolism. When sugar levels rise insulin levels also rise promoting fat storage.

Glucagon: This hormone is also produced in the pancreas and released into the bloodstream. It guards against very low blood sugars; glucagon works to increase blood sugar levels by triggering the breakdown of glycogen (stored glucose) in the liver into glucose, which is then released into the bloodstream.

Glucagon-like peptide-1 (GLP-1) is a hormone produced in the small intestine in response to food intake. This hormone is the target of the new drugs on the market that are effective in diabetes and weight management. GLP-1 is especially responsive to carbohydrates and fats, as well as other stimuli such as oral glucose ingestion, gastric distension and incretin hormones in the gut. Its role is to regulate blood sugar levels by stimulating insulin secretion and inhibiting glucagon secretion, which helps lower blood glucose levels after meals. GLP-1 also slows down gastric emptying, reduces appetite, and promotes satiety, contributing to weight loss. New drugs Ozempic (semaglutide) primarily targets the glucagon-like peptide-1 (GLP-1) receptor rather than glucagon itself. As a GLP-1 receptor agonist, Ozempic mimics the action of GLP-1, for its role in regulating blood sugar levels, appetite, and digestion.

Ghrelin is produced in the stomach when it is empty. Ghrelin communicates with the brain to let it know you want more food – the higher the ghrelin levels, the more you want to eat.

Leptin is a hormone produced in fat cells and the stomach. The job of leptin is to stop you feeling hungry. It communicates with the brain about appetite and meal satisfaction. Mostly the chat between leptin and the brain is about wanting to stop storing fat. But too much fat produces large numbers of inflammatory chemicals and blocks the positive health effects of leptin on appetite suppression. Also, high fructose foods suppress leptin release.

Melatonin rises in the brain in response to darkness, reduced levels occur with diabetes, ageing and pain. But poor sleep also increases the ghrelin levels and increases appetite.

OBESITY MANAGEMENT: DRUGS, SURGERY AND DIET

Bariatric surgery, including procedures like sleeve gastrectomy and gastric bypass, is celebrated as the gold standard for tackling obesity, offering significant weight loss and various health perks.

Sleeve Gastrectomy: This surgery removes a portion of the stomach, leaving a smaller, banana-shaped pouch. Patients feel full faster, leading to less food intake and substantial weight loss—usually around 20-30% of initial body weight, equivalent to shedding about 30-50kg.

Gastric Bypass: Here, a small stomach pouch is made, and the small intestine is rerouted to bypass part of the stomach and intestines. This leads to less food intake and nutrient absorption, resulting in considerable weight loss—typically a 50-80% reduction in initial body weight.

New Drugs: GLP-1 agonist medications have gained attention for their potential in weight loss. The craze for these drugs caused world wide shortage in 2023. Ozempic (semaglutide) mimics the action of GLP-1, in its role regulating blood sugar levels, appetite, and digestion.

- Ozempic (Semaglutide): Originally designed for type 2 diabetes, Ozempic (injection) is now approved for weight management under the name Wegovy. Trials have shown impressive results, with an average loss of 14.6% of initial body weight.

- Mounjaro: It is the brand name for a different drug called tirzepatide. This drug activates two receptors at the same time. It's a 'dual-agonist (glucagon-like peptide-1 (GLP-1) and glucose-dependent insulinotropic polypeptide (GIP)). It works in similar ways to reduce appetite and participants lost up to 20% of their weight.

Drugs vs Surgery (Ozempic vs. Bariatric Surgery): While medications like Ozempic aid in weight loss, they fall short compared to bariatric surgery outcomes. Sleeve gastrectomy and gastric bypass result in significantly greater weight loss—2-3 times more on average than Ozempic users. Additionally, bariatric surgery offers substantial health perks, including reduced mortality and resolution of obesity-related conditions like type 2 diabetes, outcomes not yet proven with medications alone.

Risks and Side Effects: While Ozempic may cause temporary side effects like nausea and vomiting, its long-term safety in weight management needs further research. Bariatric surgery carries risks like reflux symptoms and nutritional deficiencies, but advances in techniques have lowered associated mortality rates significantly, with manageable risks through proper care and supplementation.

Cost: Bariatric surgery ranging from $15,000 to $25,000. Ozempic Ozempic is available in prefilled pens containing a certain number of doses, such as 1.0 mg/0.5 mL or 0.5 mg/0.25 mL. The cost per pen can range from approximately AUD $100 to $150 or $7.30 for Concession Cardholders.

It's also worth noting that while medications and surgeries can aid weight loss, maintaining a healthy diet remains crucial for overall well-being. High fat mass increases inflammation spiraling into a whole range of diseases and disabilities.

THE MATHS OF WEIGHT MANAGEMENT: ENERGY OUTPUT VERSUS INTAKE

First, look at energy out: Here's the thing, you need to do sixty minutes a day of moderate/intense exercise to achieve any significant weight loss. Add calorie restriction to an exercise regimen and the loss a kilogram per week is possible, versus the 0.2 kg loss with just exercise alone. Put simply, exercise will *not* supplement a bad diet. Resistance training (also known as strength training or weight-bearing exercise) can help you build muscle, which in turn burns more energy. One kilogram of muscle will burn about 60 to 100 calories (equal to a thick slice of bread) per day. See Chapter 33, Exercise More.

Second, let's look at 'energy in': There's no single weight-loss diet that works best for everyone, but your chances of success will be higher if you start with realistic goals and a sensible mindset. **Calories from whatever source add to the total.** Don't choose a diet that drastically limits calorie intake or cuts out whole food groups if, for example, you're sick or pregnant. With those caveats in mind, here are a few different trendy diet options on the go:

Reduced Energy Diet: This plan lowers calorie intake to 800-1200 calories per day. You might want a dietitian or nutritionist to help initially. It involves ongoing monitoring, smaller goals, and motivational strategies.

Very Low-Energy Diet: This strict diet limits intake to only 800 calories per day, often achieved through nutritionally complete low-calorie shakes. It's for short-term use for those significantly overweight, and guarantees weight loss of 1.5-2.5 kg per week.

Keto or Low-Carb Diet (Atkins Diet): These diets restrict carbohydrates to about 5%, focusing on fats and proteins for energy. They're effective for weight loss but may lead to constipation from lack of fibre and bad breath due to ketosis.

Low Glycaemic Index (GI) Diet: This plan avoids refined carbohydrates and emphasizes protein and fiber to stabilize blood sugars and reduce snacking.

5:2 Diet: Also known as the Fast diet, it involves normal eating for five days and reduced calorie intake (25% of normal intake) for two non-consecutive days per week.

Time-Restricted Feeding: Meals are consumed within a 6–8-hour window each day, with fasting for the remaining hours, aiming to burn body fat and improve blood sugars.

Mediterranean Diet: Prioritising whole-plant foods like fruits, vegetables, whole grains, beans, and nuts, this diet is sustainable for weight loss and promotes heart and brain health.

Paleo Diet: This diet restricts carbohydrates and processed foods while permitting meats, eggs, nuts, and most vegetables.

Stop snacking: Snacking will not help weight loss. It might help keep your blood sugars in check if the food portion is small and low glycaemic, but it will do little to alter the numbers on the scales. **High insulin secretions (when we eat carbs) stop fat breakdown.** The idea is to let the insulin go down for long enough so that the fat breaks down. Remember, no fat breakdown, no fat loss.

The 'energy in, energy out' equation is a good starting point for weight loss, but not the whole story. It's complicated by differences in how macronutrients – carbohydrates, protein, fat and alcohol – behave when metabolised. It's worth understanding what each of these macronutrients do, and how they behave in the body.

THE ROLE OF THE MACRONUTRIENTS

The Energy Content in Food Per Gram

Food	Calories per gram	Kilojoules (kJ) per gram
Fat	9	37
Protein	4	17
Carbohydrate	4	17
Alcohol	7	29

Alcohol: It provides calories but not much else apart from a headache. Your body tries to ditch it ASAP because, let's face it, it's not the healthiest option. One glass of wine? That's like 40 minutes of brisk walking down the drain!

Proteins: Found in fish, meat, eggs, and more. They're the building blocks of our body, supporting everything from hormones to immunity. Aim for about a gram per kilogram of body weight, more if you're still growing.

Fats: Don't fear them, but don't overdo it either. They're like the multitaskers of nutrition, fueling your brain, boosting immunity, and helping absorb important vitamins. Focus on quality over quantity. Switching to healthier fats pays off big time for your health in the long run. And when it comes to fats, there's a good and bad side and understanding them can make your brain sore.

There are two main types of fats: saturated and unsaturated - monounsaturated, polyunsaturated and then the trans-unsaturated. Most animal fats are saturated, and most fish and plants are unsaturated. There is a mix of both saturated and unsaturated fats in many foods, animals and fish have a percentage of different types as per the graph below. Animal fats are usually solid at room temperature while unsaturated fats from plants are usually liquid. Fats are generally best in their raw state, their chemical composition can change for the worse if they're stored poorly, overheated, or overly processed. Your body can make its own saturated and monounsaturated fatty acids without help from your diet.

Fat Comparison per 100 gram

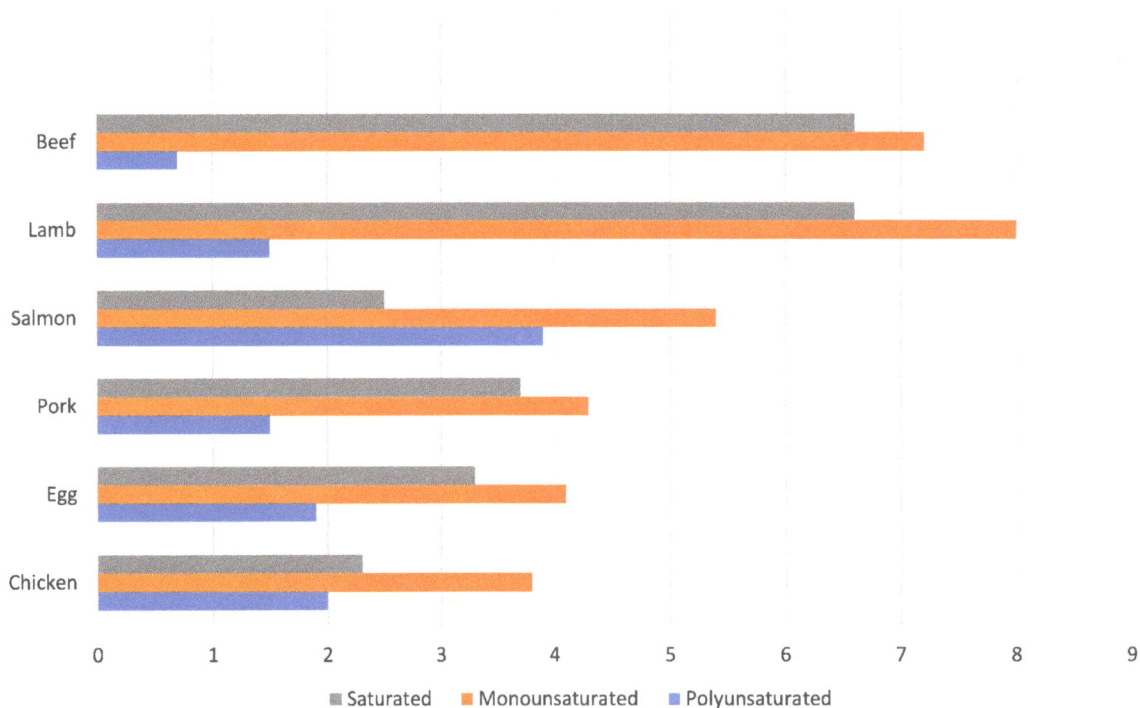

Horizontal bar chart comparing Saturated, Monounsaturated, and Polyunsaturated fats per 100 gram for Beef, Lamb, Salmon, Pork, Egg, and Chicken.

Saturated fats offer fewer health benefits than either the mono- or polyunsaturated fats. They are in dairy and meats that contain other useful nutrients. Grass fed cattle have about double the quantity of polyunsaturated fat than grain fed cattle (up to 1.0 g vs 0.4g per 100g). As you can see from our chart, fish and red/white meats, and eggs have varying types of fats.

Trans fats are unsaturated fats that have undergone a process called hydrogenation, the process is being used in food production to improve shelf life and texture. They are in fried foods, margarine, baked goods, and snacks. Unlike other types of fats, **trans fats have been strongly linked to heart disease, stroke, and inflammation.**

Monounsaturated fats: These are sourced from extra virgin olive oil, avocados, cashews, macadamias, hazelnuts, pecans, peanuts, pistachios, grapeseed, and sunflower, sesame and pumpkin seeds. Monounsaturated and polyunsaturated fats are better than saturated fats, and all are better than trans fats. Virgin pressed olive oil has been shown to significantly reduce the risk of death and illness from cardiovascular disease. The more processed forms don't have the same effects. Buy it in small quantities and store it in a dark bottle away from light.

Polyunsaturated fats: **These can't be made by your body, so must come exclusively from your diet.** They have important structural and physiological functions. They are sensitive to heat, light, and oxygen, making them prone to oxidation when exposed to high temperatures during cooking. The two main types contain omega-3 and omega-6 fatty acids:

- **Omega-3 fats** are found in fish, especially cold-water species such as salmon and mackerel. They have anti-inflammatory properties and protect against heart disease, diabetes and autoimmune diseases.

- **Omega-6 fats,** found in flaxseed oil, canola oil and walnuts, lower 'bad' low-density cholesterol (LDL), raise 'good' high-density cholesterol (HDL), and improve insulin sensitivity. The omega-3 type fats have higher anti-inflammatory capacity compared to omega-6 fatty acids, but foods high in omega-6 fats are particularly important if you're a vegetarian and don't eat fish. We have compiled the graph below showing the omega content of different oils.

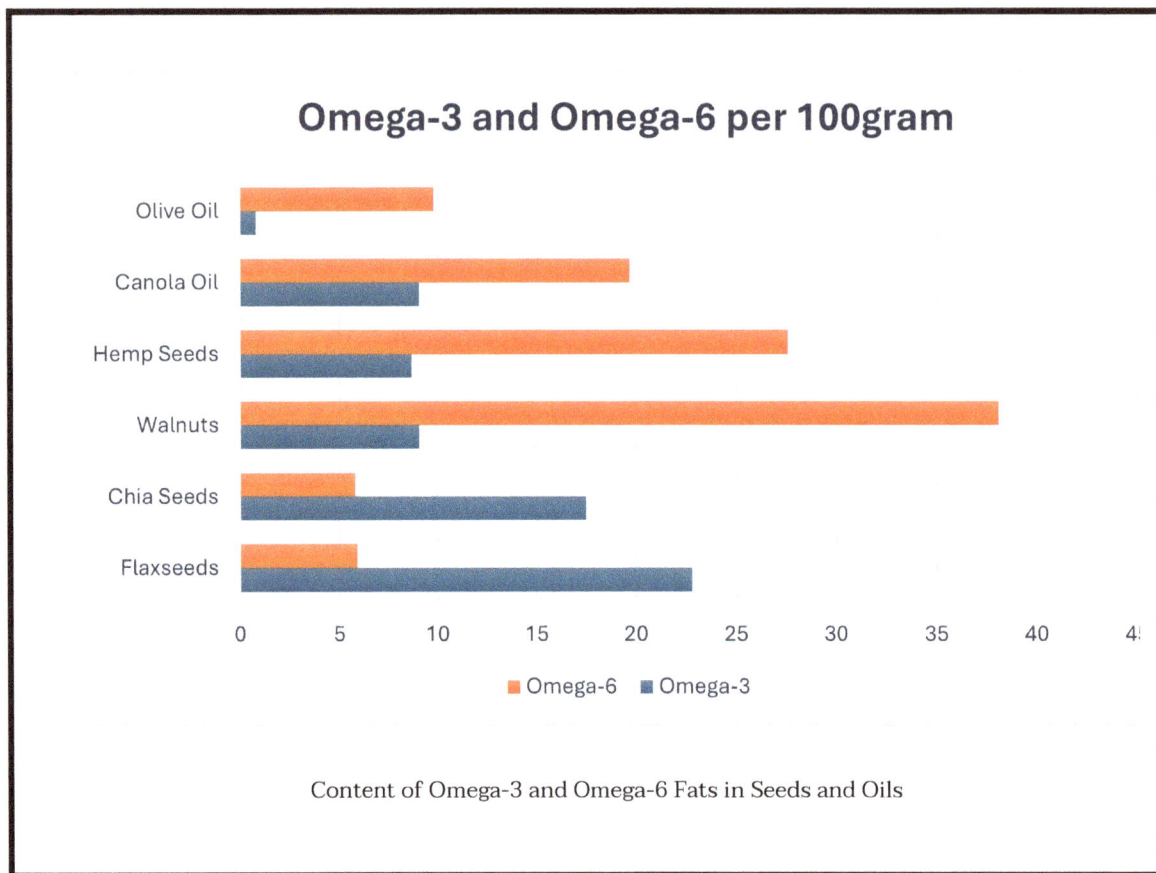

Omega-3 and Omega-6 per 100gram

Content of Omega-3 and Omega-6 Fats in Seeds and Oils

Carbohydrates: From fruits, grains, vegetables and processed sweet foods are the body's go-to source of fuel for energy. An adult can store 500-600g of carbohydrate as glycogen for energy in the muscles and liver.

Simple carbohydrates such as glucose, fructose, sucrose (table sugar) and lactose (sugar in milk) are made up of just one or two molecules. They break down easily and may cause peaks and troughs compromising blood sugar control.

Complex carbohydrates are higher in fibre and contain three or more glucose molecules, being found in beans, legumes, oats and corn. These molecules break down slowly and release their glucose gradually so you can maintain a steady flow of energy to the cells and avoid the sugar highs and lows associated with simple carbohydrates.

The Problem with Fructose: The liver is the only organ that can metabolise fructose and when large quantities are consumed excess is stored as fat. It is used widely in the food industry to make foods sweeter and occurs naturally in many fresh fruits, dried fruits and honey. High intake of fructose causes inflammation of the liver and plays a key role in fatty liver disease, but it also generates uric acid crystals that cause the painful joints of gout.

Is sugar addictive? Yes indeed. Sugar activates addictive drug-like receptors in both animals and humans. The taste of sugar sends signals to the brain which in turn signals the release of the neurotransmitter dopamine. Dopamine gives us a sense of gratification and reward whereby we would want to seek out that second slice of cake. Which all goes to show why we should never have had that first piece of cake!

On the other hand, sugar and other carbohydrates that raise blood sugars moderately seem to temporarily improve cognitive performance, memory, and reaction time - which might help your exam skills!

ARTIFICIAL SWEETENERS

If artificial sweeteners are the answer to your sugar cravings, you are on the wrong diet. Artificial sweeteners are controversial – first because of some toxicity, and second because of emerging evidence that they cause the very problems they are supposed to avoid (for example, diabetes and weight gain).

Sweetener	%Sweeter than Sugar	Sweetener	% Sweeter than Sugar
Sucralose	600%	Acesulfame K	200%
Saccharin	300–500%	Aspartame	200%
Mogrosides - (monk fruit)	300%	Glycyrrhizin -(from liquorice)	50%
Stevia	250%	Sodium cyclamate	30–50%
Xylitol	1.0%		

The most common sweeteners used to reduce our calorie counts are saccharin, sucralose, cyclamate, and stevia. Some are used in diabetic lollies. They are used world-wide in the food industry as well as in pharmaceuticals. They taste up to six hundred times as sweet as sugar – and that's part of the problem, since their intensity make them more addictive. Artificial sweeteners have been implicated in a range of health problems, including metabolic syndrome, type 2 diabetes and heart disease. Saccharin, sucralose and aspartame change the function and composition of gut bacteria and cause a rise in blood sugar - not a good idea!

OBESITY IS MOSTLY ABOUT SUGAR

ACTION PLAN – CHECKLIST

- Choose whole fresh foods from the Mediterranean diet as preference.
- Avoid foods cooked at high temperatures.
- Stop snacking.
- Reduce alcohol to one drink a day.
- Avoid high-fructose foods and low-calorie (diet) drinks.
- Exercise 30–60 minutes daily.

References:

Australian Bureau of Statistics. (2016). *Australian Health Survey: Consumption of added sugars, 2011-12*. https://www.abs.gov.au/ausstats/abs@.nsf/Lookup/4364.0.55.011main+features12011-12

Droulez, V., Williams, P. G., Levy, G., Stobaus, T., & Sinclair, A. (2006). *Composition of Australian red meat 2002. Fatty acid profile*. https://ro.uow.edu.au/hbspapers/1

Forouhi, N. G., Krauss, R. M., Taubes, G., & Willett, W. (2018). Dietary fat and cardio-metabolic health: evidence, controversies, and consensus for guidance *The BMJ*, *361*, Article k2139.

Sacks, F. M., Lichtenstein, A. H., Wu, J. H. Y., Appel, L. J., Creager, M. A., Kris-Etherton, P. M., Miller, M., Rimm, E. B., Rudel, L. L., Robinson, J. G., Stone, N. J., Van Horn, L. V., & American Heart Association (2017). Dietary Fats and Cardiovascular Disease:

A Presidential Advisory From the American Heart Association. *Circulation*, *136*(3), e1–e23. https://doi.org/10.1161/CIR.0000000000000510

Sifferlin, A. (2017). Artificial Sweeteners are Linked to Weight gain – Not Weight Loss. *Time*. https://time.com/4859012/artificial-sweeteners-weight-loss/

Strobel, C., Jahreis, G., & Kuhnt, K. Survey of *n*- 3 and *n*-6 polyunsaturated fatty acids in fish and fish products. *Lipids in Health and Disease*, *11*, 144(2012). https://doi.org/10.1186/1476-511X-11-144

Swithers, S. E. (2016). Not-so-healthy sugar substitutes? *Current Opinion in Behavioral Sciences*, *9*, 106–110. https://doi.org/10.1016/j.cobeha.2016.03.003

Taubes, G. (2017). *The Case Against Sugar*. Granta Books.

Yudkin, J. (2012). *Pure, White and Deadly* (3rd ed.). Penguin Books

Chapter 30

EAT LIKE A GREEK

"You don't need a silver fork to eat good food."

PAUL PRUDHOMME

The Mediterranean diet has been around long enough to prove its worth. This is based on the traditional cuisines of southern Europe that are among the healthiest (and tastiest) in the world. Not everyone in the Mediterranean eats the same way, but they generally have whole foods, less meat and more fish and lentils - to put it in a nutshell!

The Mediterranean diet is good for your waist and even better for your heart and your blood sugars. According to five randomised controlled studies (Romagnolo, 2017), it can reduce the risk of cardiac events by between 30 and 78%!

THE DIET

Lunch, not dinner, is the main meal of the day in Mediterranean countries – a custom worth considering. That allows you to use the energy provided over the rest of the day, and you don't go to bed with high blood sugars and reflux!

There is plenty of evidence to conclude that the Mediterranean diet guards against inflammation and chronic disease. Specifically, olive oil has been shown to reduce low density and increase high density lipoproteins which have positive effects on cardiac risk factors like obesity and high blood pressure.

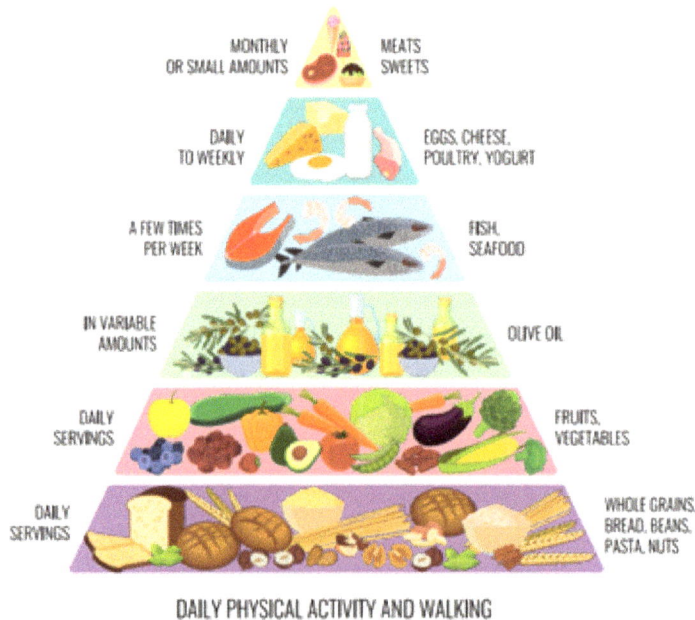

MONTHLY OR SMALL AMOUNTS — MEATS SWEETS

DAILY TO WEEKLY — EGGS, CHEESE, POULTRY, YOGURT

A FEW TIMES PER WEEK — FISH, SEAFOOD

IN VARIABLE AMOUNTS — OLIVE OIL

DAILY SERVINGS — FRUITS, VEGETABLES

DAILY SERVINGS — WHOLE GRAINS, BREAD, BEANS, PASTA, NUTS

DAILY PHYSICAL ACTIVITY AND WALKING

Mediterranean Diet Pyramid

Here is the Shopping List for Your Pantry

1. **Extra Virgin Olive Oil**: The cornerstone of Mediterranean cooking for maximum flavor and health benefits.
2. **Fish**: Choose varieties like salmon, sardines, tuna, or mackerel for a dose of heart-healthy omega-3 fatty acids.
3. **Poultry**: Chicken and turkey are versatile lean proteins perfect for Mediterranean-inspired dishes.
4. **Legumes**: Beans, lentils, and chickpeas add protein, fiber, and texture to soups, salads, and stews.
5. **Eggs**: A versatile and affordable protein option for breakfast, lunch, or dinner.
6. **Nuts and Seeds**: Almonds, walnuts, sunflower seeds, and pumpkin seeds are great for snacking or adding crunch to salads and yogurt.
7. **Whole Grains**: Quinoa, bulgur, farro, and whole wheat couscous are nutritious alternatives to refined grains.
8. **Fresh Vegetables**: Load up on colorful veggies like tomatoes, cucumbers, bell peppers, spinach, kale, and zucchini.
9. **Fresh Herbs**: Basil, oregano, parsley, cilantro, curcumin, and mint add fragrance and flavor to Mediterranean dishes.
10. **Fruits**: Seasonal fruits like oranges, lemons, berries, figs, and grapes for a sweet and refreshing treat.
11. **Greek Yogurt**: Creamy and rich in protein, Greek yogurt is a staple for breakfast or as a creamy topping.
12. **Cheese**: Feta cheese is a classic Mediterranean choice, but you can also explore other varieties like ricotta or Parmesan in moderation. Gouda, Brie, Edam, Jarlsberg, Emmental contains Vitamin K2.
13. **Olives**: Whether green or black, olives add briny flavor and healthy fats to salads, pasta dishes, and appetizers.
14. **Whole Grain Bread**: Look for hearty whole grain bread or pita bread to pair with dips, salads, or grilled meats.

By the time you have bought the goods and loaded the shopping trolley you have completed several thousand steps. So time for a siesta followed by a brisk 3km walk around the block before heading home for a glass of red wine. Enjoy some whole grain bread with a drizzle of extra virgin olive oil, top it off with some herbs, vegetable sticks, olives, grapes and feta cheese on a platter or serving board. Welcome to the good life!

EAT LIKE A GREEK

ACTION PLAN – CHECKLIST

- Shop for whole foods and whole grains, fresh fruit and vegetables.
- Use virgin pressed olive oil.
- Include fish, lentils mostly and meat every two weeks.
- Add spice, nuts and seeds.
- Drink red wine in moderation.
- Consume main meal in the mid day.
- Exercise daily.

References:

Davis, C., Bryan, J., Hodgson, J., & Murphy, K. (2015). Definition of the Mediterranean Diet; a Literature Review. *Nutrients*, *7*(11), 9139–9153. https://doi.org/10.3390/nu7115459

Romagnolo, D. F., & Selmin, O. I. (2017). Mediterranean Diet and Prevention of Chronic Diseases. *Nutrition Today*, *52*(5), 208–222. https://doi.org/10.1097/NT.0000000000000228

Chapter 31

STRESS LESS AND ADRENAL FATIGUE

"You don't develop courage by being happy in your relationships every day. You develop it by surviving difficult times and challenging adversity."

HERACLITUS

(PHILOSOPHER OF THE 4TH CENTURY BC)

Technology is changing the global workforce. The COVID-19 pandemic and the introduction of artificial intelligence (AI) has cemented the need for flexible working hours, satellite offices and the upskilling or reskilling of employees. According to Gallup (2023), some 50% of Australian, US and Canadian employees are feeling stress at work post COVID while the global average of workers' stress is 44%.

Individuals respond differently to stress. Our reactions depend on a variety of factors including our health, age, experience, coping abilities and support systems. Sometimes stress overwhelms our ability to cope: a death in the family, a relationship breakdown, COVID-19 lockdowns, the loss of a job or other financial disasters can be all too much. Times of great change – e.g. moving country or even moving house – can also test our innate resilience. Stress has its uses, but it has a price too.

THE PRICE OF STRESS

Work stress is a global issue and the price of stress refers to the economic and societal costs associated with stress-related health problems and productivity loss. Business Email Compromise (BEC) scams, where attackers impersonate company executives to trick employees into transferring funds or sensitive information, have resulted in billions of dollars in losses worldwide. The FBI's Internet Crime Complaint Center (IC3) reported BEC losses exceeding $1.8 billion in 2020 alone.

Back in Australia and according to Medibank Private and Workplace Health (Australia) the price of stress is nearly $15 billion, with 3.2 days lost per worker in a population just under 26million people. More than one-third of employees believe their job is harming their health. Phishing attacks, where fraudulent emails or websites deceive individuals into revealing personal or financial information, have also led to significant financial losses for businesses. Better technology and better cyber security are integral to business.

Aside all of the above stress has its uses. Stress isn't all doom and gloom. In small doses, it's a boost for your brain. While your adrenal glands release the hormones cortisol and adrenaline you are suddenly sharper, more alert, and ready to tackle anything. Moderate stress levels can actually boost cognitive function. Resulting in improved memory, better attention span, and increased productivity. Cellular energy is pumped up, the adrenal glands work hard, and all the gut-brain connections fire up. The problems arise when stress is maintained over a long period.

Watch for Early Signs of Stress

General Wellbeing	Infections, headaches, shallow breathing, racing heart, low libido, back pain, gut symptoms, grinding teeth, aches, pains, and fatigue.
Emotional	Worrying, crying, pessimism, depressed, over-whelmed, short-tempered, losing touch, and withdrawing socially, suffering panic attacks or nervous breakdowns.
Neurological	Experiencing tension headaches/migraines, phobias, muscle tension or weakness, altering perception of pain, 'brain fog' or chronic insomnia.
Respiratory	Feeling breathless and asthmatic.
Gastrointestinal	Suffering indigestion, nausea, reflux, difficulty swallowing, altered bowel habits, irritable bowel syndrome, gut pain, ulcers.
Cardiovascular	Recording rises in heart rate and blood pressure.
Metabolic	Rising blood sugar levels and weight gain or weight loss.
Immunological	Prone to upper respiratory tract infections, colds and flu, cold sores, dry eyes, joint aches and pains and allergies.

Hormonal	Losing sex drive due to low testosterone and other sex hormones, with raised or lowered adrenal hormone output.
Lifestyle	Drinking more, smoking, taking drugs and showing less care for self.

Unfortunately, if stress is maintained over the long term, the mitochondria and adrenal glands respond. Health suffers, relationships are strained, and life may become joyless. Long-term negative stress lowers resistance to illness, accelerates ageing, increases blood sugars, and disrupts our hormonal processes. The hit to your quality of life is bad enough, but stress can also affect *quantity* of life. Of ten leading causes of death, stress has been directly implicated in five: cardiovascular diseases, stroke, musculoskeletal disorders, suicide/homicide, and dementia. It has been indirectly associated with metabolic diseases, cancer, liver disease and lung disease.

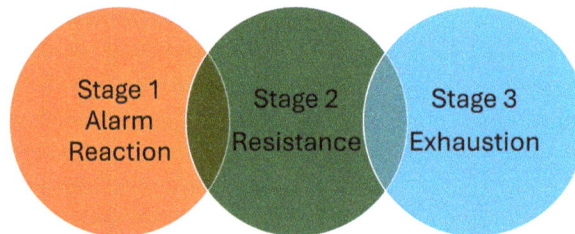

Hans Selye Model For Stress

1. **The alarm phase** triggers a fight-or-flight response. The body is drawn to a constant state of alertness or over-readiness, producing excess adrenaline. Your heart

rate increases and your muscles tense. You become apprehensive and prone to stomach upsets. Poor sleep, poor eating habits, lack of exercise, personal worries (including financial ones) can add to the collective load leading to the resistance phase.

2. **The resistance phase** occurs when the body continues to keep up its defences. Sometimes we show resilience and learn to cope. Other times we mask the symptoms of stress but remain vulnerable. Events such as a death in the family, a marriage breakdown, change of job or house move may undo any resistance, bringing forward the exhaustion phase.

3. **The exhaustion phase** occurs when our capacity to adapt is overwhelmed. Our stress hormones drive down our ability to make our 'happy' chemicals — for example, serotonin and melatonin. We cope poorly with day-to- day matters and we can end up with high blood pressure, insomnia, heartburn, headaches, muscle tension, poor immunity, and/or low sex drive.

STRESS MANAGEMENT TOOLS

Aggressive work performance goals are causing stress in an era of rising inflation and cost of living constraints. Time management in the modern tec world requires modern tools:

1. **Use productivity tools**: Take advantage of technology to streamline your work-flow and stay organised. Utilise tools like task management apps, calendar apps, and project management software to prioritise tasks and track progress.

2. **Prioritise tasks**: Identify the most important and time-sensitive tasks on your to-do list and tackle them first. This will ensure that critical deadlines are met.

3. **Break tasks into smaller steps**: Large projects can feel overwhelming, so break them down into smaller, more manageable tasks. (Swiss cheese effect) Focus on completing one step at a time to maintain momentum and **avoid procrastination.**

4. **Limit distractions**: Minimise interruptions and distractions in the workplace by setting boundaries with colleagues, **turning off non-essential notifications**, and creating a dedicated workspace free from distractions.

5. **Group similar tasks together**: Schedule specific times to respond to emails or make phone calls rather than addressing them sporadically throughout the day.

6. **Set deadlines**: Establish deadlines for tasks and hold yourself accountable for meeting them. Creating a sense of urgency can help you stay motivated and focused on **completing your work in a timely manner.**

7. **Delegate tasks**: Identify tasks that can be delegated to others and **empower your team members** to take on responsibility. Delegating effectively can help distribute workload evenly and free up time for more high-priority tasks.

8. **Take a break**: Avoid burnout by taking short breaks throughout the day to rest and recharge. Stepping away from your work periodically can help improve focus and productivity when you return.

9. **Learn to say "no" without feeling guilty** can help you manage your time more effectively.

10. **Try vagal nerve stimulation.** These exercises have a calming influence on the nervous system and have been commonly used for epilepsy and depression, but they are also useful for stress management. See Chapter 27, When All Else Fails.

11. **Reflect and adjust**: Take time to reflect on your accomplishments and identify areas for improvement. Adjust your time management strategies as needed to optimise productivity and achieve your goals.

12. **Remember, it's okay to ask for help** if you need it. Whether you're reaching out to friends and family or seeking professional guidance, there's no shame in taking care of yourself.

13. **Exercise is good for stress,** but one shouldn't overdo it. It takes about ten minutes of intense exercise or thirty minutes of brisk walking for endorphins to flow. Endorphins can also be triggered without exercise but by touch or massage, socialising (smiling, hugging, kissing or sex) and movements such as swinging and rocking.

MINDFULNESS AND STRESS

Mindfulness based therapies significantly alleviate stress and enhance overall mental health. As mentioned in Chapter 12 mindfulness assists in better emotional control and helps individuals to disengage from negativity and bring a sense of calm to distressing situations. It can assist family members by providing the skills to manage their mental, emotional and social health. The techniques of visualisation, breathing exercises (see Chapter 12) can be included in ten to fifteen minute sessions through the day.

THESE NUTRIENTS ARE SPECIFIC FOR STRESS

- **B vitamins, magnesium, zinc and vitamin C:** Alcohol is a diuretic so that vitamins and minerals may be flushed out in urine, leaving the nervous system and other organs more vulnerable.
- **Omega-3:** Found in fish, omega-3 is linked to better mood, better adaptation to stress and better overall health.
- **Gamma-aminobutyric acid (GABA):** This neurotransmitter may help hypersensitive people who feel overwhelmed by 'brain clutter' and anxiety. Women often become very anxious with depletion of GABA between ages thirty-five and forty. Low GABA is linked to low progesterone hormone levels. See Chapter 14, Women's Hormonal Health.
- **Valerian, Withania and Holy Basil** are herbal remedies traditionally used for anxiety and sleep. Valerian can be taken during the day to treat and prevent anxiety and is often as effective as prescription drugs.
- **St John's Wort:** Recognised as a mild antidepressant, it may be helpful in combatting stress and anxiety. Avoid it if you are already on antidepressants.

· **Rhodiola:** This herb works quickly and can have remarkable anti-stress, anti-fatigue and mood-enhancing effects.

POST-TRAUMATIC STRESS DISORDER (PTSD) & EMDR

Eye Movement Desensitisation and Reprocessing (EMDR) was developed by Francine Shapiro after she herself lost painful memories when she moved her eyes repetitively from side to side. She tested the process on rape, incest and Vietnam War victims and by the 1990s she had set up an EMDR institute. The process is recognised by the American Psychological Association and available on the NHS in Britain. We have found it very helpful for many who have experienced severe traumatic events, and find a marked improvement often achieved in three to four treatments.

During a consultation, the patient recalls a distressing image linked to past trauma while moving their eyes side to side, guided by the therapist's finger. This often triggers emotions and body sensations. The theory suggests trauma resides in the emotional right hemisphere of the brain, bypassing language and logic in the left hemisphere. The eye movements bridge connections between the hemispheres, processing the experience as past rather than present. One theory likens the eye movements to those in REM sleep, integrating recent events into memory.

Patients typically discuss traumatic issues with the therapist, but repetitive discussions can worsen trauma. EMDR therapy, according to the EMDR Institute Inc., resolves post-traumatic stress disorder in 84–90% of single-trauma cases after three ninety-minute sessions. It requires no homework and can be conducted on consecutive days for a swift treatment course, with minor process modifications over time.

STRESS LESS

ACTION PLAN – CHECKLIST

- Watch for early signs of stress-related symptoms.
- Prioritise daily tasks and make a list.
- Manage time-related problems with the 'Swiss cheese' effect.
- Use Mindfulness: visualisation, breathing exercises and meditation.
- Utilise tools: apps, calendar apps, and project management software.
- Prioritise tasks and track progress.
- Get psychological help for major trauma.
- Exercise daily.
- Try eye movement desensitisation and reprocessing (EMDR) for post-traumatic stress disorder.
- Supplement melatonin for sleep.

References:

Picard, M., & McEwen, B. S. (2018). Psychological Stress and Mitochondria: A Conceptual Framework. *Psychosomatic Medicine*, *80*(2), 126–140. https://doi.org/10.1097/PSY.0000000000000544

Shapiro, F. (2014). The role of eye movement desensitization and reprocessing (EMDR) therapy in medicine: addressing the psychological and physical symptoms stemming from adverse life experiences.

ADRENAL FATIGUE

" Fatigue makes fools of us all.
It robs you of your skills and your
judgement, and it blinds to to
creative solutions.
It's the best-conditioned athlete,
not the most talented, who generally
wins when the going gets tough."

HARVEY MACKAY

Adrenal fatigue isn't a disease; it's really another over-simplistic model regarding a condition where the adrenal glands are unable to produce adequate amounts of hormones, particularly cortisol, due to chronic stress. Dr James L Wilson coined the phrase 'adrenal fatigue' and described its symptoms more than twenty years ago. While it was never intended to be a scientific term, it has 'stuck' and been embraced by the public.

We believe there is a common and *reversible* condition which is influenced by how the hypothalamus and the pituitary gland react as a unit in response to long-term stress. But for ease and simplicity, let's call it 'adrenal fatigue'. **It's really about our ability to adapt when the body's stress load exceeds its capacity to secrete the necessary adrenal hormones** – not only cortisol, but DHEA and sex hormones as well. It happens usually following high demand over a prolonged period.

There is a recognised condition called 'secondary adrenal insufficiency' where low adrenal output with fatigue, weakness, weight loss and nausea are among the many symptoms. Some individuals with secondary adrenal insufficiency may experience fatigue as a result of inadequate cortisol production, which is essential for regulating energy levels and responding to stress. While chronic fatigue syndrome and secondary adrenal insufficiency are distinct conditions with different underlying mechanisms, there may be some overlap in symptoms, particularly regarding the unrelenting fatigue.

A different but uncommon condition called Addison's disease is diagnosed where there is an extreme loss of adrenal function. In Addison's disease, the adrenals are usually incapable of ever producing their hormones, and continual drug-based replacement regimes (mainly cortisone) are necessary long-term. This a severe chronic disease requiring specialist medical attention long term. Adrenal fatigue is very different.

Factors like genetics and lifestyle contribute to low cortisol levels, which can manifest as cognitive difficulties, mood swings, and sleep disturbances. If we look at Martin Picard's work on stress, we might call it 'mitochondrial fatigue'. It underscores the role of mitochondria in energy production and hormone regulation. Cortisol normally increases after the mid-thirties and can remain elevated due to sustained stress, leading to symptoms like fatigue, irritability, and insomnia.

When a stressful event elevates cortisol in the blood the levels normally fall after the stress stimulus resolves. However, levels can remain high because the feedback mechanism is faulty due to the sustained stress over a long period.

Classic Symptoms of Adrenal Fatigue

· Early morning fatigue, even after a good night's sleep.
· Difficulty getting activated in the morning.
· Needing stimulants like coffee to get started and to keep going during the day.
· Cravings for sugar and salt.
· Inability to bounce back from any setback, including illness.
· Low libido

MANAGING THE CONDITION

Treatment depends on the individual, the history, the stress load, and importantly the test results. It usually includes changes to lifestyle, diet, nutrients and hormonal supplements, with some subjective improvements usually noticeable within three to four weeks. There are several checks that need to occur to guide treatment.

· **Check hormone levels:** Check adrenal and thyroid function. Check testosterone and DHEA levels in men and add oestrogen and progesterone tests for women.
· **Check blood sugars, insulin and cardiovascular function.** Over time, stress, obesity and poor diet can lead to many lifestyle diseases.
· **Check for infections, allergens or chemical sensitivities** and other issues that contribute to his stress load.
· **Lifestyle changes:** Counselling on how to achieve effective sleep, exercise and relaxation as discussed in the beginning of this chapter. Cut down/out on caffeine, nicotine, sugar and alcohol. Start with simple things – no coffee in the afternoon and delegating the jobs at home and work. Say 'no' to increased workloads - and don't feel guilty!

Why DHEA (dehydroepiandrosterone) levels are is important: DHEA is a hormone produced by the adrenal glands and is a precursor to both testosterone and estrogen. It plays a role in various bodily functions, including energy levels and mood regulation.

Low levels of DHEA can impair the body's ability to respond to stress effectively, leading to fatigue and exhaustion. Generally, DHEA levels peak in the late 20s and gradually decline with age. We believe DHEA should have an 'ideal' level between 4 –10 µmol/L. However, 'normal' level is set by the laboratories - which we believe may be too low!

- 0.3–6.7 µmol/L for women.
- 0.9–6.8 µmol/L for men.

Blood tests aren't always the answer – testing of saliva or urine may also be necessary. Salivary cortisol, for example, indicates cortisol levels in the cells where the actions take place, rather than in serum/ blood stream, which is basically a transport system. A twenty-four-hour urinary cortisol test is ideal. It can measure not only cortisol, but other hormones made by the adrenal glands such as DHEA.

The timing of cortisol testing is essential for accurate interpretation of results. Morning cortisol levels are typically measured within the first hour after waking, to capture the peak cortisol levels. Afternoon or evening cortisol levels are typically measured around 4-6 hours after the morning sample to assess the decline in cortisol throughout the day.

Cortisol levels vary based on factors such as age, sex, individual health conditions, and the circumstances at the time the person was tested. We believe levels of cortisol in the blood should ideally range between 300 and 400 nanomoles per litre (nmol/L). The labs often support 'normal' as between 200–650 nmol/L (morning peak). This suggests than any result, in this extraordinarily wide reference range, can be 'normal' – even when one test result may be many times greater than another which we find a trifle difficult to accept!

Supplements Commonly used in Adrenal Fatigue

· Slow-release DHEA (50 mg in the morning) to boost energy.
· Slow-release melatonin (6-10mg mg in the evening) to help sleep.
· Testosterone cream (8% active ingredient) daily to improve libido and energy.
· Support the adrenal gland with herbs to improve energy such as astragalus, cordyceps and rhodiola and Siberian ginseng.
· Use calming herbs to improve sleep - valerian, withania, camomile and L-theanine from tea.
· All the B vitamins support the energy cycle with the minerals iron and magnesium.

ADRENAL FATIGUE

ACTION PLAN – CHECKLIST

- ■ Measure hormones; include cortisol and DHEA.
- ■ Measure thyroid and sex hormones.
- ■ Test blood glucose control, nutrient deficiencies, gluten sensitivity and allergy load.
- ■ Identify stressors at home, work or school, and seek help if necessary.
- ■ Identify expressions of stress – gut symptoms, migraines, musculoskeletal pains.
- ■ Engage mindful techniques. See Chapter 12.
- ■ Manage results with hormone support, diet and nutrient support.
- ■ Regularly review and make changes where necessary.

References:

Heim, C., Ehlert, U., & Hellhammer, D. H. (2000). The potential role of hypocortisolism in the pathophysiology of stress-related bodily disorders. *Psychoneuroendocrinology*, *25*(1), 1-35. https://doi.org/10.1016/s0306-4530(99)00035-9

Picard, M., & McEwen, B. S. (2018). Psychological Stress and Mitochondria: A Conceptual Framework. *Psychosomatic medicine*, *80*(2), 126–140. https://doi.org/10.1097/PSY.0000000000000544

Ryan, K. K., & Seeley, R. J. (2013). Physiology. Food as a hormone. *Science (New York, N.Y.)*, *339*(6122), 918–919. https://doi.org/10.1126/science.1234062.

Wilson, J. L. (2002). *Adrenal Fatigue: The 21st-Century Stress Syndrome*. Smart Publications.

Chapter 32

SLEEP WELL

"A ruffled mind makes a restless pillow."

CHARLOTTE BRONTE

We have argued repeatedly how important diet, stress management and exercise are to almost every aspect of health. So too is sleep! We spend about one-third of our lives asleep. We feel happier and healthier when we have a good night's sleep, and far worse when we toss and turn. Sleep is 'the biggest single contributing factor to living better' according to *The Sainsbury's Living Well Index* (2017). Sleep topped the list of beneficial lifestyle factors ahead of support networks, sex and mental health. It's not just quality of life that's affected, your quantity of life can increase as well.

About 30% of adults have some symptoms of insomnia. A chronic lack of sleep gives you a ticket to fatalities from drivers falling asleep at the wheel as well as infections, cancer, diabetes, heart attacks and even dementia.

Are You Getting Enough Sleep?

Babies	14–18 hours
Young children	10–12 hours
Teenagers	About 10 hours
Adults	7–8 hours
Elderly	10 hours

The concept of 'sleep debt' has emerged, recognising accumulated sleep loss must be "paid back" at some time, or it will be paid back in illness and chronic disease.

Non-restorative sleep: This is when you wake up mentally and physically exhausted, regardless of how long you've slept. Mental anguish disrupts sleep, but so do many diseases. Plus, to add insult to injury, non-restorative sleep has the power to crank up your sensitivity to every little ache and pain.

Chronic insomnia: This is defined as your sleeping pattern being disrupted at least three times per week for more than one month. Sleep studies show that disrupted sleep disturbs mood, and every night feels like a battle for the blankets.

Insomnia is more common in women, older people, people with anxiety and depression, those on drugs and those who are bit too friendly with the drink's menu. Sometimes it's because you are anxious, and the brain hits pause on sleep and starts playing its own late-night talk show on all your limitations - and none of this helps the mood for the new work day.

Interrupted sleep you can cope with —jet lag, all-nighters, or one night shift. But when your insomnia persists beyond a month, it's time to get a medical check-up to see if there's a bigger health problem you need to address. It's worth asking your doctor to check if the medications you're on might be contributing to your insomnia.

Signs you need more sleep: Feeling like you've been hit by the tired truck 24/7? Your body's screaming for a sugar rush to keep your eyelids from drooping. Lack of sleep can turn even the cheeriest of people into the grumpiest grinch. Forgetfulness and distraction are the side effects of sleep deprivation, and it has a knack for making even the smallest mistakes feel like major catastrophes. Once the immune system reacts and you catch more colds and flu than normal, it's time to tuck yourself in a bit earlier and give attention to the 7-8 hour sleep shift.

HORMONES THAT MAKE YOUR BODY CLOCK TICK

It turns out that all organisms have an internal body clock that is synchronised with the rotation of the planet, giving them the rhythm of day and night. The most important of these external cues, known as Zeitgebers (the German word for 'time givers'), is daylight. Our body clock resides in the hypothalamus near the base of the brain. As the sun sets and darkness descends, our brains respond by producing melatonin, the hormone that signals it's time to wind down. This natural sedative helps lower our body temperature and quietens our minds, paving the way for restorative sleep.

The hormones leptin and ghrelin respond to light: Leptin is responsible for regulating appetite and energy balance and it peaks at night. However, disrupted sleep patterns can lead to a decrease in leptin levels, potentially triggering increased hunger and cravings.

Ghrelin is secreted by the stomach and plays a role in appetite regulation. Sleep deprivation tends to increase ghrelin levels, which can lead to increased hunger and appetite. Understanding the interplay between our internal clock, hormones, and sleep patterns underscores the importance of restorative sleep for overall well-being.

Neurotransmitters like GABA work in tandem, soothing nerve activity and promoting relaxation. For those struggling with sleep, medications like Zolpidem (Stilnox) may offer temporary relief by enhancing GABA activity. However, exploring natural alternatives like GABA supplements could provide a gentler solution with fewer side effects.

STAGES OF SLEEP

The hypnogram below starts with in awake (W) phase and shows the sleep cycle of 90 minutes with four to six cycles of rapid eye movement (REM) and non rapid movement (NREM) stages that occur during a major period of sleep. The sleep cycle is an oscillation between the slow wave and REM (paradoxical) phases of sleep.

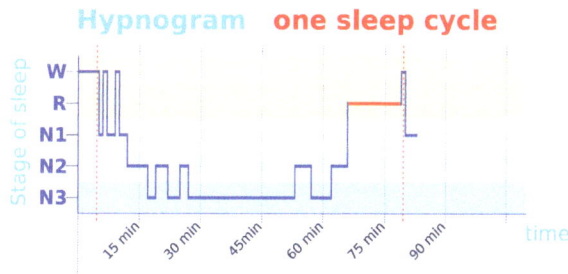

Hypnogram showing one sleep cycle (the first of the night) from NREM through REM
Schlafgut, CC BY-SA 3.0, via Wikimedia Commons

Children spend about 35% of sleep time in REM mode compared to 25% for adults. The more REM sleep they get, the better it is for children's maturing brains.

MEDICAL CONDITIONS THAT DISRUPT SLEEP

Sleep apnoea: An obstruction in the airways makes these narrow channels vibrate when breathing. Some people only snore occasionally if they drink too much or lie on their back. About 75% of regular snorers have sleep apnoea and about 40% snore occasionally. It's common among men over the age of thirty if they have a large neck (collar size over 44 cm), large tongue and other facial characteristics that contribute to the problem. Sometimes they'll have a family history of sleep apnoea, since it can be genetic. There are two kinds of sleep apnoea:

Obstructive sleep apnoea: The airways are momentarily blocked in the throat, causing difficulty breathing.

Central sleep apnoea: When the brain fails to tell the muscles to breathe, and the sleeper wakes up with a start.

Regardless of the cause, sleep apnoea has many negative effects on health:

- Poor cognition and increased accidents.
- Behavioural problems.
- Dry mouth.
- Increased heart disease and stroke.
- Depression and anxiety.
- Increased inflammation and decreased immunity.
- Increased pain.

Diagnosis of Sleep Apnoea: Sometimes an overnight stay in a sleep clinic is necessary, but devices are now portable enough to be used for home testing. These devices can make a huge difference to your quality of life. Weight is a big factor, so cutting down the calories and reducing your neck size will help enormously. A typical questionnaire can highlight areas that the individuals may *or may not* know themselves:

- Does your snoring bother other people?
- Has anyone noticed you stop breathing/ gasping/choking during your sleep?
- Are you aged fifty years or over? and do you doze off during the day?
- Are you overweight or have other medical conditions?

Restless Leg Syndrome: About 7% of the population have this problem; it disrupts sleep when one suddenly wakes up with the urge to move your legs. Those affected describe sensations such as crawling, tingling, itching, or creeping sensations/feelings deep within their legs. These sensations are unpleasant and can be mild to throbbing sensations. It can be related to nerve damage but one should check iron levels and supplement them if they're low. We also find that magnesium citrate (400 mg twice a day) may help; you can cut the dose back after a few weeks once symptoms settle.

Depression: This is more common to insomniacs, and their medications can exacerbate sleeplessness. A common class of drugs called selective serotonin reuptake inhibitors (SSRIs) is used to treat depression. These tend to initially decrease REM sleep but increase slow-wave sleep. The effects generally ease within one to three weeks, although the extent depends on dose and timing of the drug.

SLEEP HYGIENE

You can go a long way towards reducing most of your sleep problems by practising some good sleep hygiene rules:

1. **Bedroom Makeover:** Take a hard look at your sleep sanctuary. Swap out that old pillow, freshen up the bedding, and dim the lights when it's time sleep. Embrace

the face mask and earplugs if needed—keep the bedroom a peaceful oasis, free from ticking clocks, TVs, furry friends, or screens.

2. **Partner Patrol:** Is your bed mate's snoring stealing your Zzz's? It might be time for a sleep solo. It's not personal—it's all about catching those precious Z's without the background noise.

3. **Routine Matters:** Get that body clock working. Stick to a bedtime routine—same bedtime, same wake-up time every day. Steer clear of those night shifts if you can.

4. **Mind Your Booze and Pills:** Time to lay off the nightcaps. Alcohol might knock you out at first, but it's a sneaky saboteur of quality sleep. And those chocolate, coffee and cola snacks (100 and 200 mg of caffeine!), well, save them for the a.m.—no caffeine after lunch.

5. **Diet Details:** Watch what you eat before bed. Skip the spicy snacks and heavy meals; they're a one-way ticket to reflux. Ease up on the fluids closer to bedtime —no one likes waking up for bathroom breaks.

6. **Morning Moves and Sunbeams:** Rise and shine with a morning workout. Bask in the sunlight to boost your mood and set the stage for melatonin later on.

7. **Tech Timeout:** Unplug those glowing gadgets before bed—they're like little sleep thieves in disguise. No LED lights and iPad screens; we're reclaiming our melatonin levels and bidding farewell to bedtime distractions.

8. **Chill Out with Relaxation:** Stressed? Try some chill-out techniques like meditation, mindfulness, or soothing tunes to unwind. Stress less, sleep more—it's a win-win!

9. **Nana Naps:** Keep those daytime catnaps short and sweet—anything longer than thirty minutes might sabotage your nighttime snooze.

10. Remember, the real sleep secrets lie in boosting those melatonin and GABA levels. And if all else fails, there's a whole arsenal of sleep aids out there—from over-the-counter remedies to prescription picks—to help you catch those elusive Z's. Just chat with your doctor to find the right fit for your sleep style.

KEY NUTRIENTS FOR A GOOD NIGHT'S SLEEP

Tryptophan	A precursor to serotonin and melatonin, essential for calm and sleep. Requires vitamin B6 and folic acid, as well as vitamin C, zinc and magnesium for conversion. Avoid tryptophan supplements if taking antidepressant drugs.	*Source:* Red meat, chicken, turkey, fish, dairy products, nuts, seeds, oats, beans, lentils, tofu and eggs. *Amount:* 500 mg of tryptophan one hour before bed with carbohydrate foods.
Vitamin K2 and vitamin D	Vitamin K2 is required for nerve health and works hand in hand with vitamin D to promote sleep.	*Sources:* K1 (fermented soy food, natto, some meats and cheeses); K2 (green leafy vegetables).

Magnesium	Relaxes the muscles and alleviates sleep problems. Supports the chemical reactions involved in GABA and serotonin production.	*Sources:* Almonds and cashews, pumpkin seeds, wholegrain cereal, lentils, spinach, avocados, bananas, milk and fish.
Zinc	Needed for serotonin production. Fatigue is a sign of zinc deficiency.	*Sources:* Red meat, oysters, and cereals fortified with added zinc.
Melatonin	A hormone important for the sleep-wake cycle. Requires a prescription.	*Dose:* 6-10 mg one hour before sleep. Slow release is best over night
GABA (gamma-aminobutyric acid)	GABA is helpful if you have 'brain clutter'. Promotes restfulness and switches off adrenaline.	*Source:* Fermented foods. *Dose:* 400 mg 1–2 hours before bedtime.
Valerian, chamomile, passionflower and withania	Interact with GABA and reduces brain activity. Sedatives reduce the time it takes to fall asleep.	*Amount:* 400–600 mg is the usual dose for any of these herbs.
5-Hydroxytryptophan (5-HTP)	Low levels of 5-HTP have been shown to reduce REM sleep.	*Amount:* 300 mg/day taken an hour before bed on an empty stomach.

DRUGS AND OTHER THERAPIES

Zolpidem (also known by the brand name Stilnox) is a prescription drug used to induce sleep. Zolpidem is a sedative-hypnotic, so it also has a calming effect. It works within around 20 minutes.

Normison is a benzodiazepine and works to keep you asleep, as well as helping to initiate sleep, so it has a longer action than Stilnox. Most sleeping tablets are habit forming and addictive. The less medication and the more 'natural' sleep you have, the better you will feel.

Dual orexin receptor antagonists (DORAs) are a new prescription medication that work by acting as orexin receptor antagonists, which reduce the drive to stay awake, and facilitates sleep.

Acupuncture is worth trying as an alternative or as an add-on to the other options discussed in this section. We find acupuncture of most use in alleviating pain that might be keeping people awake.

SLEEP WELL

ACTION PLAN – CHECKLIST

· Have a daily routine.
· No daytime naps.
· Check if sleep apnoea is a cause.
· Avoid caffeine and alcohol and late-night meals.
· Add GABA an hour before bedtime.
· Add 6-10mg of melatonin one hour before bedtime.
· Add magnesium for restless legs.
· Avoid blue background computer screens prior to sleep.
· Practice a strict sleep hygiene night-time routine.

References:

Deloitte Access Economics. (2018). Asleep on the Job: costs of inadequate sleep in Australia (Report commissioned by Sleep Health Foundation).

Krause, A. J., Aric, A. J., Prather, A., Wager, T. D., Lindquist, M. A., & Walker, M. P. The Pain of Sleep Loss: A Brain Characterization in Humans. Journal of Neuroscience, 39(12), 2291–2300.

Oxford Economics and the National Centre for Social Research. (2017). The Sainsbury Living Well Index. Oxford Economics, UK. https://www.about.sainsburys.co.uk/~/media/Files/S/Sainsburys/living-well-in-dex/sainsburys-living-well-index.PDF

Chapter 33

EXERCISE MORE

*"Imagination grows by exercise,
and contrary to common belief, is
more powerful in the mature than in
the young."*

SOMERSET MAUGHAM

If exercise could be taken in pill form, it would be heralded as the next miracle cure. In fact, the *British Journal of Pharmacology* has suggested that exercise should be considered a drug as it has so many benefits. It's not an analogy we would offer ourselves – but let's focus our minds on the many benefits of exercise. Apart from living longer, exercise makes us feel and think and even look better! There are so many incentives to travel this road to better health.

EXERCISE CAN ASSIST THESE MEDICAL CONDITIONS

Cardiac	Gynae	Cancers	Mood	Other
Heart disease Hypertension Dyslipidaemia Stroke Respiratory problems	Abnormal periods Infertility Endometrial diseases Menopausal symptoms Pre-eclampsia	Breast Prostate Colon Lung Oesophageal Adeno-carcinoma	Alzheimer's Dementia <Cognitive Anxiety Depression ADHD Schizophrenia	Diabetes Obesity Fatty liver Gallbladder Joint disease MS Parkinson's Fatigue

When you are physically fit, your body works efficiently and effectively. It is far less likely to succumb to our most common (and costly) and preventable health problems such as heart disease, cancer, diabetes, liver disease and arthritis.

If for some reason you lose fitness, you can turn back the clock and reduce your chances of dying from heart disease. Wahid et al (2016) found that by increasing exercise by just over 11 hours per week, the chance of dying from heart disease was reduced by a whopping 23%! For cancer, moderate physical activity for about thirty to sixty minutes per day has a greater protective effect against colon, breast and endometrial cancers than low-level physical activity.

There is a notion that the number of steps taken in a day has declined by 50–70% since the inception of powered machinery, although not all populations are the same. We know exercise is good for us. But what's the 'dose' needed to stay healthy?

HOW MUCH EXERCISE IS ENOUGH?

The health benefits depend on how hard you exercise. Exercise intensity is measured by heart rate, but also by the amount of oxygen consumed. For best outcome, the intensity, the frequency, and the type of exercise all have to be taken into account. In all manner of exercise, hydration is a key factor.

Vigorous Exercise	Moderate Exercise	Low-level Activity	Strength or Resistance Training
Makes you breathe much harder than normal – include heavy lifting, digging, aerobics or fast bi-cycling.	Breathing somewhat harder than normal. Includes carrying light loads, cycling at a regular pace or doubles tennis– not walking	Doesn't change your breathing or heart rate. Includes activities such as walking and light gardening.	Builds muscle by using weights. Body weight and gravity can add resistance – push-ups, dumbbells, barbells, ankle weights or elastic bands of various tensions.

So while low-intensity exercise such as stretching or walking has its own benefits (e.g. increasing flexibility and reducing pain), don't expect miracles. Fewer than 5000 steps a day dumps us in the sedentary category, which won't improve type 2 diabetes risks, nor cardiovascular markers such as blood pressure, lipid/fat profile and weight. But push a bit harder and it's not just your blood sugars that will benefit. Both triglyceride and cholesterol levels improve when you use weights with moderate resistance.

Moderate-Intensity Activity

· We need to achieve 8,000–10,000 steps per day to be considered active.
· It takes 72 minutes per week to improve fitness levels.
· Ninety minutes per week of moderate-intensity exercise is required to increase life expectancy.
· You need thirty minutes of moderate-intensity aerobic exercise every day, or 40–45 minutes of vigorous intensity at least three days per week, as well as two to three sessions of resistance training for exercise to improve health and manage type 2 diabetes (Diabetes Australia, 2016).

High-intensity Activity: High intensity for seven to twelve weeks will give you improvements in lung function, cholesterol levels, insulin sensitivity and abdominal obesity compared to moderate intensity. But you needed to stick with it; training programs of six weeks or less have little effect! Guidelines have traditionally favoured moderate-intensity exercise for people with coronary heart disease however, doctors will often make recommendations for patients who want to regain their previous level of fitness.

Resistance Training: Resistance training improves strength and bone mineral density. Physical fitness researcher and author Wayne Westcott wrote a great paper on resistance training back in 2012 for the American College of Sports Medicine, and many of the important points below have been taken from his review.

Muscle loss can occur with ageing due to hormonal factors. Less muscle contributes to a decline in metabolism, which is why you gain weight easily and have difficulty losing weight after fifty years. You can regain muscle strength using weights or resistance bands, cycling and climbing stairs. Ideally aim for twelve to twenty sets of exercise two to three times per week on non-consecutive days – so spread it out and give the muscles a bit of a rest after the workout. The other good news is that you can add about 1.4 kg of lean weight after about ten weeks of resistance training. But before you start, make sure you have your resistance training supervised by an exercise physiologist or certified personal trainer.

RESISTANCE TRAINING

Resistance Exercise: Perform eight to ten multi-joint exercises for the major muscle groups (chest, shoulders, back, abdomen, arms, hips and legs).

Frequency Training: Train each major muscle group two to three non-consecutive days/ week.

Training Sets: Perform two to four sets of resistance training for each muscle group.

Resistance Repetitions: Use resistance that can be performed for eight to twelve repetition.

Training Technique: Perform each repetition in a controlled manner through a full range of motion. Exhale during lifting actions and inhale during lowering actions.

Source: Wayne L. Westcott, PhD. *Resistance Training is Medicine: Effects of Strength Training on Health.*

For those who think they can't commit to an exercise regime, think again. Try standing instead of sitting – consider a stand-up desk at work. We see colleagues and friends at work do this intermittently, and they seem to like it. Even two minutes of light-intensity exercise can be beneficial, especially if you are really out of shape, walking up the stairs at work is even better. Short bursts of exercise, such as a two-minute stair climb five to eight times, can increase cardiac fitness.

EXERCISE FOR WEIGHT MANAGEMENT

Time	Intensity	Weight Loss/Gain
150–250 minutes per week (20–35 minutes per day).	Moderate to vigorous	To prevent weight gain.
225–420 minutes per week (~60 minutes per day).	Moderate to vigorous	To achieve any significant weight loss.
200–300 minutes per week.	Moderate to vigorous	To prevent weight gain after weight loss.
Add calorie restrictions to an exercise program: For realistic weight loss burn 300–400 calories per workout session. Through regular physical activity and calorie monitoring: Create a daily calorie deficit of approximately 500–1000 calories.	Moderate to vigorous	1 kg per week loss is possible.

Source: Swift et al. (2013).

Exercise in a Hurry: If you really want the best return on the time you 'invest' in exercise, consider high- intensity training – an approach advocated by Dr Michael

Mosley in his book *Fast Exercise* (2014). Being time poor but keen to live to a healthy old age, he looked for an alternative and found it in high-intensity training. High-intensity training eschews the 'moderation in all things' approach. Instead of plodding away on a treadmill or cycling at a steady pace, you do a few extremely short bursts of exercise, intense enough to get your heart rate soaring, interspersed with a couple of minutes for recovery.

Done properly, it is safe, effective and surprisingly enjoyable. It burns more fat than conventional exercise and, best of all, it's over in less time than it takes to drive to the gym.

When To Say "NO" to Exercise: For starters, don't exercise if you're having difficulty breathing. If you have high blood pressure of about 180/105, steer clear of exercise until levels are normal. Don't exercise if your blood sugars are very low or if you have cancer and your blood count is down or cancer has spread into the bones. As good as exercise is, it can't be 'prescribed' for everyone.

EXERCISE MORE

ACTION PLAN – CHECKLIST

- Aim for at least 150 minutes per week of moderate to vigorous exercise.
- Aim for 10,000 steps per day.
- Use high-intensity exercise for cardiovascular health.
- Your doctor will recommend the intensity if you have a medical condition.
- Improve muscle mass and bone density with muscle resistance training.
- Add short bursts of high- intensity exercise on days with time restriction.
- Keep well hydrated.

References:

Booth, F. W., Roberts, C. K., & Laye, M. J. (2012). Lack of exercise is a major cause of chronic diseases. *Journal of Comparative Physiology*, *2*(2), 1143–1211. https://doi.org/10.1002/cphy.c110025 Mosely, M., & Bee, P. (2013) *Fast Exercise*. Short Books.

Vina, J., Sanchis-Gomar, F., Martinez-Bello, V., & Gomez-Cabrera, M. C. (2012). Exercise acts as a drug; the pharmacological benefits of exercise. *British Journal of Pharmacology*, *167*(1), 1–12. https://doi.org/10.1111/j.1476-5381.2012.01970.x

Wahid, A., Manek, N., Nichols, M., Kelly, P., Foster, C., Webster, P., Kaur, A., Friedemann Smith, C., Wilkins, E., Rayner, M., Roberts, N., & Scarborough, P. (2016). Quantifying the Association Between Physical Activity and Cardiovascular Disease and Diabetes: A Systematic Review and Meta-Analysis. *Journal of the American Heart Association*, *5*(9), Article e002495. https://doi.org/10.1161/JAHA.115.002495

Westcott, W. L. (2012). Resistance training is medicine: effects of strength training on health. *Current Sports Medicine Reports*, *11*(4), 209–216. https://doi.org/10.1249/JSR.0b013e31825dabb8

Swift, D. L., Johannsen, N. M., Lavie, C. J., Earnest, C. P., & Church, T. S. (2014). The role of exercise and physical activity in weight loss and maintenance. *Progress in cardiovascular diseases*, *56*(4), 441–447. https://doi.org/10.1016/j.pcad.2013.09.012

Chapter 34

OSTEOPOROSIS

"To succeed in life you need three things: a wish bone, a back bone and a funny bone."

DR KAVANAGH

Osteoporosis is a disease in which the bones become thin and fragile and tend to break easily. Normally old bone is replaced with new bone, but in osteoporosis the new bone does not keep pace with the demand. Bone tissue is continuously remodeled by the actions of bone cells. **Osteoclasts** dissolve old and damaged bone tissue so it can be replaced with new, healthier cells created by **osteoblasts**.

Normal bone structure looks like a honeycomb, but in osteoporosis the holes become larger, and the bone becomes more porous and fragile and starts to resemble holey Swiss cheese. Osteoporosis doesn't discriminate—it's something both men and women must watch out for. But it tends to pop up more often in women after menopause, mostly related to long break from oestrogen. Hormones, minerals and vitamins as well as weight-bearing exercises help to create a healthy density. Protein makes up half the volume and a third of the mass – thus keep in mind as we age we need to consume at least a gram per kilo body weight of protein per day.

Risk Factors for Osteoporosis

· Postmenopausal women.
· Oestrogen-deficient females.
· Testosterone deficiency in men.
· Family history of osteoporosis.
· Heavy smokers or alcohol drinkers.
· Autoimmune diseases.
· Steroid users, e.g. asthmatics and arthritics.
· Vitamin D deficiency.
· Poor diet, excess salt.
· Lack of exercise.
· High homocysteine interfering with collagen.
· Inflammatory bowel disease.

DIAGNOSING OSTEOPOROSIS

Diagnosing osteoporosis involves a bone density test, which uses X-rays to assess the concentration of calcium and other essential minerals within specific bone segments like the spine, hip, and forearm.

One common method is DEXA (Dual energy X-ray absorptiometry). The machine uses two different X-ray beams—one for soft tissue and one for bone. By analysing the difference, we can gauge the bone mineral density and keep track of any changes over time.

There are other tests which gather information about hormonal levels, bone health markers, and potential underlying conditions that can impact bone density. Here's why each test is important:

1. **Female Menopause Tests (FSH and Testosterone):** Menopause can affect bone health due to hormonal changes. Follicle-stimulating hormone (FSH) levels can indicate menopause status, while testosterone levels may affect bone density in both men and women.

2. **Testosterone Deficiency (Men):** Low testosterone levels in men can contribute to bone loss, making it important to check for deficiency.

3. **Blood Calcium Levels:** Calcium is crucial for bone strength, so measuring blood calcium levels helps assess whether the body has enough calcium available for bone health.

4. **Vitamin D and Vitamin K2:** Vitamin D is essential for calcium absorption and bone mineralisation. Low levels can lead to weakened bones, making it important to check for deficiency. Vitamin K2 assists Vitamin D transport calcium into the bone.

5. **Thyroid Tests:** Thyroid disorders can affect bone metabolism, leading to either bone loss or excessive bone formation. Each cycle of bone 'turnover' takes about 200 days and excess thyroid hormone will hasten this rate of bone turnover. On the flip side, overt hypothyroidism induces a low bone turnover with a prolonged bone remodeling cycle,

6. **Parathyroid Hormone (PTH):** PTH regulates calcium levels in the blood and bone. Abnormal levels can indicate conditions affecting bone density such as hyperparathyroidism or hypoparathyroidism.

7. **Alkaline Phosphatase (ALP):** ALP is an enzyme involved in bone formation. Elevated levels may indicate increased bone turnover, which can occur in conditions like osteoporosis.

PROTECTING BONE DENSITY IN AGEING

1. **Calcium-Rich Foods:** Incorporate a variety of calcium-rich foods into your diet, including kale, spinach, broccoli, dairy products, Brazil nuts, almonds, and sesame seeds. Don't forget about the bones in tinned salmon or tuna.
2. **Boron:** Boron influences the metabolism of calcium, magnesium, and vitamin D, which are all important for bone health. It helps enhance calcium absorption and utilisation in the body.
3. **Phosphorus:** Phosphorus works alongside calcium to form hydroxyapatite crystals, which are the main mineral component of bone tissue. Phosphorous is in a wide variety of food.
4. **Magnesium:** Magnesium influences the activity of osteoblasts and osteoclasts, the cells responsible for building and breaking down bone tissue. It also helps regulate calcium levels in the body. Sources include nuts, seeds, avocado and wholegrains.
5. **Zinc:** It helps stimulate bone-building cells and plays a role in collagen synthesis, which is important for bone structure.
6. **Copper:** It is involved in the formation of collagen and connective tissue, which are integral components of bone. It also plays a role in bone mineralisation and maintenance. Sources: shellfish, legumes, chocolate, dark leafy greens.
7. **Silicon:** Enhances bone mineral density and strength.

8. **Vitamins and Minerals Synergy**: Vitamin C enhances mineral absorption by increasing stomach acidity, while vitamin D (found in fatty fish, eggs, and cheese) and vitamin K2 help transport calcium into bones.

9. **Dietary Habits and Bone Health**: Diets rich in fish show more positive effects on bone density compared to those a high red meat intake.

10. **Stomach Health**: Keep an eye on acid reflux, especially as you age. Insufficient hydrochloric acid (HCl) in the stomach can affect protein and mineral absorption. Consider supplements like Betaine HCl or Hydrozyme to restore HCl levels.

11. **Exercise for Strength**: Engage in regular weight-bearing exercises such as walking, jogging, stair climbing, and weightlifting to maintain bone strength.

12. **Hormonal Balance**: Hormones play a significant role in bone health throughout life. Pay attention to hormone levels, especially during adolescence and menopause. Progesterone, oestrogen, and testosterone all contribute to bone stability.

13. **Stress Management**: High cortisol levels and stress can negatively impact bone health by increasing bone resorption. Manage stress effectively and maintain adequate vitamin D levels.

14. **Osteoporosis Medications**: Discuss medications like Prolia and Fosamax with your healthcare provider if necessary.

15. **Sun Exposure and Vitamin D**: Sun exposure and vitamin D-rich foods can help maintain optimal vitamin D levels, especially post-menopause.

16. **Vitamin K2** plays a crucial role in regulating calcium for healthy bone structure, particularly in conjunction with vitamin D. It's a complex process, which we will attempt to explain.

WHY VITAMIN K2 IS SPECIAL

Vitamin K2 together with vitamin D play a crucial role in managing optimal bone health. Vitamin K2 directs calcium to the bones preventing its deposition in soft tissues such as blood vessels, which can lead to arterial calcification and cardiovascular issues.

To understand its significance, let's explain some of its complex biochemistry. Vitamin K is fat-soluble and exists in two primary forms:

- **Vitamin K1 (phylloquinone)**, derived from plants like leafy greens, aids in blood clotting.
- **Vitamin K2 (menaquinones Mk-2 to Mk-14)** comprises a group of compounds pivotal for bone formation and protection against chronic diseases. Vitamin K2 enhances the activity of osteoblasts, the cells responsible for bone formation, and regulates bone metabolism. While some forms of K2 are synthesised by bacteria, others, like MK-4 and MK-7, play key roles in bone health:
    - MK-4, found in various foods like fish, liver, and dairy, is the primary form in the human body, influencing genes related to energy metabolism and calcium balance.
    - MK-7, abundant in natto (fermented soy), boosts osteoblast function and is better absorbed than MK-4. Cheese products also contain MK-8, MK-9, and MK-10.
- Despite its importance, our bodies store only small amounts of vitamin K1 and long-chain K2 forms in the liver.

The Japanese researcher Iwamoto found that 45mg/day was the minimum effective dose for improving bone mass parameters in postmenopausal women with osteoporosis. The dose is best delivered in 3 separate doses of 15mg per day for optimum utilisation. In Chapter 22 on heart disease, we deal in detail with the evidence that vitamin K2 can also serve a major role in decreasing calcium deposits in arteries protecting against hardening of the arteries.

OSTEOPOROSIS

ACTION PLAN – CHECKLIST

- Check out your risk factors for osteoporosis.
- Check hormonal profile.
- Get a bone mineral density test if risk factors are moderately high.
- Use diet and pharmacological agents to increase bone mass.
- Use weight-bearing exercises.
- Add vitamin D, vitamin K2 and boron.
- Consider using a mineral formula specific for osteoporosis.

References:

Nieves J. W. (2013). Skeletal effects of nutrients and nutraceuticals, beyond calcium and vitamin D. *Osteoporosis international : a journal established as result of cooperation between the European Foundation for Osteoporosis and the National Osteoporosis Foundation of the USA*, *24*(3), 771–786. https://doi.org/10.1007/s00198-012-2214-4

Iwamoto, J. (2014). Vitamin K_2 therapy for postmenopausal osteoporosis. *Nutrients*, *6*(5), 1971–1980. https://doi.org/10.3390/nu6051971

Rheaume-Bleue, K. (2015). *Vitamin K2 And The Calcium Paradox: How a Little-Known Vitamin Could Save Your Life*. Harper Collins.

Chapter 35

VITAMIN D AND THREE MIGHTY MINERALS

"All truths are easy to understand once they are discovered; the point is to discover them.

GALILEO GALILEI

1. VITAMIN D – DON'T SHUN THE SUN

Vitamin D has two sources. It is a fat-soluble vitamin we consume from food and a hormone produced in the skin in response to sunlight. It's so important that vitamin D receptors are found in numerous cells and tissues, including those in the immune system, bones, kidneys, intestines, and skin. They are also present in cells of the cardiovascular system, brain, and certain endocrine organs. This wide distribution underscores the importance of vitamin D in various bodily functions, such as calcium and phosphate homeostasis, immune response, and cell growth. At least nine hundred different genes use vitamin D to produce proteins and other chemicals necessary for health.

Recent recommendations have focused on the risks rather than the many benefits of sun exposure. Vitamin D is more than just a vitamin; a Swedish study found that the death rate from all causes doubled amongst avoiders of sun exposure compared to those with the highest sun exposure.

Notably, the sun affects serotonin activity and serenity; low sun levels are linked to depression and Alzheimer's disease. Greater sun exposure increases our overall immune health. Studies have also shown that sun exposure lowers the risk of breast, colorectal and prostate cancers, and the favourable effects were not just due to better vitamin D levels.

When the sun's UV-B radiation levels fall during winters at latitudes >40°, the risk of vitamin D deficiency increases the rate of flu infections. Unsurprisingly, we find there was a higher rate of fatality from COVID-19 infections in areas of Europe with vitamin D deficiency (less than 30 ng/mL). Additionally, vitamin D deficiency intensifies the severity of COVID-19 infections.

Yes, we know that skin cancer is a risk from ultraviolet radiation, but there are two sides to this coin. Non-burning sun exposure is associated with a reduced risk of melanoma, while sunburns are associated with a doubling of the risk of developing melanoma. Confusing the story even more is the observation that outdoor workers who get used to sun exposure have a lower incidence of melanoma than indoor workers. Add to that is the fact that many of our defences against such damage are related to vitamin D produced by exposure to UV-B!

You're at particular risk of vitamin D deficiency if you're older, have naturally dark skin, don't consume enough vitamin D in your diet, work night shifts, cover up for religious reasons or spend too much of your time indoors.

Sun Exposure Guidelines

Vitamin D3 is formed through the action of ultraviolet B (UV-B) radiation (wavelength 290–315 nm) on 7-dehydrocholesterol in the skin. The guidelines for sun exposure are thus:

Expose 15% of the body (arms, face and hands) * every day:
  Summer (Fair skin): 5–10 minutes most days.
  Summer (Dark Skin): 15–60 minutes mid-morning and mid-afternoon.
  Winter (Fair skin): 7–30 minutes most days depending on latitude.
  Winter (Dark skin): 30 minutes to 3 hours mid-morning and mid-afternoon.

  * Experimental data indicates that exposure of around 15% of the body surface (arms and hands or equivalent) near the middle of the day will result in the production of about 1000 IU (25 µg) of vitamin D. This is enough to attain a slight red flush on the skin.
  Source: Vitamin D and health in adults in Australia and New Zealand (a position statement article in *The Medical Journal of Australia*, June 2012).

SOURCES OF VITAMIN D

Vitamin D_3 (Cholecalciferol): D_3 is really a hormone the skin produces in response to sun exposure. **Some 90% of your vitamin D comes from sun exposure.**

The remaining 10% comes from your diet;

Foods high in D_3 : fatty fish and cod liver oil.

Foods High in Vitamin D$_2$ (Ergocalciferol): Found in shiitake mushrooms and fortified food.

How much vitamin D is enough?: Blood levels below 75 nmol/L for adults and 50 nmol/L for a child reflect deficiency. With a deficiency comes a risk for almost every inflammatory disease. If you believe, as we do, that almost every disease starts with inflammation, it makes sense to aim for an optimal – not just adequate – intake of vitamin D.

Adults should have 800 international units (IU) of vitamin D per day, although up to 4000 IU per day is considered safe. If levels are low, expect a prescription of 1000–2000 IU per day. Children should have around half the adult amount (400 IU per day).

VITAMIN D AND DISEASE PREVENTION

Our genetics can influence your vitamin D receptors. Many people have different binding affinities, so some have increased risk of inflammatory diseases.

Bones and muscle: Vitamin D helps the body absorb calcium, phosphate and magnesium to protect and build bone. It is also necessary for connective tissues such as collagen and elastin.

Immune system: Vitamin D protects against autoimmune diseases such as multiple sclerosis (MS), fibromyalgia, type 1 diabetes, and corona and retroviruses. Respiratory tract infections, influenza and chronic obstructive pulmonary disease are linked to vitamin D deficiencies. COVID 19 falls within this category.

Cancer: Many forms of cancer are associated with vitamin D deficiency, including four of the most common: prostate, breast, colon and ovarian. Vitamin D lowers the risk of death in those who have cancer. Those at risk of cancer benefit from a daily dose of 1000 IU of vitamin D supplementation for over three years.

Diabetes: Deficiency is linked to insulin resistance and metabolic syndrome. Children with type 1 diabetes have a high rate of vitamin D deficiency. Supplementing vitamin D in the first year of life has been linked to 80% decreased risk of type 1 diabetes in later life.

Brain: Vitamin D receptors are distributed throughout the brain. They may help prevent and treat learning disorders, memory problems, mood and neurodevelopmental conditions such as autism. Deficiencies are linked to a decline in cognition.

Gut: Vitamin D supports friendly bacteria in the gut. It reduces inflammation and protects the intestinal barrier. Low levels are associated ulcerative colitis, Crohn's disease and chronic gastritis.

Hormones: Vitamin D can help boost testosterone in middle-aged men. Low levels are linked to low libido and pre and postmenopausal symptoms in women. Higher levels protect against preterm births, asthma, pre-eclampsia and gestational diabetes.

References:

Hoel, D. G., Berwick, M., de Gruijl, F. R., & Holick, M. F. (2016). The risks and benefits of sun exposure 2016. *Dermato-endocrinology*, *8*(1), Article e1248325. https://doi.org/10.1080/19381980.2016.1248325

Nowson, C. A., McGrath, J. J., Ebeling, P. R., Haikerwal, A., Daly, R. M., Sanders, K. M., Seibel M. M., & Mason, S. (2012). Vitamin D and health in adults in Australia and New Zealand: a position statement. *The Medical Journal of Australia*, *196*(11), 686–687. https://doi.org/10.5694/mja11.10301

2. IRON – A VEGAN CONUNDRUM

According to the World Health Organization (WHO), about 24.8% of the global population, were affected by anaemia in 2016. Around 10% of non-pregnant women in Australia are anaemic. Vegetarianism is increasingly common in the community and vegetarians are particularly at risk of low iron stores and need to be vigilant with their diet. To this end we dive quite deeply into the complexity of low iron stores and ill health.

The body is unable to make iron, so it must be consumed in the diet. There are over ninety functions of iron and lots of things that can wrong when iron is in short supply. People just don't 'get' how important iron is for pregnancy, for the baby's brain and development and for strength of the mum – but also for children, teenagers, the middle-aged and for the centenarians.

Functions of Iron: Iron is required to produce haemoglobin in the red blood cells, which binds oxygen and then delivers it to the brain, tissues, muscles and many other cells. Iron is necessary to generate the energy molecule ATP in the cells, without which we cannot function. We need iron to manufacture our DNA, for the neurotransmitters dopamine and serotonin that regulate mood and motivation, for brain function, immunity and detoxification. We also need it to produce oestrogen and testosterone.

If you look at the list of features of iron deficiency, it is no surprise that poor supply and absorption can negatively influence growth, mood, behaviour and cognition into adulthood. It is best to act on signs of iron deficiency before lasting damage is done.

Vegans, vegetarians or anyone on a restricted diet, including young fussy eaters, can easily end up being deficient in iron. Dietary intake should balance iron losses of about one to two milligrams per day.

Features of Iron Deficiency

Impaired growth

Poor immunity (frequent colds and infections)

Fatigue and lethargy, weakness

Cold hands and feet

Breathlessness

Dizziness

Poor concentration and lack of motivation

Reduced performance, poor behaviour

Mood swings

CAUSES OF IRON DEFICIENCY

1. **You don't absorb iron properly:** Drugs for heartburn, reflux or ulcers can reduce gastric acid, lowering iron and other nutrient absorption. Your levels of hydrochloric acid necessary for protein breakdown also often fall with age.

2. **You lose blood** due to injury, medical conditions (e.g. haemorrhoids, colitis, diverticulitis or cancer) or side effects e.g. (bleeding) caused by anti-inflammatory medications.

3. **You are a woman:** Women can lose up to 3 ml of blood per day during menstruation if your hormones are out of kilter and you have heavy periods. Pregnancy and childbirth increase demands for iron. Women need up to three times more iron towards the end of the pregnancy.

4. **You are a child:** As children grow, their demand for iron increases. The demand can outpace supply if they were born underweight or don't have enough iron.

Milk products can negatively affect iron absorption. Too much dairy can replace foods high in iron in toddlers.

5. **You are an elite athlete:** Strenuous exercise can see iron lost in sweat and blood due to injuries at a time when it is needed to grow and repair tissue.

6. **You are in an institution or have ill health:** Iron is more likely to be lacking in groups with poorer diets and poor absorption.

Yes, too much iron is toxic in high doses, but it's hard to overload on iron from dietary sources. Excessive stores of iron tend to build up due to other causes, such as repeated blood transfusions or a hereditary condition called haemochromatosis, where iron overload can damage the liver, heart and spleen.

There it is a misconception that low serum iron equals iron deficiency. For children, we need to be aware that:

· Serum iron is a poor measure of iron status in the body.
· Low serum ferritin is a good marker for total body iron status.
· Low serum ferritin is mostly seen in iron deficiency.

IRON DEFICIENCY AND ANAEMIA DEFINITIONS

Iron Deficiency	Anaemia	Iron-deficiency Anaemia	Iron Deficiency Without Anaemia
Too little iron in the body may be present without anaemia. Blood levels indicate decreased ferritin.	A decrease in the total haemoglobin or the number of red blood cells. Iron dependent functions are compromised.	An advanced stage of iron deficiency. Low ferritin stores, reduced red cell volume and reduced haemoglobin concentration occurs.	More common than iron-deficiency anaemia. Vitamin B12 and folic acid deficiency can also cause anaemia.

The bottom line: Low ferritin and raised transferrin signal iron deficiency, and serum iron can be normal in iron deficiency.

- Lack of adequate iron can have a negative influence on growth, mood, behaviour and cognition into adult life. The more iron-deficient the child, the stronger the symptoms of impulsivity, inattention and hyperactivity. See Chapter 16.
- Four very common features of iron deficiency in children are very often not associated with pallor and anaemia. Our mnemonic to help recall these features is F.I.M.E: Foggy brain, Immune deficit (frequent infections), Mood disorder and Energy deficit. Irrespective of the presence of anaemia, check ferritin in a child with those symptoms. Although not necessarily associated with anaemia, problems may exist with the other ninety-two enzymes that require iron for activity so that the child may flourish.

· Low serum ferritin, not low serum iron, is a reliable marker of uncomplicated iron deficiency. The common range is 30–300 µg/L. Our experience is that some people function better at a level of 100 µg/L.

Iron Absorption: Haem iron: From animal sources. We absorb around 20% of haem iron, but that rate is reduced by lengthy cooking. **Non-haem iron:** From green leafy vegetables and supplemented cereals. We absorb around 7–11% of non-haem iron.

Sources of Iron in Haem and Non-Haem Foods *Source:* https://www.dietitians.ca/Your-Health/Nutrition-A-Z/Minerals/Food-Sources-of-Iron.aspx			
Food per 75g	Haem Iron Content (mg)	Food	Non-haem Iron Content (mg)
Beef, cooked	1.4–3.3	Spinach, ½ cup	2.0–3.4
Chicken, cooked	0.4–2.0	Tomato purée, ½ c	2.4
Pork, cooked	0.5–1.5	Broccoli, ½ cup	1.7
Liver (chicken)	6.2–9.7	Cereals, 30 g	4.0–4.3
Kidney, cooked	2.3–4.4	Tofu, ¾ cup	2.4–8.0
Salmon, raw	0.96	Eggs, 2 large	1.2–1.8

Vegetarians may sometimes require supplementation. For others, the best option is to have a mixed diet of meat, seafood, fruit and vegetables. Vitamin C greatly increases both haem and non-haem iron absorption, so think of vitamin C (citrus and berries, etc.)

Iron Requirements

Age	Male (mg/day)	Female (mg/day)	Age	Male mg/day	Female mg/day
7–12 mths	11.0	11.0	14–18 yrs	11.0	15.0
1–3 years	9.0	9.0	19–70 yrs	8.0	18.0
9–13 years	8.0	8.0	Pregnancy		27.0

Foods and Medication that Reduce Absorption

· Phytates found in grains, seeds and nuts decrease absorption, but heat treatment, soaking, germination and fermentation can help degrade phytates.
· Tannins, principally in tea retard absorption.
· Oxalates in spinach, rhubarb, kale and beet bind to the non-haem iron.
· Calcium negatively affects both the haem and non- haem iron absorption. Looking at babies with high milk intake here.
· Medications that inhibit iron include antacids such as Zantac, Nexium and Pariet; Neomycin and Tetracycline (antibiotics); and Allopurinol (drug for gout).

References:

Lam, Q. (2013). Common Sense Pathology – Interpreting Serum Ferritin. Royal College of Pathologists of Australasia. *Australian Doctor.* https://www.rcpa.edu.au/getattachment/d2521e16-e5c3-46e8-abca- 652d6838f527/Interpreting-Serum-Ferritin.aspx

3. HAVE A VIRUS? THINK ZINC

Out of the many nutrients studied for their antiviral activity in the pandemic, zinc is one of the most efficacious against coronaviruses. Zinc inhibits the replication of a variety of viruses in both humans and animals. It assists with degrading the virus and it has also been shown to impair the replication of coronaviruses.

You might have used zinc shampoos or creams when treating dandruff, eczema or ringworm. A zinc (pyrithione) complex helps treat tinea, dermatitis, *Streptococcus* and *Staphylococcus* by interfering with cell division. Zinc lozenges work for a sore throat and the zinc creams protect against sunburn.

Zinc is a mineral. In human terms it can be considered as a hard-working project manager and one of our great communicators. It plays a huge role in cell signalling and transport, enabling reactions within the cells and regulating their many functions. It has a good old gossip with another cell communicator – calcium.

Zinc is a constituent of some three thousand proteins and has an action in nearly ninety enzyme systems – not far behind iron. 85% of zinc is found in bone and muscles, about 11% in the skin and liver, and the rest in the prostate and the eye. About 25% of the world's population is zinc-deficient, and much of this has to do with malnutrition, low protein intake or malabsorption.

It is important to have some zinc each day because it has a fast turnover. This is difficult for vegetarians and children who are fussy eaters. Zinc deficiency causes them to be even more fussy as they end up feeling miserable and an easy target for colds and flu.

Food Sources	Zinc mg per 100 grams	Food Sources	Zinc mg per 100 grams
Sun-dried tomatoes	13.6	Egg, cooked	1.2
Wheat cereals	2.0	Pumpkin seeds	7.5
Milk	0.4	Lentils, almonds, Pecans, Brazil nuts	3.0–4.3
Cheddar cheese	3.6	Sunflower seeds	5.8
Beef	7.8	Prawns, crabmeat	1.6-2.2
Pork	2.4	Oysters, raw	47.9

Functions of Zinc

The main biological functions of zinc have to do with growth and development, immunity and metabolism. It is part of the structure of many proteins, including our DNA. Zinc accumulates in bone and plays a role in the structure, strength and maintenance of bone tissue.

As zinc is an antioxidant, it protects cells and membranes, but it also has a major function in detoxification. In the brain we need zinc to make serotonin, melatonin and GABA, which all guard against depression, anxiety and Alzheimer's disease.

Zinc competes with iron and copper for binding to cell membranes and displaces these more reactive metals. This can be a good thing but zinc itself may get displaced by other metals such as cadmium and copper.

ZINC DEFICIENCY

A common nutrient deficiency in general medical practice is zinc deficiency. It's common for patients who present with fatigue, poor appetite, regular infections and/or skin complaints. Children are often pale, fussy eaters, cranky, anaemic and perhaps allergic.

Zinc deficiency is linked to a host of diseases such as cancer, cardiovascular disease, dementia, dermatitis, osteoarthritis and diabetes. The manufacture, secretion and actions of insulin are zinc dependent.

Sometimes malabsorption may be due to low hydrochloric acid (HCl) in the stomach. It can be a bit of a merry-go-round since zinc deficiency causes low HCl, and low HCl causes zinc deficiency via malabsorption. Add to the absorption problem is the fact that calcium, magnesium, iron and zinc all use the same transporters in the gut, so there is competition for absorption. Low levels may also be secondary to stress and ageing, drugs or infections such as *Helicobacter*.

Proving Zinc Deficiency: This is more difficult than one would expect because circulating levels fluctuate as much as 20%, and as zinc is predominantly in the cells, it can be low without showing up in serum blood tests. Levels are also lowered with infection, so check the C-reactive protein and other markers for infection or inflammation.

Low protein levels must also be taken into consideration as zinc is bound to albumin. So, there are two tests that may be more helpful than the serum blood tests:

1. Red cell zinc tests, which have a reference range between 145 and 245 (big range – aim for the higher level).

2. Hair mineral analysis, which measures the cellular levels of both the favourable and the toxic minerals.

Supplementing Zinc

Often the best way to work out if zinc deficiency problem is to have two weeks' supplementation and see if the problem diminishes! Parasitic infections, poor protein intake and high phytic acid from grains hinder absorption and in turn cause deficiency. The best way to supplement is to take zinc in a watery solution while fasting which increases absorption to around 60–70%. However, the taste may be an issue for some, so then split the dose and have it with meals. Too much zinc is a very rare event because we can adjust levels by excretion through the gastrointestinal tract, urine, skin and sweat.

The dose for children: Generally, 10–20 mg/day, depending on the age.
Adult dose: 45mg/day.

References:

te Velthuis, A. J. W., van den Worm, S. H. E., Sims, A. C., Baric, R. S., Snijder, E. J., & van Hemert, M. J. (2010). Zn2+ Inhibits Coronavirus and Arterivirus RNA Polymerase Activity *In Vitro* and Zinc Ionophores Block the Replication of These Viruses in Cell Culture. *PLOS Pathogens*, *6*(11), Article e1001176.

Zhu, M., Zhou, J., Liang, Y., Nair, V., Yao, Y., & Cheng, Z. (2020). CCCH-type zinc finger antiviral protein mediates antiviral immune response by activating T cells. *Journal of Leukocyte Biology*, *107*(2), 299–307. https://doi.org/10.1002/JLB.1AB1119-314RRR

4. MIGHTY MAGNESIUM

We went hunting through the research papers to see just how many enzymes were influenced by magnesium. Who counts these anyway? Most stay on the safe side and suggest it has a function in over 300 enzymes – one brave soul suggested 400!

Some people call magnesium 'amazing'. Dr J.J Ryan would summarise by saying 'magnesium is the mineral that tells all the other minerals what to do.' indicating its essential role in the body's mineral balance and overall health. So let's just get a handle on some of the facts: where it is, what it does and where we get this 'amazing' mineral.

Only about half of the magnesium in the diet gets absorbed, and less if there are gut problems. It is stored in the bone, and any excess is excreted by the kidneys which have the most control of magnesium balance. The body content of magnesium is around 20 mmol/kg of fat-free tissue and 99% of this is in bone. Excretion follows the body clock (the circadian rhythm), with most excretion at night. Red cell magnesium better reflects the cellular magnesium, and hair mineral analysis is more predictive of body stores.

Functions of Magnesium

Magnesium enzymes are involved in energy/glucose reactions, fat and protein production, and muscle contraction and relaxation - to name a few! Any dietary restriction of magnesium promotes osteoporosis and starts the slippery slope to fractures, hospitals, and possible death in the elderly. Apart from good bone structure, magnesium is important in blood pressure and heart rhythm, but it also has a huge influence on neurological function as the release of all neurotransmitters are magnesium dependent. For every 100 mg/day increment in magnesium intake, the overall risk of having metabolic syndrome is lowered by about 17%. You may also recall the vital importance of magnesium in the Krebs Energy Cycle to assist in overcoming chronic fatigue syndrome and fibromyalgia. (See Chapter 25). Enzymes necessary to metabolise vitamin D are magnesium-dependent, so there are not many functions where magnesium does not have a role.

Signs of Low Magnesium

Too little magnesium may give subtle symptoms of fatigue and weakness, and perhaps nausea. The symptoms may escalate to cramps, poor pain threshold, tremors, agitation and anxiety or depression, or cardiac symptoms. Very low magnesium may be associated with numbness and tingling, and (rarely) severe deficiency may be seen in seizures or abnormal cardiac function, though of course these symptoms can occur in other medical conditions unrelated to magnesium deficiency. Endurance exercise can lower magnesium with problems of muscle cramps and insomnia, so it is always worth a trial of magnesium supplementation for 2–3 weeks. Other conditions where magnesium is useful are ADD, ADHD, arthritis, insomnia, premenstrual syndrome, psoriasis, colitis, depression and epilepsy.

Excess Magnesium

Excess magnesium, if present, usually follows magnesium infusions. Flushing, nausea and low blood pressure may occur. If levels are seriously high, cardiovascular effects may result with increased heart rate and possible other cardiac events. Fatigue, drowsiness and confusion, poor muscle tone, and inhibition of bone calcification by displacing calcium in the bone are all possible complications of high magnesium content in the body. Having noted all this, such events are exceedingly rare.

Magnesium is found in a wide variety of whole foods, unfiltered drinking water accounting for about 10% of daily magnesium.

Source: Dietitians of Canada (https://www.unlockfood.ca/en/Articles/Vitamins-and-Minerals/What-You-Need-to-Know-About-Magnesium.aspx).

Food	Serve Size	Magnesium (mg)
All-Bran	30 g	83–111
Wheat Germ	30 g (⅓ cup)	96
Soy cheese	50 g	114
Spinach	125 ml (½ cup)	83
Pumpkin or squash seeds	60 ml (¼ cup)	307
Tofu (prepared with magnesium chloride)	175 ml (¾ cup)	55–99
Almonds	60 ml (¼ cup)	88–109
Spinach	125 ml (½ cup)	83
Potatoes with skin	1 medium	47–52

SUPPLEMENTING MAGNESIUM

The recommendation is about 400mg per day for an adult. It is best taken on an empty stomach for better absorption, but if it causes loose bowel motions, take it with food. You get better absorption when the elemental magnesium is bound (chelated) to a carrier.

Magnesium citrate is well absorbed and good for constipation.

Magnesium glycinate (diglycinate) is useful in anxiety and poor sleep, cardiac conditions and diabetes.

Magnesium sulphate is also used primarily as a laxative, and the hydroxide forms are also used in antacid preparations.

VITAMIN AND MINERAL

ACTION PLAN – CHECKLIST

· Expose your body to the sun daily.
· Consume foods with vitamin D daily – fish, cheese and eggs.
· Consider both the risks and symptoms of iron deficiency, and test where appropriate.
· Supplement iron when blood levels are low and consider the cause of low iron.
· Consume red meat, eggs or fish, spinach, hummus and fortified cereals if iron is deficient.
· Test for zinc deficiency if there are immune, skin or digestive complaints.
· Supplement zinc for 3 months, then retest.
· Add foods with high zinc – oysters, red meat, baked beans and pumpkin seeds.
· Add 400 mg magnesium per day for three weeks for symptoms of cramping, muscle aches and pains.

References: Gröber, U., Schmidt, J., & Kisters, K. (2015). Magnesium in Prevention and Therapy. *Nutrients*, *7*(9), 8199–8226. https://doi.org/10.3390/nu7095388

Chapter 36

JUST ADD WATER

*"Man cannot discover new oceans
unless he has the courage to lose
sight of the shore."*

ANDRÉ PAUL GUILLAUME GIDE

From regulating body temperature to the digestion, absorption, transport and eventual elimination of other nutrients and hormones, water does it all. It accounts for approximately 60% of your body weight as an adult and 75% at birth.

Even before you sweat, you lose about 4% of your body weight in water per day, half of it through the skin and lungs. That's almost 2.5 L per day if you weigh 60 kg. You make about 250 ml water per day through metabolic processes (eating and digesting food), so you need to drink water to make up the difference.

If you ever feel a bit sluggish or dizzy, it might just be your body giving you a nudge to grab that water bottle. Once you hit that 6% water loss mark, it's your body's gentle reminder to take a hydration pit stop. Athletes can experience water loss of up to 10% in extreme conditions, so rehydration is key. If the water lost isn't replenished, its delirium and a bad end to all your hard work.

Function of Water in the Body

- Transport nutrients and oxygen to the cells.
- Convert food into easily absorbed molecules.
- Eliminate waste products through the kidneys.
- Grow and repair cells.
- Regulate the body's temperature.
- Cushion body joints by preventing friction between bones and ligaments.
- Keep the nose, mouth, eyes and lungs moist.
- Prevent constipation.
- Assists glycogen storage in a soluble form.

How Much Water Should You Drink

Water Intake	Adult Men	Adult Women
Australian Guidelines	3.4 litres per day	2.9 litres per day (> pregnancy)
US Dietary Guidelines, 2010	3.7 litres per day	2.7 litres per day
European Guidelines, 2010	2.5 litres per day	2.0 litres per day

You get 80% of the water you need from fluids including tea, coffee and juice, and 20% from solid foods. All these are counted in your water intake per day. Fruit, vegetables, milk and yoghurt all have high water content. Your intake will depend on your age, gender, activity level, health and environment.

As a rule, you'll need to up your intake if you are larger, male, physically active, in a hot climate, at a high altitude or experiencing fever or diarrhoea. Dehydration, whether acute or chronic, can affect your brain, heart, skin, kidneys, joints and energy levels.

Children heat up more quickly because they have a greater surface area to body mass ratio, but they don't cool down as efficiently because they sweat less than adults. The elderly are less sensitive to thirst, and up to 30% are estimated to be dehydrated, so get into the habit of drinking water as the birthdays increase.

Organ	Health Effects of Water
Brain 70% of the brain is water	Brain receptors detect change and send messages to make you feel thirsty and hungry. They are less efficient in the elderly.
Heart 80% of blood is water	Reduced blood volume and blood pressure can make you feel dizzy when you stand up quickly. Just one glass of water has been shown to help relieve these symptoms.
Skin 64% water	Water makes skin look and act younger and healthier. Sadly, you won't avoid wrinkles by drinking more water, since those come with ageing, genetics and sun exposure.
Kidneys 79% water	Your kidneys filter blood to get rid of waste materials, including toxic chemicals and drugs. Kidney stones are less likely to occur if you drink plenty of water.

Joints 80% water in cartilage, 79% in muscles surrounding the joints	Water cushions the joints and protects the spinal cord. Pain is more likely when dehydrated. Hydration helps with nutrient and waste product exchange.
Cells 70% water	Chemical reactions need water to work properly. Low energy can be a symptom of dehydration.

What Not to Drink: Alcohol is a diuretic, which increases the amount of water you lose in urine. Alcohol reduces levels of the hormone vasopressin, which normally help the body reabsorb water rather than pass it out. By comparison, caffeine (in coffee and tea) is only a very mild diuretic. Some herbs act as diuretics, the most common is dandelion, known in Ireland as 'piss the beds'! Celery is a mild diuretic.

JUST ADD WATER

ACTION PLAN – CHECKLIST

· Drink six glasses of water per day and more in hot climates.
· Limit alcohol and cut down on coffee.
· Be aware that all sources of food are counted in fluid intake, e.g. yoghurt, fruit and vegetables.

Reference: Armstrong, L. E., & Johnson, E. C. (2018). Water Intake, Water Balance, and the Elusive Daily Water Requirement. *Nutrients*, *10*(12), 1928. https://doi.org/10.3390/nu10121928

Chapter 37

MEDICATE CAREFULLY

*"However beautiful the strategy,
you should occasionally look at the
results."*

WINSTON CHURCHILL

According to the United Nations, the number of people aged 60 years or older is growing faster than any other age group. By 2050, it is projected that one in six people in the world will be over the age of 65. The aging population also has social implications, including increased demand for eldercare services. Three in every five Australians aged over sixty-five years have two or more chronic conditions.

Medication Problems in the Ageing Patient: In their initial assessment of elderly patients facing medical challenges, geriatricians often discover a concerning trend: some individuals may be prescribed a staggering *nine* medications, while half are simultaneously receiving care from multiple physicians. It's not a new problem. In some cases, the geriatrician may get rid of everything but one or two critical drugs. They find that the patient is often a whole lot better, with a sharper mind, happier and much more agile.

Harm from medications can arise from unintended consequences as well as medication error – wrong medications, wrong time or wrong dose. Medications that reduce stomach acid reduce nutrient absorption –not a good idea in the elderly. Diuretics lower blood pressure, but they also excrete potassium and other nutrients. Cramping, muscle weakness and fatigue may be avoided by adding high potassium foods or a tablet daily. Statins drugs reduce cholesterol, but they also are well known for precipitating muscle fatigue and muscle pain, not to mention poor memory. Pain medications, alcohol abuse and adverse reactions to drugs are just the ticket to falls and delirium common in the elderly.

Younger Patients Also Have Problems: Medications for bipolar disorder, ADHD, schizophrenia, depression and anxiety abound. Difficult clinical situations often result in prescriptions of tranquillisers for anxiety, antidepressants for mood disorders and hypnotics for sleep etc. The problem is that the medicines and their dose together with their interactions make the clinical issue quite difficult to treat precisely. Reviewing a patient's needs becomes particularly complicated if the patient is 'doctor shopping' because of dependence on addictive pain medication.

It's a global issue with the misuse of prescription drugs such as benzodiazepines, as well as stimulants, barbiturates and sedatives relatively common. Paracetamol overdose can occur accidently, but it is often used by those who attempt to harm themselves.

THE PROBLEM WITH FILLERS

Excipients (such as fillers, binders and lubricants, etc) constitute up to 90% of the total volume of a medicine. Their job is to impart stability to the drug and participate in delivery, absorption and timely release, plus the subsequent therapeutic action of the active ingredient/s. Excipients can cause problems because people have different metabolic effects or excretion rates.

Donald Birkett from the *Australian Prescriber* (2003) explains that individual patients could have idiosyncratic sensitivity to colourings that are in the generic, often cheaper products, but not in the innovator product.

Henry Osiecki is an Australian biochemist of his family-owned nutritional manufacturing company Bio Concepts. He goes to great lengths to explain why the company limits fillers and excipients in their products. He recognises that colours and additives, including gluten and corn, can cause reactions in many sensitive individuals.

GENETIC TESTS CAN HELP

Our genetics have a big part to play in our response to drugs. A pharmacogenomic profile is a test that provides information on potential drug interactions, and the ideal medicines and dosages suitable for you and your condition. The test involves mostly blood but may require saliva or cells from your cheek. The test will determine how rapidly these drugs are metabolised and whether the drug is likely to give benefit or may possibly give side effects. The cost is about $197 in Australia but it is not covered by Medicare. Other factors, including illness, nutrition and concurrent medication, can affect the results.

'QUACKS, HACKS AND BIG PHARMA FLACKS'

Dr. Ben Goldacre, a medical doctor and journalist, has written two books criticizing the medical and pharmaceutical industries. In "Bad Science," he targets quacks, hacks, and Big Pharma, expressing disdain for nutritionists and the pharmaceutical industry.

The book reached number one on the nonfiction charts, sold over half a million copies, and was translated into 25 languages. His second book, "Bad Pharma," exposes how drug companies mislead and harm patients by hiding unflattering data. It's widely read in the medical community, though not always accepted.

Goldacre is generally kind to doctors but criticises their prescribing practices, possibly due to their lack of experience and time to navigate the complex relationships between pharmaceutical companies, academics, physicians, and consumer health groups lobbying for government-subsidised drugs.

Richard Horton, editor of The Lancet, stated in 2015 that much of the scientific literature might be untrue. Another prominent figure who has expressed similar concerns is John Ioannidis, a professor of medicine and epidemiology at Stanford University. In his highly influential 2005 paper titled "Why Most Published Research Findings Are False," Ioannidis argued that a large proportion of published research findings are likely to be incorrect due to various biases, methodological issues, and statistical problems in scientific research. This paper has been widely cited and has sparked ongoing discussions about the reliability of scientific literature.

The COVID-19 pandemic highlighted daily scientific disagreements. In March 2022, British Medical Journal authors Jureidini and McHenry argued that evidence-based medicine has been corrupted by corporate interests, failed regulation, and academic commercialsation. Instead of acting as independent, disinterested scientists and critically evaluating a drug's performance, key opinion leaders become what marketing executives refer to as "product champions."

Our magic potion remains elusive!

MEDICATE CAREFULLY

ACTION PLAN – CHECKLIST

- Let your doctor know of all your current medications.
- Advise the doctor of supplements you may be taking.
- Confirm the reason for your prescription, the dose and the timing.
- Discuss medications that produced side effects in the past.
- Outline allergies and sensitivities to avoid side effects of fillers.
- Pharmacogenomic tests can predict suitability of drugs if adverse reactions persist.

References:

Birkett, D. J. (2003). Generics – equal or not? *Australian Prescriber*, *26*, 85–87. Goldacre, B. (2008). *Bad Science*. Fourth Estate.

Horton, R. (2015). Off line: What is medicine's 5 sigma? *The Lancet*, *385*(9976), 1380. Lilienthal, C. (2019). Drugs, side effects and how they changed me. *Australian Doctor*.

Jureidini, J. McHenry, L B. (2022) The illusion of evidence based medicine BMJ ; 376 :o702 doi:10.1136/bmj.o702

Ioannidis J. P. (2005). Why most published research findings are false. *PLoS medicine*, *2*(8), e124. https://doi.org/10.1371/journal.pmed.0020124

Jureidini. J,. McHenry, L. B,. (2022) The illusion of evidence based medicine. *BMJ*; 376 :o702 doi:10.1136/bmj.o702

Chapter 38

AGEING GRACEFULLY

"Discard me not in my old age; as my strength falls, do not abandon me."

PSALM 71

Degenerative ageing is insidious – not obvious in the early years, but blatant later in life. It's not much fun and having fun in life is important. The optimistic live longer than the pessimists, the communicators live longer than the hermits, and those with passion surpass the apathetic. Good relationships can be just as important as your family. To live longer and healthier lives we need to stay connected. Resolving conflict will give you a bit more time. Being less neurotic will help, and so will a glass of wine! So, what are the keys to improved quality and quantity of life, outside of having a good time?

In this chapter we're diving into the secrets of extending our time on this planet. We're all about maximising our 'quantity of life' by tapping into essential tools and lifestyle tweaks. By embracing good nutrition and creating an environment that fosters longevity, we're not just adding years to our lives; we're also sprinkling some joy and vibrancy into each day.

We will deal with this under the following headings:

1. Basic lifestyle factors in disease prevention.
2. The 'God' molecule, glutathione: levels decrease as we age.
3. Longer telomeres are signs of a longer life. We present ways to help lengthen those telomeres – and avoid some factors that shorten them.

1. LIFESTYLE FACTORS IN DISEASE PREVENTION

Three Caribbean islands have more centenarians per capita than any other nation. The fourth place goes to Japan with Australia behind Canada, France and the UK. "Blue Zones" have been coined by Dan Buettner who travelled to places where people live exceptionally long lives - Costa Rica, Loma Linda in California, Okinawa in Japan, Sardinia in Italy and Icaria in Greece. The diet of these populations is rich in plant-based foods; beans are consumed regularly, and they have a little meat, fish or eggs. They have active daily lives and live in a relaxed atmosphere where they connect with family and friends.

The oldest person alive as we write this book is María Branyas Morera, born in 1907. She has lived through two world wars, the Spanish civil war, the 1918 flu pandemic and recovered from COVID in 2020. Although she is not strict about her diet, she believes in the positive effects of natural yoghurt. She also believes her longevity is attributed to luck and genetics. She attributes her long life to "order, tranquillity, good connection with family and friends, contact with nature, emotional stability, no worries, no regrets, lots of positivity, and [staying] away from toxic people." All which loosely ties in with our opening paragraph.

Genetics are believed to count for about 25% of this story. Long lived people often come from families who also live into old age. Modern medical technology, access to healthcare and improved living conditions play a role in longevity. Most centenarians worked physically hard in their early years, they ate less food and had lower body weight. Good sewerage and good clean water have made a big impact, but obviously the health advancements in nutrition and pharmaceuticals have contributed. Social and environmental factors have influenced the increasing number of centenarians today. The question now is how long we can live ?

2. THE 'GOD' MOLECULE – GLUTATHIONE

Glutathione (GSH) is found in every cell in the body. Its first job is to protect the cells against oxidation/ageing as they go about their normal metabolic processes. And secondly, it detoxifies and eliminates any of the toxic chemicals (including that extra glass of wine) which occur during the process. Glutathione is the "go to" molecule for anti-ageing.

The cleansing and binding/chelating powers of glutathione protect you while you accumulate toxins, acid residues, chemicals, fungi, bacteria and cancerous agents. It acts as a double agent, switching states between the oxidised (loss of electrons) and reduced forms (with a net gain of electrons) as it gets bombarded with the need to do multiple reactions.

This multitasker has been likened to a Kamikaze pilot performing suicidal crashes on enemy targets! You need over 90% of the glutathione in a reduced state – which can be difficult to supply when inflammation sets in.

Supply chains are a problem because glutathione is easily digested in the stomach, and it doesn't survive long enough to be absorbed in the gut. To overcome this issue it's now available in a mouth spray.

Foods with good amounts of glutathione, such as cruciferous vegetables, garlic and onions, often fail to deliver the goods in times of high body stress/infection. The best way to provide glutathione is to provide the requirements for its production; it's a relatively simple molecule with only three building blocks: glycine, cysteine, and glutamine:

1. **Glycine:** The body makes glycine which makes it non essential in the diet. Food sources are meat, chicken and pork, seeds and lentils.

2. **N-acetyl cystine (NAC):** NAC supplies the key sulphur molecule – cysteine. It's found in turkey, cheese, eggs, lentils and yoghurt, and readily available via supplementation.

3. **Glutamine:** This nutrient removes excess waste (ammonia) and repairs tissues. It has a major role in immunity and is required for normal digestions and brain function. Glutamine is found in protein based foods such as beef, milk and eggs but also in rice and corn. Doctors quite often use supplemental glutamine to prevent post-operative complications.

α-lipoic acid (ALA): ALA is a scavenger of free radicals and helps regenerate glutathione. Small amounts are found in green vegetables, red meat and tomatoes. A study of protein malnutrition in children found glutathione supplementation reduced the risk of dying by 69%, followed by ALA (54%) and NAC (18%) - not a bad effort!

3. LONGER TELOMERES ARE GOOD

In the nucleus of each cell, your DNA is packed tightly into coiled thread-like structures called chromosomes. They store your genetic information. The ends of the chromosomes are capped by telomeres; and just as plastic caps keep your shoelaces from fraying and falling apart. Telomeres protect the DNA structures from fraying. As the cells divide, telomeres become progressively shorter, losing a bit of DNA each time. The only part of the chromosome that is lost is from the telomere, and the rest is left undamaged.

The structure of DNA is made up of molecules with nitrogen bases (guanine-cytosine and adenine-thymine). Each of us has about three billion bases, with more than 99% being the same. The telomeres at the ends of the DNA strands have much less. We start off with about 10,000 base pairs at birth, and they decline by around twenty to forty base pairs each year.

Telomere length may be a measure of biological age. Cardiovascular disease, stroke, cancer, arthritis, osteoporosis, cataracts, type 2 diabetes, hypertension, mental diseases, chronic obstructive pulmonary disease and dementia are all associated with shorter telomeres. The telomeres of obese women are shorter than those of their leaner counterparts. If you smoke cigarettes, for each pack/year subtract another five base pairs off your telomeres. Shorter telomeres have three times the risk of heart disease, and if your diet is low in fish and seed oils (DHA and EPA) expect your telomeres to shorten even more quickly. Shorter telomeres are linked to depression, chronic stress and poor sleep. White cells fight infections, and if the telomeres in your white cells are short, you have an eight-fold risk of death from infectious disease! Exercise is a positive factor in longevity. Adults who had little exercised (16 minutes per week) had 200 fewer base pairs compared to people who are active.

Telomere length is related to age and ethnicity, and each person has significant individual differences at birth. On average, female telomeres are just slightly longer than males. The longest telomeres are found in the heart muscle tissue (myocardium), and the shortest in the liver and kidneys (renal cortex). Some tissues have a greater loss – human liver tissue has a loss of about 55 base pairs of telomeric DNA per year.

The common denominators in the whole scenario are increased oxidative stress and inflammation. While it may sound depressing, the upside of this research is that lifestyle changes, omega-3 fish oil, the nutrient vitamins B12, C, D, E, K, folic acid and α-lipoic acid (ALA) have been shown to be protective. It's the balance between lengthening and shortening that determines the mean length and distribution of your telomeres. Genetics, pregnancy, early adversity, current stress and lifestyle factors all compromise adult telomere length.

Factors That Decrease Telomere Length	Factors That Increase Telomere Length
	• Exercise
• Chronic stress	• Low-calorie diet and reduced protein
• Prenatal neglect	• High-fibre diet
• A younger age at conception	• Lower waist circumference
• Low socioeconomic status	• Lower stress and stress reduction
• Low education	• Reduced depression
• Depression	• Mindful eating for overweight women
• Caregiving	• Yoga
• Anxiety	• Later gestational age
• Neuroticism	• Meditation and social support
• Being overweight	• Vitamins C, E, D, K1 and K2
• Abdominal obesity	• Good sleep
• Sedentary lifestyle	• Omega-3 free fatty acids
• Smoking	• Lower blood ratio of omega-6 to omega-3
• Insulin resistance	polyunsaturated fatty acids
• Low vagal tone	

Measuring the Telomere Length

The most accurate telomere test is called a flow-FISH test and is advertised in the USA. White blood cells (leukocytes) are isolated from a blood sample and mixed with fluorescent peptide nucleic acid (PNA) probes that bind specifically to the telomere repeats. The test cost in the USA is in the order of $400.

AGEING GRACEFULLY

ACTION PLAN – CHECKLIST

- Protect your cells against oxidation with fruit and vegetables and a lean body mass.
- Reduce the risk factors for disease, e.g. smoking and non-essential drugs.
- Sleep well and exercise daily.
- Engage socially with friends, family and community.
- Learn new things.

References:

Ames, B. N. (2018). Prolonging healthy aging: Longevity vitamins and proteins. *Proceedings of the National Academy of Sciences of the United States of America*, *115*(43), 10836–10844

Cai, D., Zhao, S., Li, D., Chang, F., Tian, X., Huang, G., Zhu, Z., Liu, D., Dou, X., Li, S., Zhao, M., & Li, Q. (2016). Nutrient Intake Is Associated with Longevity Characterization by Metabolites and Element Profiles of Healthy Centenarians. *Nutrients*, *8*(9), 564. https://doi.org/10.3390/nu8090564

Farzaneh-Far, R., Lin, J., Epel, E. S., Harris, W. S., Blackburn, E. H., & Whooley, M. A. (2010). Association of marine omega-3 fatty acid levels with telomeric aging in patients with coronary heart disease. *JAMA*, *303*(3), 250–257

Wu, G., Fang, Y., Yang, S., Lupton, J. R., & Turner, N. D. (2004). Glutathione Metabolism and Its Implications for Health, *The Journal of Nutrition*, *134*(3), 489–492

Blackburn, E. H. (2001). Switching and Signaling at the Telomere. *Cell*, *106*, 661–673

Hajjar, I., Hayek, S. S., Goldstein, F. C., Martin, G., Jones, D. P., & Quyyumi, A. (2018). Oxidative stress predicts cognitive decline with aging in healthy adults: an observational study. *Journal of Neuroinflammation*, *15*(1), 17. https://doi.org/10.1186/s12974-017-1026-z

Lin, J., Epel, E., & Blackburn, E. Telomeres and lifestyle factors: roles in cellular aging. *Mutation Research*, *730*, 85–89

Chapter 39

COVID-19, THE UNWELCOME VISITOR

"Gentlemen, it is the microbes who will have the last word."

LOUIS PASTEUR

The Coronavirus Disease 2019 (COVID-19) is primarily a respiratory infection caused by the coronavirus SARS-CoV-2. Like all viruses, SARS-CoV-2 has incurred random genetic errors when replicating (mutations) and ultimately we had the Alpha and Delta variations predominant in 2020 and 2021 until the emergence of the Omicron variant in 2022. For most of us, we just name the group as COVID.

When the time came to protect against the new virus all common sense went out the window and the vaccine was considered the magic potion that could save the world while other effective drugs were sidelined. Doctors now turned influencers hit the airways with the mantra "safe and effective". The Lancet tried to "calm the farm" and published an article on July 2021 about the safety and effectiveness of the vaccines which got very little airtime while we were all bathed in fear.

Early in the pandemic Olliaro (2021) posted a paper in *The Lancet* which explained the difference between relative risk reduction (RRR) and absolute risk reduction (ARR) for the vaccine efficacy. RRR showed impressive numbers: 95% for Pfizer-BioNTech, 94% for Moderna-NIH, 91% for Gamaleya, and 67% for both J&J and AstraZeneca-Oxford.

However, ARR, which looks at the whole population, was much lower: 1.3% for AstraZeneca-Oxford, 1.2% for Moderna-NIH and J&J, 0.93% for Gamaleya, and 0.84% for Pfizer-BioNTech. Basically, to protect one person you need to vaccinate 81 for the Moderna–NIH, 108 for the Gamaleya, and 119 for the Pfizer–BioNTech vaccines.

HISTORICAL EXPERIENCE

On 11 March 2020 the World Health Organization (WHO) declared COVID-19 to be a pandemic. Most countries took the WHO advice on board and followed its public health directives; one Nordic country (Sweden) refuted the strict WHO directives and instead had some limited measures on social distancing.

Sweden had no state emergency, no lockdowns of schools or restaurants or offices, nor were there mask mandates. However, vaccinations became available by December 2020. In short, the Swedish Government was on the road to herd immunity and their messaging lacked the alarm of the WHO. While the world looked on, the death rates rose well above their Nordic neighbours. Internationally, Sweden became the "pariah state" and respectful debate around scientific evidence gave way to mudslinging. The Swedes held firm and continued to support their government's stance.

Some minor adjustment to Sweden's public health advice followed the spike in deaths; vaccine passports were introduced late in 2021 but by February 2022 almost all restrictions were abolished and by April 22 the virus was no longer considered a danger to society at large. Sweden's economy did well, there was no suicide increase and importantly by 2023 the death rate from COVID-19 was similar to many other countries and lower than the rates in the USA, UK, and Southern Europe.

Hindsight is a wonderful thing, and not all countries have been happy with their government's response to the pandemic. Apart from Sweden only Singapore and Israel felt their countries handled the outbreak well. The Pew Research Data (2022) indicate just 36% of Americans had a positive view of Biden's handling of the coronavirus outbreak and 60% felt confused by changes in recommendations. Americans were the most ideologically divided about the importance of COVID vaccines and 82% say the country is more divided since the pandemic.

The release of the Pfizer papers after a court ruling in January '22 threw a spanner in the works with the identification of 1223 deaths from the vaccine in the two months between December 1, 2020 and 28 February 2021. Regarding the vaccine use in pregnancy and lactation, there were 413 cases of which 84 serious and 329 non-serious.

COVID enquiries in UK, France, Italy have generally centred around preparedness and response, mandates, masks and lockdowns and whether the policies have reflected scientific knowledge or political shortcomings. The UK Inquiry is expected to run until 2026 covering the impact on health systems, vaccines and therapeutics and political governance. Not all information will be viewed by the public which do not have access to the same data provided to the vaccine manufacturers, for "commercial sensitivity reasons".

In Australia, the government enquiry has also generally centred around preparedness and response, but issues of public concern has been the lack of public awareness of the genetically modified organism (GMO) vaccine technology and the consent relating to the promise that the vaccine would "prevent it from multiplying in other cells", that it would be "restricted to the vaccine site" and it "does not cause disease in humans and other organisms other that apes".

According to Gigi Foster, Professor of Economics, UNSW Business School, the cost of Australia's COVID lockdowns has been at least 68 times greater than the benefits they delivered. "Since April 2020, government responses to the COVID pandemic have had little to do with public health promotion, and everything to do with political incentives, money and power," see: LockdownCBA_1Aug2022-ExecSummary.pdf (the-greatcovidpanic.com)

LASTING HEALTH DEFICITS

By 2024 COVID (Omicron strain) showed more transmissibility but fortunately caused less severe disease than previous strains. Predominant symptoms start 2-14 days after infection and include cough, nasal congestion, loss of taste or smell, muscle aches and pains, headaches, and gastrointestinal symptoms. The problem with this and other viruses is the increased ill effects in those with underlying health conditions which happen most commonly in the aged population. Most people recover from the virus relatively quickly but not everybody is so well served. Long-COVID can be broadly defined as persistent symptoms for more than 6 months after the initial infection. It is also more likely in those with a history of infection from the Delta strain and those who have needed to seek medical treatment.

That said, more than 200 symptoms have been linked to long-COVID. Symptoms can fluctuate and last more than a year after the initial infection. Researchers have likened the symptoms of long-COVID to that of chronic fatigue syndrome which is a complex and debilitating medical condition that can occur after a severe viral infection such as glandular fever and stress. (See Chapter 25).

Here we compare some 16 of the main symptoms from these two conditions.

Symptoms	Long-COVID	Chronic Fatigue Syndrome
Persistent and profound fatigue	Yes	Yes
Headache	Yes	Yes
Poor memory & concentrations	Yes	Yes
Sleep difficulties	Yes	Yes
Joint and muscle pains	Yes	Yes
Gastrointestinal problems	Yes	Yes
Flu symptoms, cough, sore throat	Yes	Yes
Dizziness or light headedness	Yes	Yes
Problems with temperature regulation	Yes	Yes
Chronic lung problems and shortness of breath	Yes	Shortness of breath with exertion
Cardiovascular problems, chest pain, and fast pounding heart	Yes	Not generally
Loss of smell and taste	Yes	Not generally
Sensitivity to noise and light	No	Yes
Food and chemical sensitivities	No	Yes

Both conditions share the catalyst of a viral infection with fatigue, 'brain fog', light-headedness and sleep problems. The big difference is that the respiratory, cardio-vascular and taste symptoms are more specific to the COVID-19 virus and vaccine. Another outcome of severe COVID-19 infections is the greater risk of contracting other health conditions such as diabetes, kidney disease, pulmonary embolism (lung clots) and myocarditis (inflammed heart) following the onset of COVID-19 infection.

TREATMENT AND PREVENTION OF COVID-19

Omicron, the current COVID-19 strain, has had many mutations since 2021, making it tricky by evading existing immunity and challenging both our natural defenses and vaccination protection. The CDC mentioned in a March 15, 2023, update that reinfections can happen just weeks after a previous infection. This is why over-the-counter medicines can be helpful in protecting against the virus and also treating the symptoms.

Research (Arregocés-Castillo et al., 2022) indicates that vaccines can be less effective for older folks with pre-existing conditions (Nordstrom et al., 2022). This is similar to what we've seen with the flu, where vaccines offer 30%-50% protection for the elderly (Murasko et al., 2002). Boosting our immune system is key since stress, chronic illnesses, and aging can make us more vulnerable to infections.

Keeping weight, blood sugars and blood pressure in healthy ranges are of particular importance in seeking to guard against a poor outcome from any viral contact. Then again, if you do have the virus, there is an increased demand for some micronutrients – specifically vitamins D, A and C, the B group vitamins, and the minerals zinc, iron and selenium. They favourably influence not only susceptibility to infectious diseases, but also the course and outcome of the infection as well.

Repurposing low-dose naltrexone (LDN): Hyperinflammation and thrombosis (blood clotting) are hallmarks of severe COVID-19. Naltrexone is a drug used to address alcohol and drug addiction at doses of 50mg/day. It works on your endorphins which affect mood, and it also has anti-clotting and anti-inflammatory effects while managing pain at low dose. Doses (1–5mg) has been used in many inflammatory conditions and has the added advantage of enhancing the blood brain barrier, thus protecting against damage in the brain. LDN has recently been shown to be an effective treatment for some people with both chronic fatigue and long COVID. Naltrexone is also discussed in Chapter 3.

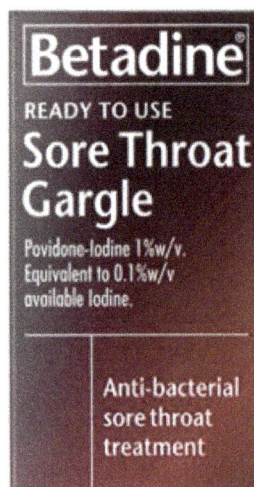

BETADINE GARGLE

The cheap effective povidone-iodine gargle should be in all our medicine cabinets. This *Betadine Sore Throat Gargle* has been proven to reduce the viral load for those with COVID in-fection and it helps prevent infection if taken as a precaution. Studies have confirmed that 0.5% PVP-I is effective in reducing SARS-CoV-2 in the nasal cavity, nasopharynx and oropharynx. It costs around AU $15.00 and it has the instructions on the packet.

Zinc and viral protection: Zinc reduces viral replication and protects against severe inflammation (cytokine storm). Many of the health issues that put people at risk during the pandemic are related to inadequate zinc levels. Low levels of zinc are often present in the elderly, and infection rates in general are lowered when zinc is supplemented to the tune of 45 mg per day over twelve months. It's worth having blood levels of zinc checked when the opportunity presents. Recent research had focused the effects of zinc on calcium ion channels and its relation to long COVID and chronic fatigue. See Chapter 35.

Vitamin D and virus protection: We emphasise that there are specific benefits that adequate vitamin D may bring to serious infections such as COVID-19. For each 10 nmol/l (160 IU) increase in vitamin D, you can expect a 7% lower risk of infection.

The risk of pneumonia has been shown to be nearly four times greater where low levels of vitamin D coexist. The more severe the deficiency, the greater the risk for intensive-care hospital admission. These statistics prevailed even before the COVID-19 pandemic. We recommend a dose of 800 IU per day. Unless you have oily fish frequently, it is very difficult to obtain vitamin D from dietary sources. Sensible sun exposure and fatty fish are required in stressful times. Vitamin D is also helpful in treating fatigue and depression. (See Chapter 35).

Vitamin C (ascorbic acid): Vitamin C reduces those inflammatory signalling molecules associated with severe inflammation. It does this by helping to prevent tissue damage which assist healing. Thus, it is an ideal fit for both the prevention and treatment of viral symptoms. To prevent infection we need to optimise cellular and tissue levels. In contrast, to treat established infections we need higher (gram) doses of the vitamin to compensate for the increased demand.

For example, the recommended intake in Australia and Europe is 45 mg and 90 mg respectively, but to guard against infection vitamin C intakes of 100–200 mg per day is needed to optimise cell and tissue levels. As vitamin C is a water-soluble vitamin, it doesn't interact well with cell membranes, so only about 50% absorption is achieved. Nanotechnology (72–100 Nm) allows better absorption. One Nm (nanometre) is one-millionth of a millimetre, thus a 5mg teaspoon dose results in around 1650 mg of vitamin C per day because of the 90% absorption. The cost is significantly higher at nearly fifty dollars for about two weeks' supply, but this form of vitamin C transcends any digestive and absorption problems associated with normal high-dose vitamin C tablets.

Melatonin: This hormone is secreted during darkness, mainly from the pineal gland in the brain. It has a key role in your sleep-wake cycle. It is an antioxidant, but the reason we are adding melatonin is because of its ability to increase oxygen, decrease inflammation and enhance the immune system. Experience with the SARS-CoV virus suggests that sufficient amounts of this hormone protect against sepsis/infection, with notable anti-inflammatory effects in the brain where significant damage can be done with COVID-19. Hyperinflammation is a major feature in COVID-19 patients due to overreaction of the immune system, damaging the heart, kidneys and intestines, as well as the lungs and brain. Melatonin is safe, nontoxic, and available in pure form for human use as a supplement. You do need a prescription, and it is best taken at night to avoid a side-effect of sleepiness during the day.

Quercetin is another useful nutrient against respiratory viruses. Quercetin is a flavonoid used commonly in bronchial asthma for reducing mucus and inflammation. It is found in onions, grapes, cherries, citrus and leafy vegetables. The dose is 250–500 mg per day.

Useful herbs and the coronaviruses: Out of 200 Chinese medicinal herb extracts screened for antiviral activities against earlier SARS-CoV, *Lycoris radiata* was the most potent. *Bupleurum chinense* and the more common *Glycyrrhiza glabra* or liquorice were also effective against certain aspects of coronaviruses.

Liquorice has anti-viral, anti-inflammatory, antiallergic and anticancer activities, and liquid extracts had positive effects when tested on SARS-infected monkeys. Liquorice assists by making it difficult for the virus to attach to target cells and hinders viral reproduction slowing its spread. It also showed positive results against herpes, HIV, Epstein-Barr virus and the shingles virus (Herpes Zoster). But be careful with liquorice if you have high blood pressure, as it may raise it.

Turmeric supports your liver, enhancing its ability to rid your body of toxins, including those from viruses. Add black pepper (piperine) to increase turmeric absorption by up to 2000%, or nanotechnology which impart a 95% curcumin release. Both have powerful antioxidant capacity, as well as having anti-inflammatory, wound healing, and antimicrobial activities.

Black cumin seeds, otherwise known as *nigella sativa*, have been used for centuries for its antibacterial, antiviral, antiparasitic and antifungal properties.

Probiotics and prebiotics: COVID-19 has been found in the faeces of people infected with the virus. A strong gut barrier is a defence against infection while a permeable barrier can trigger local inflammation. Gut bacterial diversity is reduced in older age.

COVID-19

ACTION PLAN – CHECKLIST

- Keep weight, blood pressure and blood sugars within normal range.
- Ensure adequate zinc and supplement 30–40 mg if levels are low.
- Use Betadine Gargle for viral protection and treatment.
- Add probiotics, antibacterial and antiviral herbs and spices.
- Keep up vitamin D intake and get adequate sunshine when possible.
- Add vitamin C 500 mg twice a day to guard against the virus.
- Add 500 mg of quercetin if there are chest or sinus complaints.

References:

Olliaro, P., Torreele, E., & Vaillant, M. (2021). COVID-19 vaccine efficacy and effectiveness-the elephant (not) in the room. *The Lancet. Microbe,2*(7), e279–e280. https://doi.org/10.1016/S2666-5247(21)00069-0

Arregocés-Castillo, L., Fernández-Niño, J., Rojas-Botero M., Palacios-Clavijo,A., Maryory Galvis-Pedraza, M., Luz Rincón-Medrano, L., et al. (2022). Effectiveness of COVID-19 vaccines in older adults in Colombia: a retrospective, population-based study of the ESPERANZA cohort. *The Lancet, Health & Llongevity*. https://doi.org/10.1016/S2666-7568(22)00035-6

Ashour, H. M., Elkhatib, W. F., Rahman, M. M., & Elshabrawy, H. A. (2020). Insights into the Recent 2019 Novel Coronavirus (SARS-CoV-2) in Light of Past Human Coronavirus Outbreaks. *Pathogens*, *9*(3), 186. https://doi.org/10.3390/pathogens9030186

O'Kelly, B., Vidal, L., McHugh, T., Woo, J., Avramovic, G., & Lambert, J. S. (2022). Safety and efficacy of low dose naltrexone in a long covid cohort; an interventional pre-post study. *Brain, behavior, & immunity - health*, *24*, 100485. https://doi.org/10.1016/j.bbih.2022.100485

Berry, D. J., Hesketh, K., Power, C., & Hyppönen, E. (2011). Vitamin D status has a linear association with seasonal infections and lung function in British adults. *British Journal of Nutrition*, *106*(9), 1433–1440.

Murasko, D.M., Bernstein, .ED., Gardner, E.M,, Gross, P., Munk, G., Dran S, Abrutyn, E. (2002). Role of humoral and cell-mediated immunity in protection from influenza disease after immunization of healthy elderly. *Exp Gerontol*. 2002 Jan-Mar;37(2-3):427-39. doi: 10.1016/s0531-5565(01)00210-8. PMID: 11772530.

Pfizer Documents. (2021) 5.3.6 Cumulative Analysis of Post-authorization Adverse Events Reports of PF-07302048 (BNT162B2) Received Through 28-Feb-2021 Post Marketing Experience, p6 -p12; Tables 1 &6.BNT162b2 Reportshttps://phmpt.org/pfizers-documents/

Seow, J., Graham, C., Merrick, B., Acors, S., Steel, K., Hemmings, O., O'Bryne, A., ..., & Doores, K. (2020). Longitudinal evaluation and decline of antibody responses in SARS-CoV-2 infection [Preprint].*medRxiv*, Article 20148429. https://doi.org/10.1101/2020.07.09.20148429

Nordström, P., Ballin, M., Nordström A. (2022). Risk of infection, hospitalisation, and death up to 9 months after a second dose of COVID-19 vaccine: a retrospective, total population cohort study in Sweden. *Lancet*. 2022 Feb 26;399(10327):814-823. doi: 10.1016/S0140-6736(22)00089-7.

Chapter 40

WHERE TO FROM HERE

"Success is Not Final, Failure is Not Fatal: it is the Courage to Continue that Counts."

WINSTON CHURCHILL

There is little doubt that Australia has one of the best health systems in the world. The Therapeutic Goods Administration (TGA) regulates complementary medicines, as it does conventional medicines and medical devices, so that individuals are reassured of safety when choosing both complementary and conventional medicine to manage acute and chronic diseases. Approximately 70% of Australians use complementary medicines.

The most commonly used complementary medications are vitamins and minerals – which have no government subsidy. Close behind are pain relievers, followed closely by heart or blood pressure medications which are heavily subsidised.

The high demand for complementary medicine products is driving growth, with the industry reaching $5.2 billion in revenues in 2018. Australian brands are recognised and trusted internationally, with China importing more complementary medicines from Australia than almost anywhere else in the world. The Chinese themselves have a thriving industry that manufacture complementary medicines including most of the vitamin C used all over the world. The brand Centrum is owned by Pfizer and made in China.

In North America, many medical schools include complementary and alternative medicine in their undergraduate courses, and some hospitals (Yale, Duke and Johns Hopkins) offer acupuncture, meditation and massage therapies. Some hospitals include vitamin D, coenzyme Q_{10} and omega-3 fatty acids and now zinc in their treatment protocols. But in general, medical and pharmacy undergraduates receive very little training in nutrition, let alone herbal medicines.

Back in 1965 it was suggested that folic acid (vitamin B9) deficiency could be a risk for neural tube defects at birth. It took almost twenty years for the Medical Research Council (MRC) Vitamin Study (1983) to be initiated. Opponents expressed horror at the very thought of such a trial. Was it ethical? Could any vitamin, let alone folic acid, prevent such a major medical condition? Sir James Gowans (MRC Secretary) stood fast against a barrage of hostile press and political commentary, and by April 1991 conclusive results had emerged to warrant ending the trial early. The study showed that about 80% of neural tube defects could be prevented by taking just 4 mg folic acid daily, commencing before pregnancy.

That a simple cheap vitamin could have such far-reaching consequences seemed unbelievable, as was the case with iodine and vitamin B3. The guidelines now recommend routine supplementation of folate, iodine and perhaps iron in pregnancy as a preventative measure to support optimal growth and prevention of chronic diseases later in life. Vitamin D is now recommended for everybody in the UK in the winter months.

Yes, things are changing, albeit if slowly. Still, many of you will be aware of the slogans that vitamin intake ends up with expensive urine output, but not if you are pregnant, an athlete, prone to coronavirus, are old, young, living in England ...!

The body of research supporting the use of these complementary medicines is growing – albeit slowly. There are plenty of classic studies proving the value of ancient herbal medicine such as St John's wort, feverfew and curcumin, and there is genuine interest in the potential of probiotics to assist in many complex medical conditions. Very little funding research goes in Australia go towards cheap natural medicines. One reason is a turf war between the pharmaceutical industry and those that make the supplements. Indeed, we observed government support for pharmaceutical companies and their products during the coronavirus era. Expensive medicines like Paxlovid, costing $1390 per dose, were recommended, while cheaper and effective alternatives such as povidone-iodine gargle (Betadine), costing $15, were not mentioned. Similarly, zinc and vitamin D were also not recommended.

The Pharmaceutical Benefits Scheme (PBS) consumed around 16% of the total government healthcare expenditure for 2022-23. There is some concern that the pharmaceutical industry in Australia is far too closely involved with the Health Department for the latter to be independent. This is hardly surprising, with the amount of money and lobbyists thick on the ground in government corridors. But a dearth of funding shouldn't act as a barrier. Traditional herbal medicine has helped people for hundreds of years with comparatively few ill effects.

IN SUMMARY

Personal responsibility for our health requires us to take a good hard look at our lifestyle choices, of which diet, exercise and sleep are paramount. Compare this to the way we'd care for a valued motor car, regularly servicing it to make sure it stays in top condition. Your electric vehicle has coolants with water, lubricants and other additives to improve the efficiency and longevity. Add fuel and tyres to your standard "service". Surely your body should receive better care than your car.

Water: May we suggest about six glasses of water/fluid a day. If relying on town water and you don't like the chlorine, it is easy to get rid of by boiling the water. Reverse osmosis gets rid of most of the toxic fluoride, but unfortunately takes out the good minerals, too.

Oil: Essential fats are those that must be consumed in the diet from fish, nuts and seeds. Your brain is 60% fat. Fats are necessary for hormone production and lubrication of all tissues. And if you don't eat sufficient fats you miss out on the fat-soluble vitamins A, D, E and K.

Fuel: We've summarised the importance of diet at some length in Chapter 30, along with the benefits of the fresh, wholesome food of the Mediterranean diet; but we should not forget the benefits of sunlight with the delivery of vitamin D to almost every cell in the body. We've discussed how your shrinking telomeres are associated with lifestyle factors and how poor nutrition is connected with many degenerative diseases.

Regular use: As the old saying goes, 'use it or lose it.' Every week we receive more information on the benefits of exercise, which we have summarised in Chapter 33. There's hardly a condition we have discussed in this book that isn't helped by regular exercise. It's a great pity that, as we age, our activity tends to diminish significantly, just as all those diseases start becoming more prominent.

Regular health checks: If you have a family history of cancer of the colon, regular colonoscopies are wise. Check your breasts for lumps. If you have chest pain, get a medical opinion on this.

If you're drinking alcohol in excess, have your liver functions checked. If you are exhausted, don't just put up with it – seek out the opinions of different health professionals until you are satisfied with the answer.

If your cognitive performance, or that of a relative, is failing, don't just think 'which nursing home?' Review medications, push hard to find causes and aim for early intervention. If you're a forty-year-old woman recently overtaken by significant anxiety, or a fifty-year-old similarly with onset of depression, think of progesterone and oestrogen deficiencies respectively; check them out and seek remedies to enhance your neuro-transmitters, GABA and/or serotonin.

Don't accept irritable bowel syndrome for a final diagnosis – find out what's making it cranky. And if you have unexplained weight loss, make sure cancer anywhere has been excluded.

LESSONS FROM PREVIOUS GENERATIONS

Contentment and productivity are integral to wellness and this hasn't changed over the generations. In our consulting work over many years, and particularly at our own residential health centre, we have been exposed to some exceptionally interesting presenters, asking such philosophical questions as "What is the meaning of life?" rather than simply, "What are the tricks to keep living, and trying to feel well while you are around?" We thought you would be interested in some modern and ancient thoughts on the matter:

Aristotle: Born in 384 BC into a medical family from northern Greece, he was a student of Plato, who had studied under Socrates. Aristotle taught Alexander the Great, who came to the throne of Macedon at the age of twenty and built an empire by the age of thirty. Aristotle looked deeply into the meaning of life. In Nicomachean Ethics he 'set the pace' in his tract on excellence: '... for as it is not one swallow or one fine day that makes a spring, so it is not one day or a short time that makes a man blessed and happy.'

John Locke (1632–1704) was an English philosopher who embraced Aristotle's teachings and the concept of happiness. His writings on equality were inspirational for both the French Revolution and the American Constitution. His teachings suggested that while happiness and liberty travel together, one must be careful not to confuse imaginary happiness that comes with momentary desires with true happiness that comes from taking care of ourselves and our moral obligations.

Abraham Maslow wrote *A Theory of Human Motivation* (1943), describing the basic stages of motivation through which we move: our 'hierarchy of needs'. Each level of the hierarchy must be met in order to move forward to the next level, until finally we achieve our full potential, which he called 'self-actualisation'. His hierarchy of needs included:

1. The most basic needs are food, air and water. We would also add sleep.
2. Safety is the next basic need, where we need shelter and funds to get by.
3. Love and belonging are crucial needs; community spirit is important.
4. Self-esteem – we need to have control and a recognition of who we are.
5. Self-actualisation – to be able to grow and develop, to have a dream, to be creative. In Maslow's hierarchy these are of lesser importance, whereas Aristotle and Locke had argued that these were the 'main deal'.

Dr Stephen Covey (1932–2012), a corporate guru in the USA and a disciple of Aristotle, suggested that the meaning of life was: *to Live, to Love, to Learn, and to Leave a Legacy.*

- **To Live** – Covey was on message with Aristotle's teachings: to experience all aspects of life.
- **To Love** – self, God, partner, family, friends, community, planet earth and country.
- **To Learn** – both from experience and education.
- **To Leave a Legacy** – Aristotle had a desire for wisdom and knowledge and truth, and this was mirrored by Covey (1989) in his book *Seven Habits of Highly Effective People (First Seek to Understand then Seek to Be Understood).*

When discussing 'legacies' at our own health conferences, mothers (in particular, those who were not into setting up business dynasties) felt they had missed out. We pointed out that not many businesses survive even a few generations, but parents who impart good values to their children pass on enormous legacies which can last forever! Some women who were unable to have children felt they missed out, until one pointed out that there are many ways to love and be loved.

Dr Peter Baldwin and Dr Vered Gordon published a paper in September 2019 in the *Australian Doctor*, introduced with the following: 'A sense of self: living with chronic disease'. A diagnosis of chronic disease can profoundly impact a person's perception of who they are. By understanding how people adjust to a diagnosis, doctors can be important partners in the journey to physical and emotional wellbeing. They summarised: "By clarifying the areas that give the patient a sense of meaning and purpose, their GP can work with them to consider ways they can continue to be involved in valued activities".

Garry Egger, as Professor of Health Sciences at Southern Cross University, proposed less obvious determinants of human health are ignored. What we now know as Lifestyle Medicine relates to both micro (immediate surroundings) and macro (the country, the world) – the benefits of good sleep, our interactions with technology, and our existing and future socioeconomic status. Major determinants include the lack of meaning in life, alienation and loss of culture being drivers of chronic disease.' He referred to the Austrian neurologist and Holocaust survivor Viktor Frankl, whose pursuit of happiness was more concerned with satisfaction and fulfillment in life. In Frankl's classic World War II study *Man's Search for Meaning,* Frankl suggested 'meaninglessness' in life was strongly linked to criminal behaviours, addictions and depression, with purpose in life being a major positive health determinant.

While "meaninglessness" is another word for isolation and loneliness, it is a common inducer of inflammation – something that is particularly common in displaced communities. Meaning doesn't have to be religious or ethereal, but can come down to day-to-day purpose, implicating a significant psychological component in chronic disease.

In saying goodbye, and giving thanks to you for joining us in this book, we leave you with a quote from an India guru, Sathya Sai Baba:

Life is a song – sing it.

Life is a game – play it.

Life is a challenge – meet it.

Life is a dream – realise it.

Life is a sacrifice – offer it.

Life is love – enjoy it.

www.ingramcontent.com/pod-product-compliance
Lightning Source LLC
Chambersburg PA
CBHW041605260326
41914CB00012B/1390